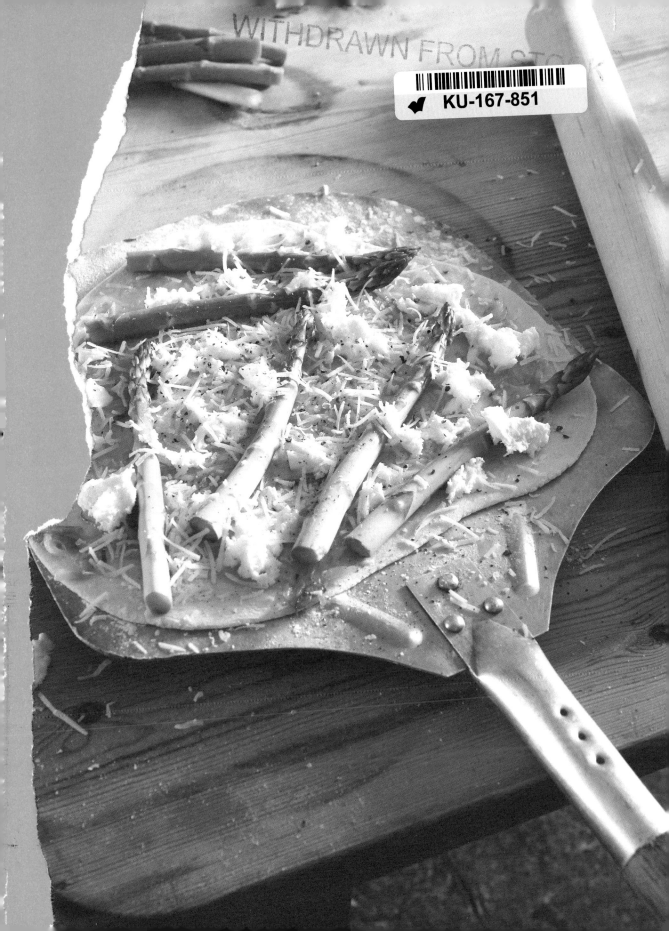

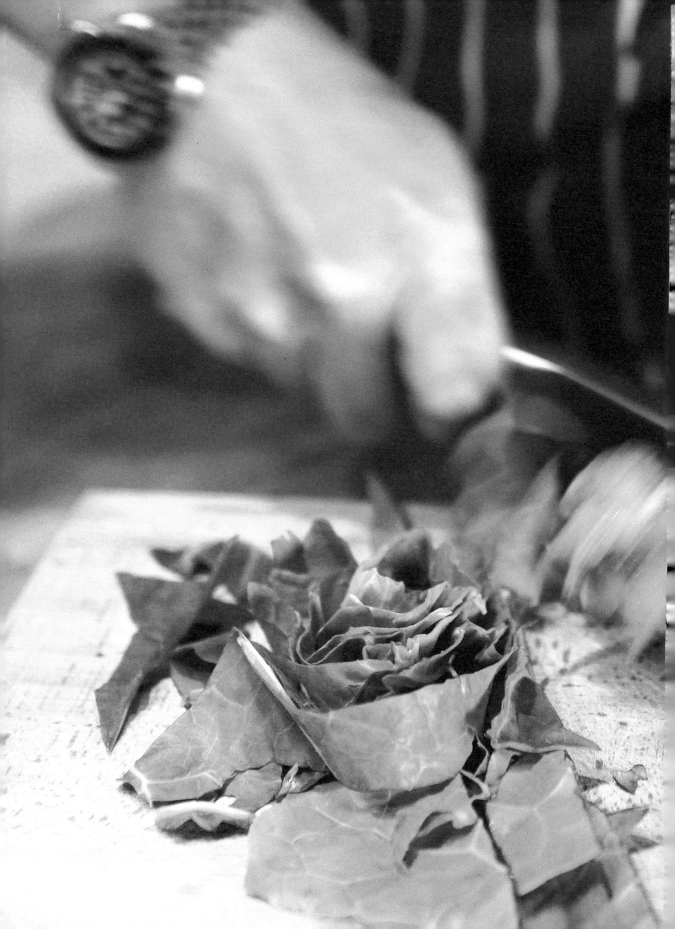

River Cottage
veg
everyday!

Hugh Fearnley-Whittingstall

Photography by Simon Wheeler
Illustrations by Mariko Jesse

BLOOMSBURY PUBLISHING
LONDON · OXFORD · NEW YORK · NEW DELHI · SYDNEY

For Louisa

Hugh Fearnley-Whittingstall *is an award-winning writer, broadcaster and food campaigner with an uncompromising commitment to seasonal, ethically produced food. He has been presenting programmes for Channel Four for over fifteen years, and this is the seventh River Cottage book he has written. His previous work includes* The River Cottage Cookbook, *for which he won the Glenfiddich Trophy and the André Simon Award,* The River Cottage Meat Book *and* The River Cottage Fish Book, *both of which also won the André Simon Award,* The River Cottage Family Cookbook, *which was the Guild of Food Writers Cookery Book of the Year, and* River Cottage Every Day. *He writes a weekly recipe column for the* Guardian. *Hugh and his family live in Devon, not far from River Cottage HQ, where Hugh and his team teach and host events that celebrate their enthusiasm for local, seasonal produce.*

First published in Great Britain 2011

This edition published in 2018

Text © 2011 by Hugh Fearnley-Whittingstall
Photography © 2011 by Simon Wheeler
Illustrations © 2011 by Mariko Jesse
The moral right of the author has been asserted

Bloomsbury Publishing Plc, 50 Bedford Square, London WC1B 3DP

Bloomsbury Publishing, London, Berlin, New York and Sydney

A CIP catalogue record for this book is available from the British Library

ISBN 978 1 4088 8852 0

10 9 8 7 6 5 4 3 2 1

Project editor: Janet Illsley
Designer: Lawrence Morton
Photographer and stylist: Simon Wheeler (www.simonwheeler.eu)
Illustrator: Mariko Jesse (www.marikojesse.com)
Printed and bound in Italy by Graphicom

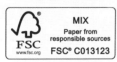

bloomsbury.com
rivercottage.net

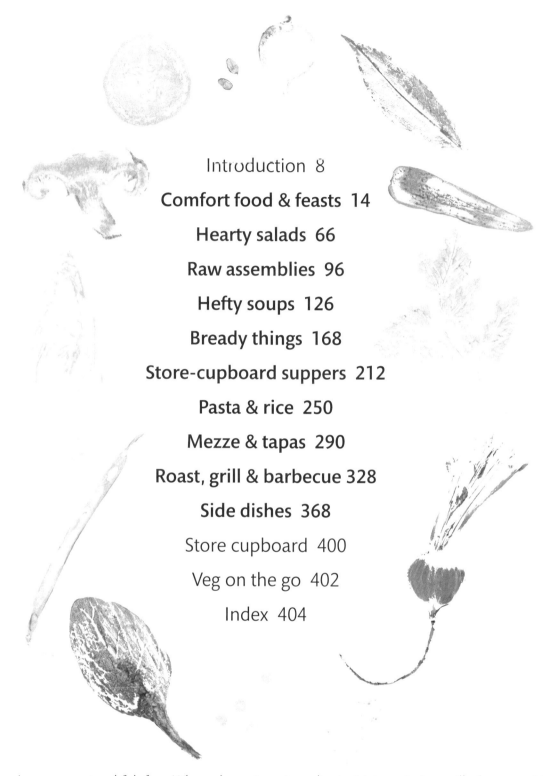

All recipes are meat and fish free. Where cheese is an ingredient, strict vegetarians will of course wish to source a vegetarian cheese. Recipes marked 🟍 are suitable for vegans, provided optional non-vegan ingredients listed are excluded and vegan options for ingredients such as mustard and wine are used.

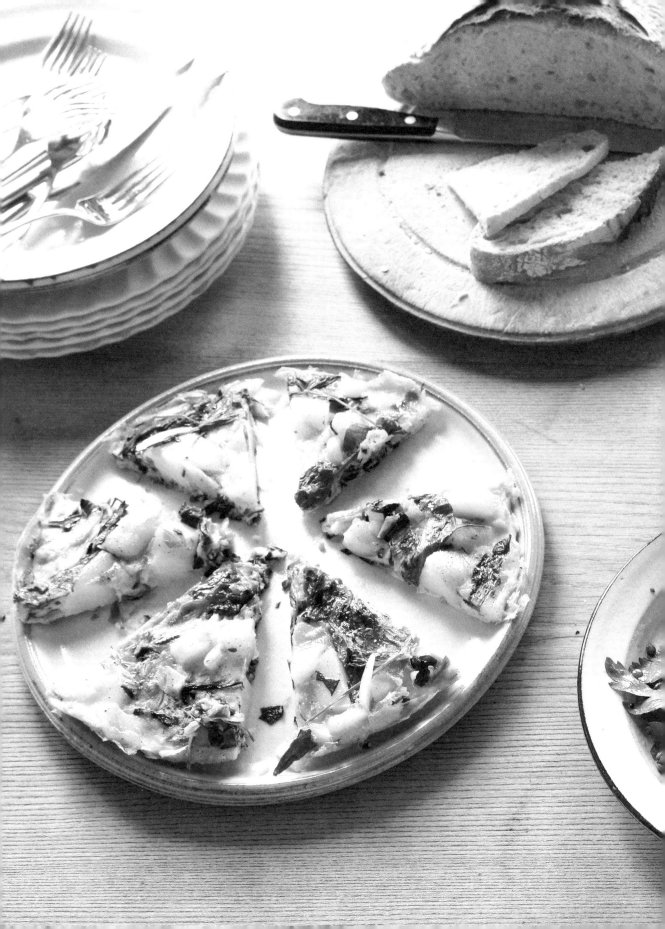

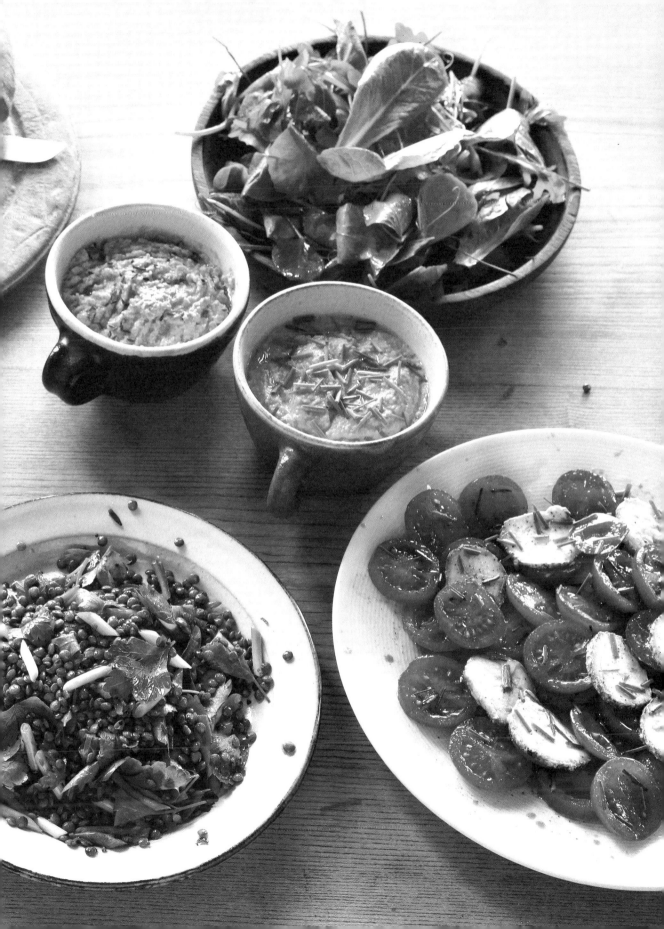

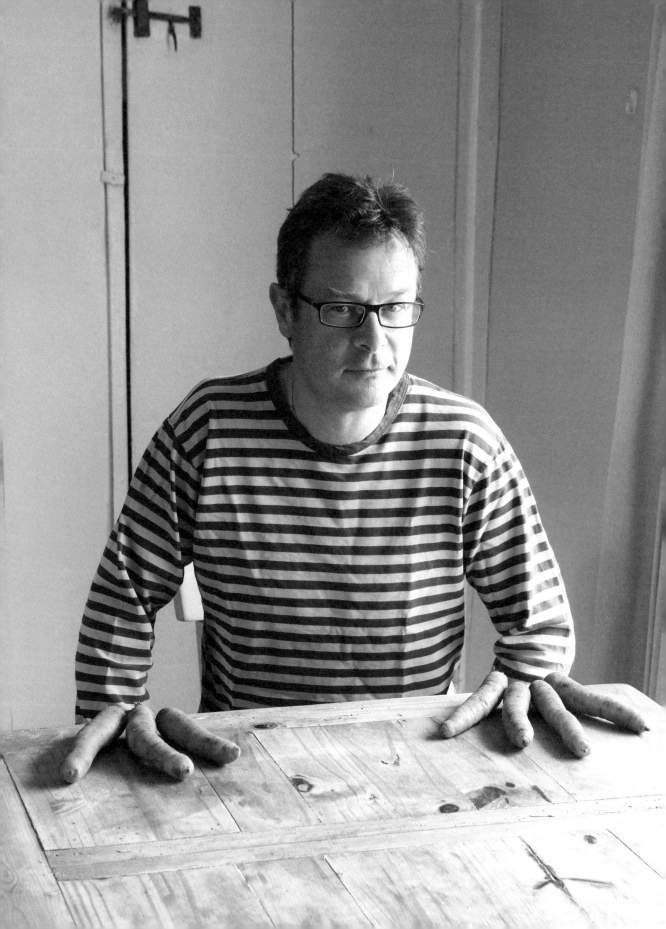

This is a vegetable cookbook. Whether or not it's a *vegetarian* cookbook depends perhaps on your point of view, and your food politics. It's not written by a vegetarian, or with the intention of persuading you or anyone else to become a vegetarian. But in the sense that not one of the recipes here contains a scrap of meat or fish, then it is indeed quite strictly vegetarian. I certainly hope that many vegetarians will buy it, use it and enjoy it.

And it is also, I would like to think, evangelical. Call me power-crazed, but I'm trying to change your life here. The object of the exercise is, unambiguously, to persuade you to eat more vegetables. *Many* more vegetables. Perhaps even to make veg the mainstay of your daily cooking. And therefore, by implication, to eat less meat, maybe *a lot* less meat, and maybe a bit less fish too. Why? We need to eat more vegetables and less flesh, because vegetables are the foods that do us the most good, and our planet the least harm. Do I need to spell out in detail the arguments to support that assertion? Is there anyone who seriously doubts it to be true? Just ask yourself if you, or anyone you know, might be in danger of eating *too many* vegetables. Or if you think the world might be a better, cleaner, greener place, with a few more factory chicken farms, or intensive pig units scattered about the countryside. Surely it's close to being a no-brainer...

So, to be absolutely clear, all the recipes that follow are suitable for vegetarians. Since I have used dairy products and eggs, they are not all appropriate for vegans. But over a third of them are (those marked ❥), and another third easily could be, if suitable substitutes for butter and milk were used. If you're a vegan, you'll know what to do.

I can certainly appreciate that if you've seen my shows, and used my books, you may be feeling a bit baffled to be holding in your hand a near-as-damn-it vegetarian cookbook written by that notorious carnivore Hugh Fearnley-Whittingstall. But if you know my work a little more intimately, if you've probed and dabbled beyond the recipes and into the more discursive text, this should come as no great surprise – I've visited this territory before. Only now I'm at the vegetable end of the meat argument, and it's a very refreshing place to be.

But let me recap my core thinking on this subject anyway – I'll try and keep it pithy. In my meat book I argued that we eat far too much meat in the West – too much for our own health, and far too much for the welfare of the many millions of animals we raise for food. I believe that factory farming is plain wrong – environmentally and ethically. So it saddens me to say that, despite some recent significant gains in the UK on poultry and pork welfare, the problems associated with the industrial production of meat are, globally speaking, as bad as ever. I've been similarly forthright about fish. I believe it's a wonderful food, which I like to catch and love to eat. But I have also pointed out that we are in ever-increasing danger of eradicating this amazing source of food altogether.

Good reasons, you might think, for becoming an out-and-out vegetarian. But that isn't my plan. I still believe in being a selective omnivore, casting a positive vote in favour of ethically produced meat and sustainably caught fish. However, I now understand that in order to eat these two great foods in good conscience, I have to recognise, control and impose limits on my appetite for them.

But why, I hear some of you remonstrating, given that I still eat meat and fish, would I want this book to exclude them *entirely*? What's wrong with a *soupçon* of meat and fish? Perhaps, like me, you've already become adept at making a little meat go a long way. You've embraced the notion that a few shards of bacon, or a sprinkling of chorizo crumbs, or some scraps of leftover chicken, are a perfect way to give a lift to a big salad, or add interest, spice and texture to a creamy vegetable soup; that an anchovy here and there gives a lovely salty tang (especially, as it happens, to vegetables).

So why will I not allow such sound and thrifty strategies, where a modest amount of meat is used as a perk or spice in a dish, to season and punctuate the vegetable recipes in this book? Because it would be a cop out, that's why! That approach, useful though it is at times, is ultimately the wrong mindset for serious change. It suggests you're *clinging on* to meat; that you feel any meal is incomplete without it. And that's the feeling I think we all need to let go of.

The way I see it, if we are remotely serious in our commitment to eat less meat and fish, we will want to make plenty of meals – perhaps even the majority of them – *completely without* meat and fish. For many of us, this is quite a big concept to swallow, but I want to tackle it head on. We may be increasingly aware of the good reasons to eat less meat, but our cooking culture is still largely based around flesh. The idea of a fridge entirely free of sausages, bacon, chops or chicken can strike fear into the heart of many a cook – even a resourceful one. Meat is so familiar, so convenient, the easy route to something that we instantly recognise as a 'proper meal'. I want to show you how straightforward it can be to embrace vegetables in the same way.

Changing your prime culinary focus from meat to veg will require a shift in attitude – but not, I would argue, a very big or difficult one. It's true that if you eschew meat and fish, you have to look at other ingredients with fresh eyes. You have to take a new, more creative approach to them. But once you become accustomed to cooking vegetables as main meals it will soon seem like the most natural thing. This book is your starter pack on that mission.

I have to admit that when making my own commitment to cook and eat more veg, and indeed to write this book, it was a little hard to shake off the meat lover's niggling prejudices. But I can honestly say that my own anxieties – about cooking without meat being somehow less satisfying, less flavoursome or less easy – have proved groundless. I have actually found it all to be very liberating. I think the kind of vegetable cookery I've embraced here is more democratic – there's no longer a tyrannical piece of meat dominating the agenda, making everything else feel like a supporting act.

In contrast, the recipes that follow are often a harmonious blend of several different vegetables – and a meal based on them often gives equal weight to several different dishes. Much as I enjoy the generous one-pot or one-plate vegetarian curries, hotpots or lasagnes (of which plenty are coming up), I find there's something *particularly* enticing and satisfying about a meal made up of several 'small' dishes, such as you get with Middle Eastern mezze or Spanish tapas. Vegetable cookery really lends itself to such delicious, pick-and-mix spreads, where you can try a little (or a lot) of whatever takes your fancy. I love the slight lawlessness of this way of eating. It's all so much less predictable and more fun than being a slave to meat.

If you *are* a vegetarian, and a keen cook, I'm sure you'll already have your own repertoire of favourite dishes. Perhaps you're wondering whether this book is for you? Well, I hope I can offer you something new, too. My view is that vegetarians have not been as richly catered for in the cookery book market as they deserve. Ironically, I think there's been a little too much emphasis (consciously or unconsciously) on *replacing* meat. Whereas I think, when we turn our attention to veg, we should feel pretty relaxed

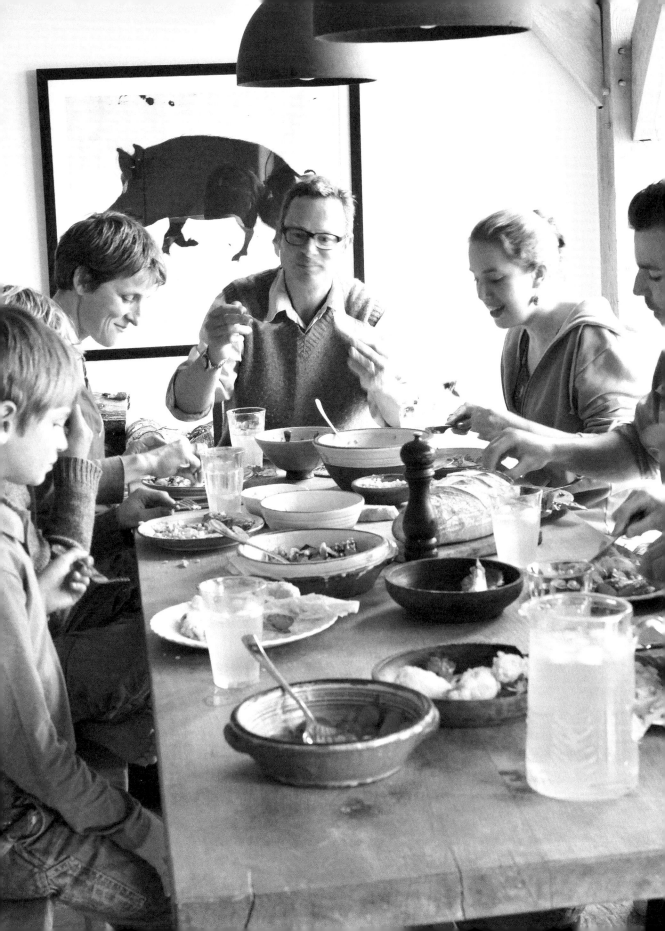

about simply *ignoring* meat. Then we can get on with the life-enhancing business of enjoying the extraordinary range of fresh seasonal vegetables we can buy (and indeed grow), by cooking them in a whole range of new and exciting ways. Much as I see the vital food value and great culinary potential of pulses and grains, I've little time for veggie sausages, nut cutlets and TVP. I'd rather break that mould, and muddle my chickpeas, kidney beans and quinoa with fresh leaves, crunchy roots and sun-ripened fruits: squashes, peppers, courgettes, aubergines and tomatoes, to name but five.

The truth is I really don't need to be talked into a conversation with the nation's vegetarians. I've been having that conversation, and enjoying it, for years. I have a lot of time for vegetarians (though apparently not *all* of them have a lot of time for me), and that's because I respect anyone with principles about food. One of the silliest spectacles I have ever seen in the brash world of 'TV chefs' is that of colleagues, who really should know better, goading vegetarians as if they were somehow not to be taken seriously in the kitchen. (Or even out of it – one of them actually said that if any of his children grew up to be vegetarians he'd shoot them. I'm secretly hoping that one of them does, so I can see their dad eat his words.)

In some quarters it's even been assumed I might harbour similar feelings towards vegetarians. Of course I don't. In fact – and I can't say this without smiling – *some of my best friends are vegetarians*. When it comes to the recipes in this book, I hope it's very much a two-way street, not least because I learned some of my favourite dishes from my vegetarian friends. I also feel I am a better cook now than I was when I set out to write this book. I feed my family better, with more vegetables, than I did before. I am less reliant on that freezer full of home-grown meat, and self-caught fish (fantastic as those ingredients are) than I used to be. I enjoy my cooking, and my eating, more than ever. And that feels wonderful.

So here you are: more than two hundred River Cottage veg recipes. And for those who just love to get on and cook, here's the best bit. The philosophising and moralising is done. I'm climbing down off my soapbox. Because this is not a book of caveats and cautions. It's not an argumentative case for not eating something bad or rare or threatened. In fact, it's not a book about problems at all. Quite the opposite: it's full of solutions. And the main solution is, quite simply, to eat more vegetables!

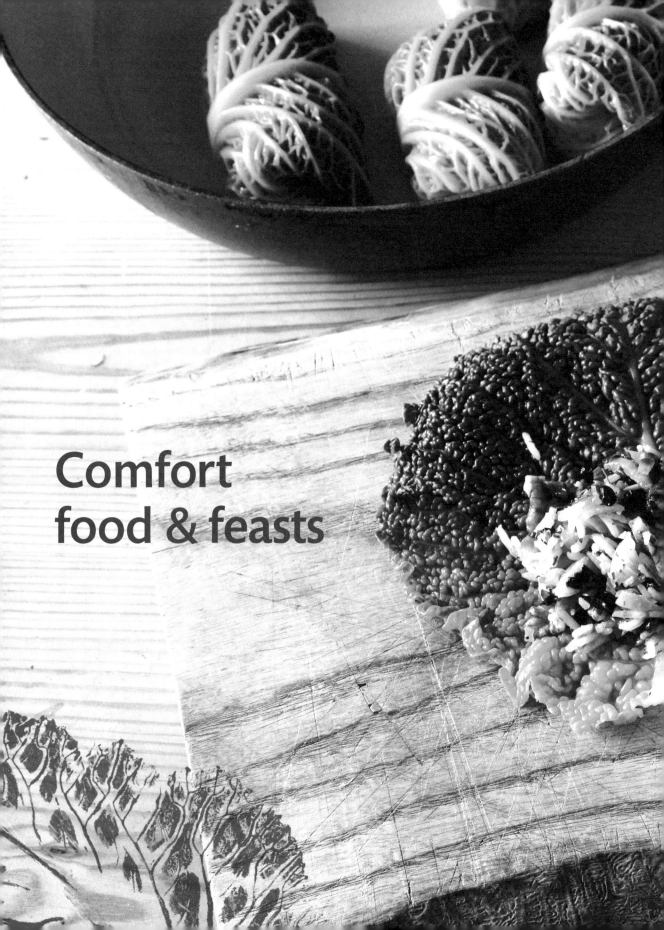

Comfort
food & feasts

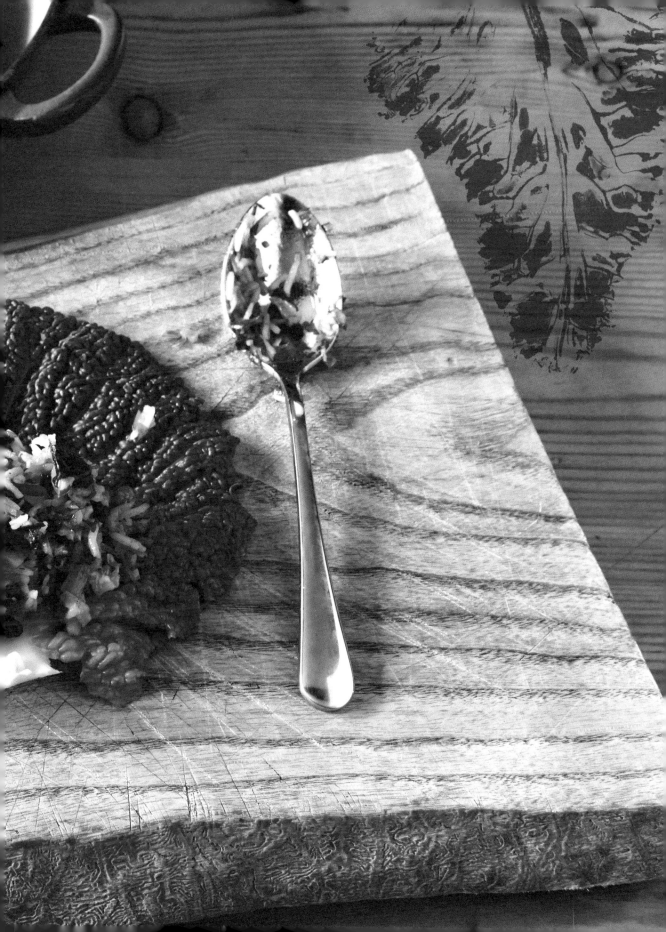

With this chapter, right from the off, I want to lay to rest any fears you may have about veg-based meals being insubstantial, lacking in flavour or somehow not 'proper food'. These recipes are the first to turn to if you want to eat less meat but are a little bit wary about the prospect – perhaps because you can't help feeling some degree of sensory deprivation may ensue. It needn't. Pile into these recipes, and your tummy will be filled, your craving for flavour fully satisfied. They are fulfilling in every sense – they will not only sate your hunger, but their tastes, scents and textures will both tempt and gratify you.

The dishes here are multi-layered and multi-faceted, with strength and depth of both flavour and texture. You'll find saucy, sweet and spicy curries and stews; crisply crusted pies and tarts; starchy staples enlivened with unexpected twists; and a host of tempting vegetarian classics from around the world – re-interpreted for the busy modern family. This is where your decision to serve up more meals without meat really takes root – with a bunch of reliable regulars you'll always be proud to present and delighted to share.

These recipes all meet the important criteria of being able to stand up as main courses comfortably in their own right. That doesn't necessarily mean you would want to serve them entirely on their own (although in some cases, you most certainly could). But each of them can clearly be the principal offering of a meal. They are, dare I say it, among the 'meatier' dishes of the book. Indeed many of them can be brought out as the kind of abundant, generous, celebratory centrepieces you might choose to serve for a Sunday lunch, a birthday supper, a bonfire night party or any other kind of festive gathering. Yes, it really is possible to celebrate such occasions without cooking flesh!

This chapter also bears out a truth you'll find me repeating more than once through these pages: that if you decide to eat less meat, and at some meals, no meat, then you have to take a fresh look at all the other ingredients you're cooking with. Many of them will need to appear centre stage, where the meat used to be. Don't worry about it. Root vegetables, beans and pulses, fleshy stems and even full-flavoured green leaves, can all take the strain, holding their own in stews, hotpots, curries and pies. The recipes that follow have been chosen to prove the point.

I'll also be asking you to re-assess a certain style of dish that you might previously have regarded as a complement to, rather than a replacement for, meat. You may be used to eating comforting things like a classic potato dauphinoise (see page 60), or the more quirky sweet potato and peanut gratin (see page 63), 'on the side'. However, if you shunt them into the middle of your plate and build around them with a few simple accompaniments, they will satisfy in a whole new way.

If you doubt this, ask yourself how often is it that the lovely potato and celeriac gratin, or even the perfect roast spud or tender, sweet parsnip, is actually the most delicious thing on the plate that it just happens to be sharing with some not-so-great meat and less-than-inspired gravy? Now imagine what is possible when, from the outset, you aim to make that gratin, or those roasted roots, the focal point of the feast. A bit of extra spice perhaps, a cheesy, nutty, crumby topping, something unexpected hiding in the middle... As soon as you lavish a bit of attention on the veg you'll find you're richly rewarded.

As you might expect, there are plenty of what could be called cold weather dishes in this section – lots of lovely, bubbling root gratins, beany chillies and curries, and rich savoury lasagnes. But food doesn't have to be wintry to be comforting and filling, and you'll also find a roughly equal number of summery dishes, such as the lettuce, spring onion and cheese tart (see page 44), or the gorgeous tomato and pepper stew known as chachouka (see page 20). These will help to convince you, I hope, that veg-based meals can deliver top-notch contentment at any time of year.

I've given suggestions for how to serve the dishes at the end of most of the recipes, but they are just ideas. Common sense and your own personal tastes will prevail. Sometimes, you might feel that a helping of pasta or rice, or perhaps a baked potato or a pile of creamy mash, is required in order to soak up the sauce, round them out and make a meal of them. Conversely, you might hanker for a crisp, light salad to cut their richness. It'll depend on your mood, the weather, who you're feeding and how hungry you all are. This is the kind of food where I hope the lion will sit down and tuck in with the lamb, the old with the young, the hungry with the light of appetite. In other words, there's elasticity here to cater for all comers on all occasions. And they will all be special occasions, I promise.

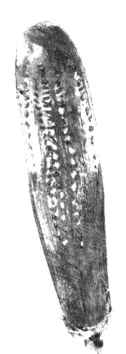

Aubergine parmigiana

This is one of my favourite ways to cook large aubergines, and it's one of those dishes with few ingredients that seems to be greater than the sum of its parts. It is one to take your time over – ideal for a rainy afternoon in the kitchen – but once assembled it can be chilled or even frozen and cooked later on.

SERVES 6

4 medium aubergines (about 1kg)

4–5 tablespoons olive oil

2 balls of buffalo mozzarella (125g each), torn into pieces

About 35g Parmesan, hard goat's cheese or other well-flavoured hard cheese, finely grated

FOR THE TOMATO SAUCE

2 tablespoons olive oil

2 onions, chopped

3 garlic cloves, chopped

4 x 400g tins plum tomatoes, roughly chopped, any stalky ends and skin removed

1 bay leaf

A little sugar

Sea salt and freshly ground black pepper

Trim the aubergines and slice lengthways into 3–5mm thick slices. Layer the slices in a colander, sprinkling each layer with a little salt. Leave to draw the juices for an hour or so.

Meanwhile, make the tomato sauce. Heat the 2 tablespoons olive oil in a very large, wide pan over a medium heat. Add the onions and garlic and fry gently for about 10 minutes, stirring occasionally, until soft. Add the tomatoes with their juice and the bay leaf. Bring to a simmer, then simmer briskly, stirring often, for about half an hour, or until the sauce is thick and rich. Season well with salt and pepper, and a little sugar to taste.

Quickly rinse the aubergine slices and pat dry thoroughly with kitchen paper or a tea towel. Heat a large frying pan over a medium-high heat and add 1 tablespoon oil. When the oil is hot, fry a batch of aubergine slices for about 2 minutes each side, until golden and tender. Remove and set aside. Repeat with the remaining aubergine slices, adding a little more oil to the pan before you fry each batch.

Preheat the oven to 180°C/Gas Mark 4. Lay a third of the aubergine slices over the bottom of an ovenproof dish, roughly 25 x 20cm, and at least 5cm deep. Cover with a third of the tomato sauce. Dot a third of the mozzarella over the sauce, then scatter a thin layer of grated cheese over that. Repeat with the remaining ingredients, so you have three layers in the dish.

Bake for 30–40 minutes, until bubbling and golden on top. Serve with lots of fresh green salad – and bread, if you like.

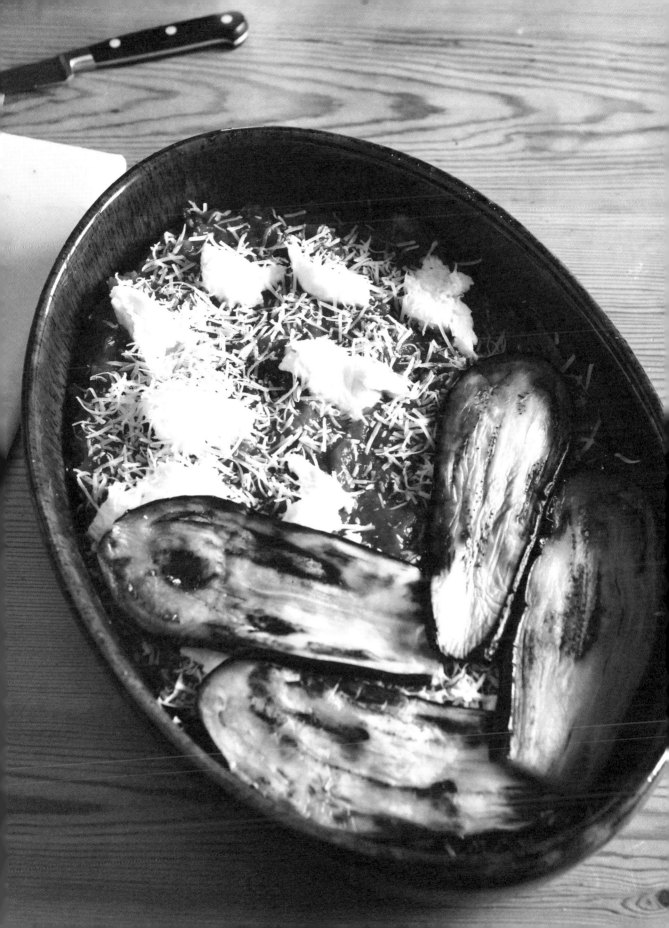

Chachouka

This spicy North African pepper and tomato stew with eggs baked on top makes a lovely, lazy supper. The classic Italian peperonata (see below) is prepared in the same way but without eggs or spices – it is equally good.

SERVES 4

3 tablespoons olive oil

1 teaspoon cumin seeds

1 large onion, halved and finely sliced

1 garlic clove, crushed

1 red pepper, cored, deseeded and finely sliced

1 yellow pepper, cored, deseeded and finely sliced

½ teaspoon hot smoked paprika

A pinch of saffron strands

400g tin plum tomatoes, roughly chopped, any stalky ends and skin removed

4 eggs

Sea salt and freshly ground black pepper

Heat the olive oil in a large, preferably ovenproof, frying pan over a medium heat. Add the cumin seeds and let them fry gently for a couple of minutes. Add the onion and cook gently for 8–10 minutes, or until soft and golden.

Add the garlic and peppers and continue to cook over a low heat for at least 20 minutes, stirring often, until the peppers are soft and wilted. Add the paprika, crumble in the saffron, then add the tomatoes with their juice and some salt and pepper. Cook gently, stirring from time to time, for 10–15 minutes. Preheat the oven to 180°C/Gas Mark 4.

Taste the mixture and adjust the seasoning if necessary. If your frying pan isn't ovenproof, transfer the mixture to a baking dish. Make 4 hollows in the surface and carefully break an egg into each one. Sprinkle with salt and pepper. Bake for 10–12 minutes, until the egg white is set and the yolk still runny.

VARIATION

Peperonata

Simply leave out the cumin, paprika, saffron and eggs, serving the stew after simmering – with bread and/or a crisp green salad.

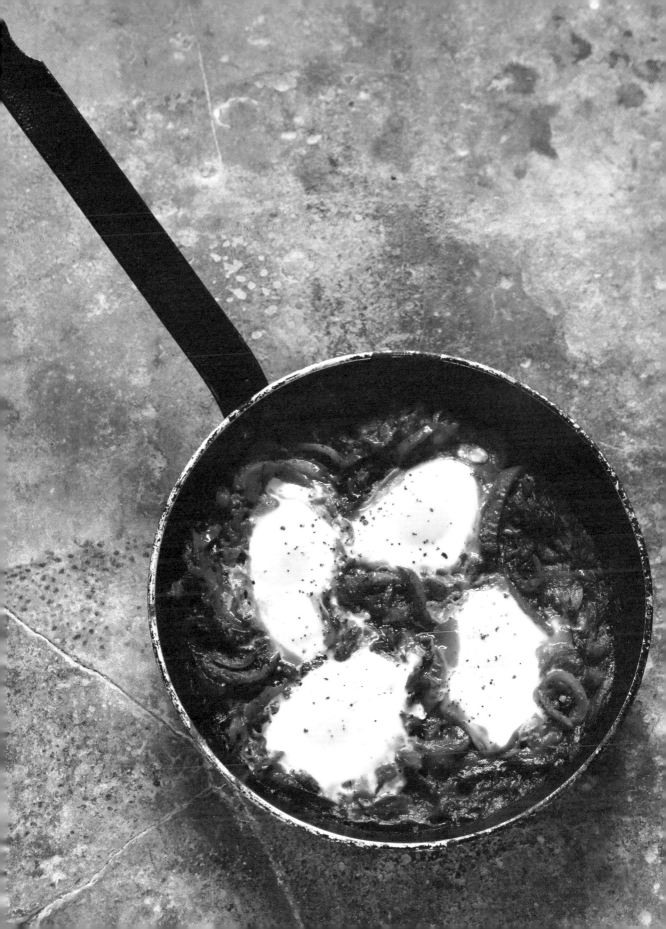

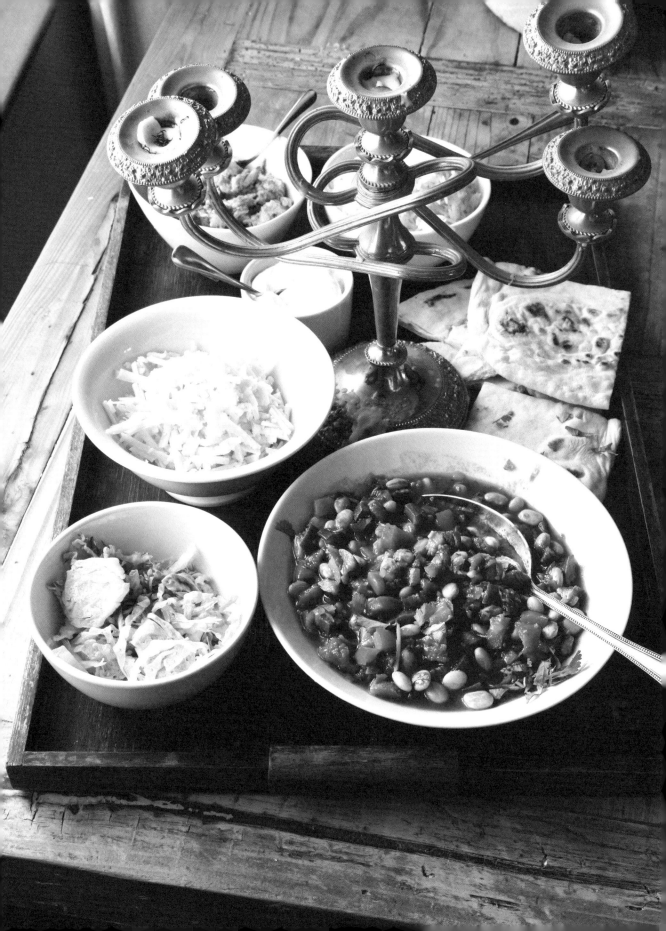

Pinto bean chilli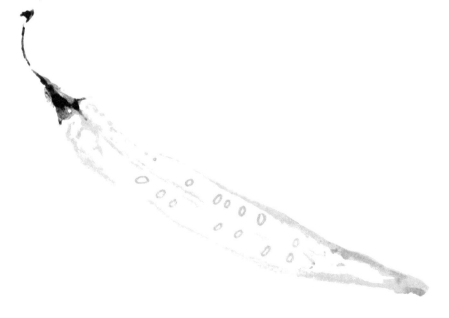

You can adapt this easy, fiery chilli to the seasons, swapping summer's courgettes and peppers for autumn's mushrooms and squash, for instance. And you can easily double or triple the quantities if you want to feed a crowd (it's perfect for bonfire night), or lay some down in the freezer.

SERVES 4–5

2 tablespoons olive, sunflower or rapeseed oil

3 onions, chopped

2–3 green chillies, to taste, deseeded and finely chopped

2 garlic cloves, finely chopped

2 teaspoons ground cumin

1 teaspoon cayenne pepper

¼ teaspoon allspice

2 courgettes, cut into 1cm dice

1 red pepper, cored, deseeded and cut into 1cm dice

2 tablespoons tomato purée

400g tin plum tomatoes, roughly chopped, any stalky ends and skin removed

400g tin pinto beans, drained and rinsed

100ml red wine

A good handful of parsley, finely chopped

A good handful of coriander, finely chopped, plus extra to serve

A handful of oregano, finely chopped

Sea salt and freshly ground black pepper

TO SERVE

Lemony guacamole (see page 296)

Shredded lettuce

Soured cream (optional)

Grated Cheddar (optional)

Heat the oil in a saucepan over a medium-low heat, add the onions and sweat, stirring from time to time, until very soft and just starting to take on some colour. Add the chillies, garlic, cumin, cayenne and allspice and stir for a minute.

Add the courgettes and red pepper and stir to coat in the spices. Add the tomato purée, tinned tomatoes with their juice, pinto beans, red wine, parsley, coriander and oregano. Pour over 200ml water and add some salt and pepper. Simmer gently for 25–30 minutes, stirring from time to time, until the veg are all tender and everything is thick and saucy. Taste and adjust the seasoning, adding a little more salt and/or pepper if you think it needs it.

To serve, put the guacamole, shredded lettuce, soured cream and cheese, if using, into small serving bowls. Scatter more chopped coriander over the chilli and accompany with rice and/or flatbreads (see page 176) or tortillas and the various toppings, for everyone to help themselves.

Chard and new potato curry

This hearty curry is fantastic in late summer or early autumn. If you want to make it ahead of time and refrigerate or freeze it, leave out the yoghurt and add it at the last minute, just before serving.

SERVES 4

About 500g Swiss chard

2 tablespoons sunflower oil

1 onion, halved and finely sliced

3 garlic cloves, peeled

1 green chilli, deseeded and finely chopped

3cm piece of ginger, peeled and chopped

1 teaspoon garam masala

½ teaspoon mustard seeds

½ teaspoon ground cumin

¼ teaspoon ground turmeric

3 cardamom pods, bashed

350g new potatoes, quartered

250g plain (full-fat) yoghurt

1½ tablespoons tomato purée

A small bunch of coriander, roughly chopped

A small handful of almonds, cashews or pistachios, toasted and chopped

Sea salt and freshly ground black pepper

Separate the chard leaves from the stalks. Cut the stalks into 2–3cm pieces and roughly chop the leaves.

Heat the oil in a large saucepan over a medium heat, add the onion and fry until just golden. Meanwhile, pound the garlic, chilli and ginger together with a pinch of salt to a paste. Add to the onion and cook, stirring, for a couple of minutes. Tip in the rest of the spices and stir for a minute or two.

Add the potatoes and chopped chard stalks and fry, stirring frequently, for 5 minutes, so that they are well coated with the spice mixture. Pour in about 400ml water – enough to just cover the veg. Bring to a simmer, cover and cook for 10–12 minutes until the potatoes are just tender. Add the chard leaves, stir and cook until just wilted.

In a bowl, whisk together the yoghurt, tomato purée and some of the hot liquid from the curry. Remove the curry from the heat, stir in the yoghurt mixture, return to the heat and warm through very gently (if it gets too hot, the yoghurt will curdle). Stir in most of the coriander.

Taste and add salt and pepper if needed. Scatter over the toasted nuts and remaining coriander, then serve with rice and naan or chapattis.

VARIATIONS

Spinach and new potato curry
Use 600–700g spinach in place of the chard. Remove any tough stalks and add the leaves to the curry once the potatoes are done. Cook for a minute or two before adding the yoghurt mixture.

Winter kale and potato curry
Use maincrop potatoes, peeled and cut into bite-sized chunks, rather than new potatoes, and replace the chard with kale. Discard the kale stalks, roughly shred the leaves, and add them when the potatoes are nearly done. Simmer for 2–3 minutes, or until tender.

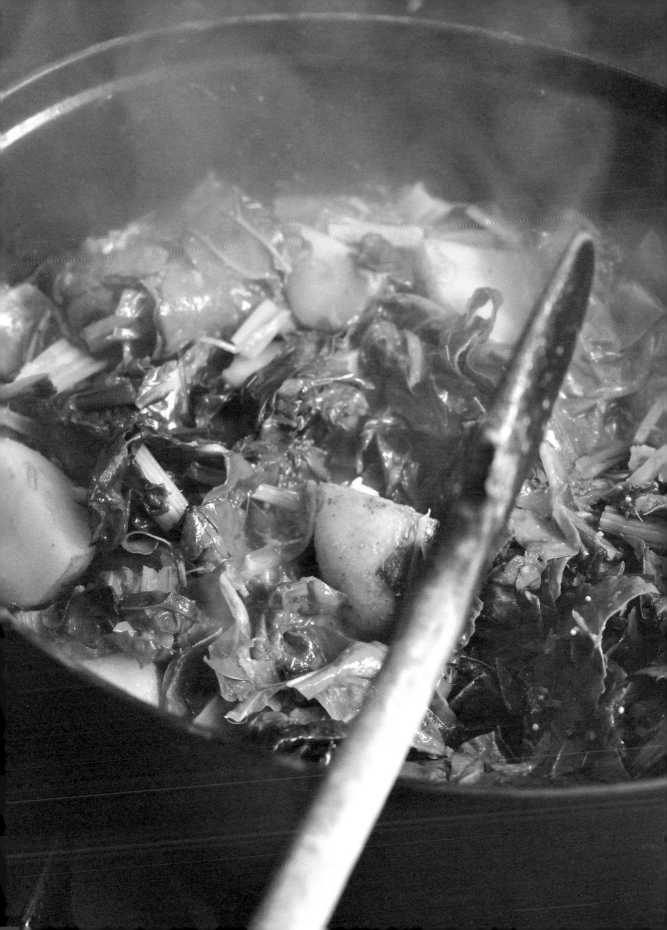

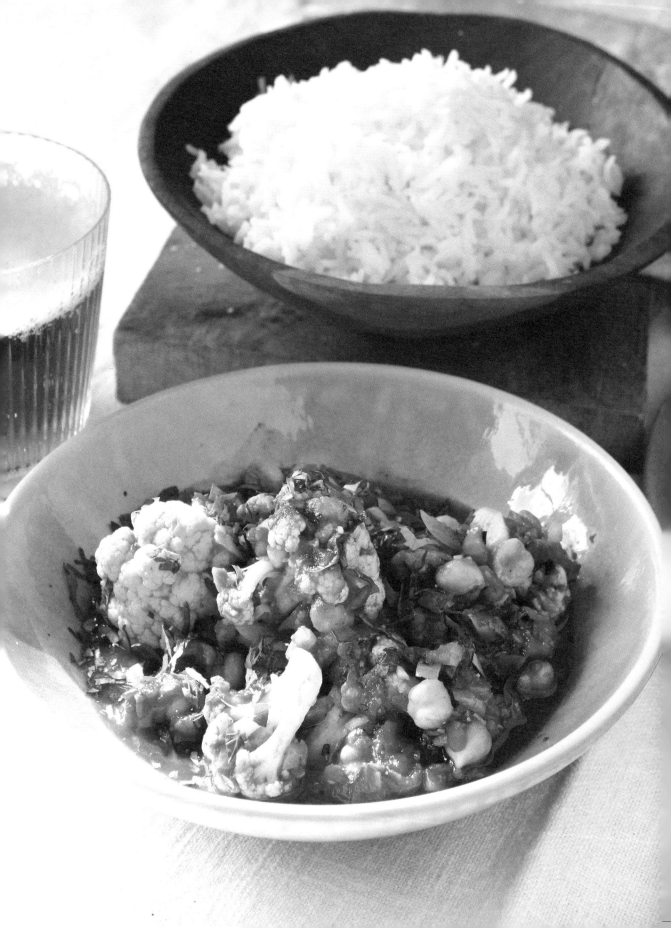

Cauliflower and chickpea curry ♥

This beautifully simple, light curry is closely based on a wonderful recipe from chef Angela Hartnett. It's always preferable to use some carefully selected ground and whole spices in a recipe like this but, if you're in a hurry, use a ready-made curry powder instead of the dry spices.

SERVES 4-6

1 medium-large cauliflower (about 800g), trimmed

2 tablespoons sunflower oil

3 onions, chopped

4 garlic cloves, chopped

1 teaspoon freshly grated ginger

2 teaspoons ground coriander

2 teaspoons ground cumin

A large pinch of dried chilli flakes

2 star anise

400g tin plum tomatoes, chopped, any stalky ends and skin removed

400g tin chickpeas, drained and rinsed

2 teaspoons garam masala

A good handful of coriander, chopped

Sea salt and freshly ground black pepper

Cut the cauliflower into medium florets. Put into a large pan, cover with cold water, add some salt and bring up to a rolling boil. This will part-cook the cauli. Take off the heat straight away, drain well and keep warm in the pan.

Heat the oil in a large saucepan over a medium heat. Add the onions, garlic and ginger and sauté for about 10 minutes, stirring often.

Add the ground coriander, cumin, chilli flakes, star anise and some salt and pepper and cook for a further 5 minutes.

Add the tomatoes with their juice and the chickpeas. Stir well, then add the cooked cauliflower. Pour in enough cold water to almost but not quite cover everything (100–200ml) and bring to a simmer. Simmer for 5–10 minutes, stirring once or twice, until the cauliflower is tender.

Stir in the garam masala and half the chopped coriander, then check the seasoning. Serve scattered with the remaining coriander and accompanied by rice, flatbreads (see page 176) or naans.

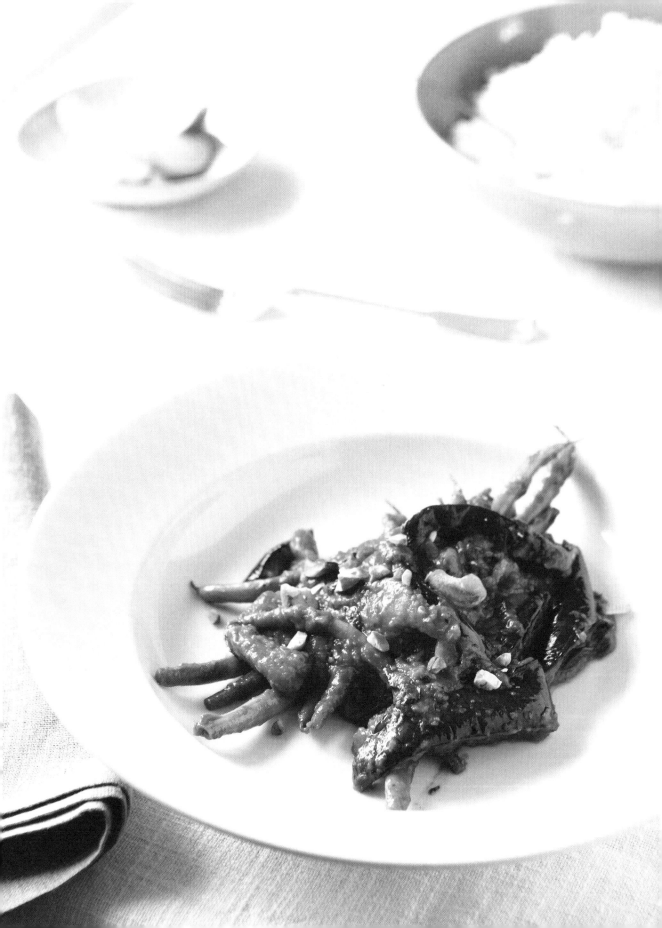

Aubergine and green bean curry^v

This gorgeously rich curry uses my roasted tomato sauce as a base, though a good-quality passata would work well too. I've deliberately made twice as much curry paste as you need for the recipe – partly because it's easier to blend that way, but also because it's so useful to have a second batch either to make this again or for any other veg curry. Alternatively, use a well-sautéed blob of it as the base for a simple noodle soup or laksa. You can keep the paste, covered, in the fridge for up to a week, or freeze it.

SERVES 6–8

5 large aubergines (about 1.7kg)

About 6 tablespoons sunflower oil

300ml roasted tomato sauce (see page 366) or passata

400ml tin coconut milk

300g French beans

A good handful of coriander, chopped

75g cashews or almonds, toasted and coarsely chopped (optional)

Sea salt and freshly ground black pepper

FOR THE CURRY PASTE

5–6 shallots or 2 medium onions, finely chopped

6 garlic cloves, roughly chopped

2 thumb-sized pieces of ginger, peeled and roughly chopped

2 lemongrass stalks, tough outer layer removed, finely sliced

5–6 medium green chillies (medium-hot), deseeded and roughly chopped

2 teaspoons ground cumin

2 teaspoons ground coriander

1 teaspoon ground turmeric

TO SERVE

Lime wedges

Put all the curry paste ingredients into a blender with 2 tablespoons water and whiz to a coarse paste. Stop a few times to scrape down the sides if necessary.

Halve the aubergines lengthways. Cut each half into three lengthways, then halve each piece, so you have 12 wedges from each aubergine.

Heat 2–3 tablespoons of the oil over a medium-high heat in a large, non-stick frying pan. Sauté the aubergines, in batches, until lightly browned, adding more oil as needed. As you remove them from the pan, lay the aubergine wedges on kitchen paper to drain.

Heat 1 tablespoon oil in a large, deep saucepan and add half the curry paste (refrigerate the rest for another use). Fry over a medium heat, stirring constantly, for 3–4 minutes. Add the aubergines to the pan and stir for a minute or two until coated with the spice mixture.

Now add the tomato sauce or passata and the coconut milk. If the tomato sauce is very thick, you can add a little water now too. Simmer, partially covered, for 10 minutes. Add the French beans and simmer until they are tender, about 5 minutes.

Season well with salt and pepper and stir in the chopped coriander. If using the toasted nuts, scatter them over the curry, then serve with lime wedges and accompanied by rice.

North african squash and chickpea stew

This richly spiced combination of squash, tomatoes and pulses is based around a traditional Moroccan recipe, harira. That dish is actually a soup but, whenever I make it, I find myself veering towards such a thick and chunky texture that 'stew' seems a more appropriate description. It hardly matters – it's a delicious, belly-filling, one-pot dish.

SERVES 6

2 tablespoons sunflower oil

2 large onions, diced

2 garlic cloves, finely chopped

1 celery stalk, finely diced

1 teaspoon freshly ground black pepper

1 teaspoon ground turmeric

½ teaspoon ground cinnamon

½ teaspoon ground ginger

100g red lentils

400g tin chickpeas, drained and rinsed

8 saffron strands, toasted and crushed

500ml roasted tomato sauce (see page 366) or passata

A good handful of parsley, roughly chopped

A large bunch of coriander, roughly chopped

300g squash or pumpkin

1.2 litres vegetable stock (see page 130)

1 bay leaf

50g vermicelli, orzo or other small pasta

Dates, to serve (optional)

Heat the oil in a large saucepan over a medium heat. Add the onions and sauté until just starting to turn golden. Turn the heat down to medium-low and add the garlic, celery, pepper, turmeric, cinnamon and ginger. Sauté for a couple of minutes.

Now add the lentils, chickpeas, saffron, tomato sauce or passata, parsley and about half the coriander. Cook over a low heat for 15 minutes.

Meanwhile, peel and deseed the squash or pumpkin and cut into large cubes. Add to the pan with the stock and bay leaf. Cover and simmer gently for about 30 minutes. Add the pasta and simmer until it is cooked. Season with salt and pepper to taste.

Serve immediately, scattered with the remaining coriander leaves and with a few dates on the side, if you like.

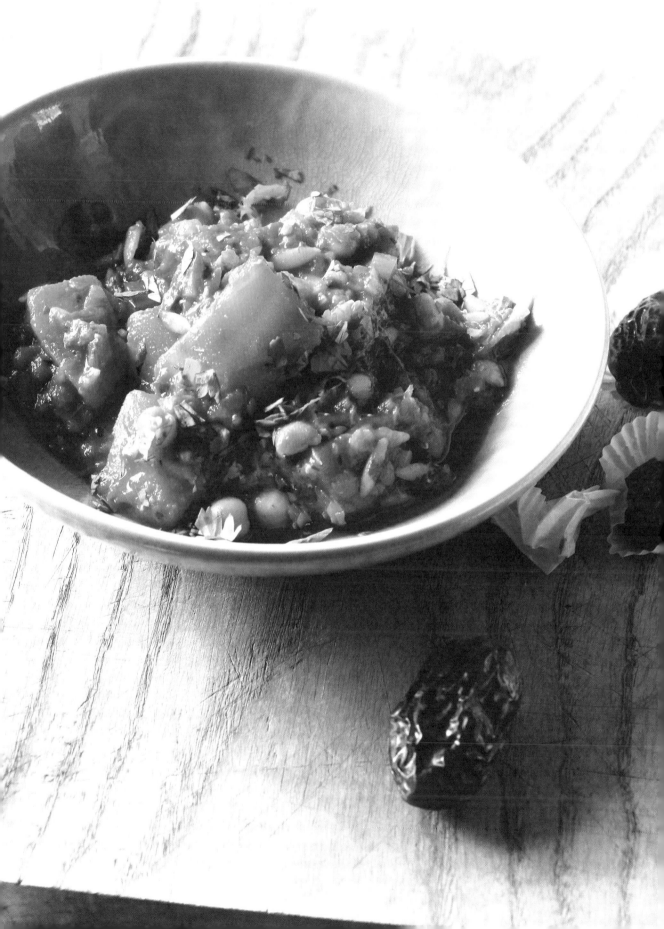

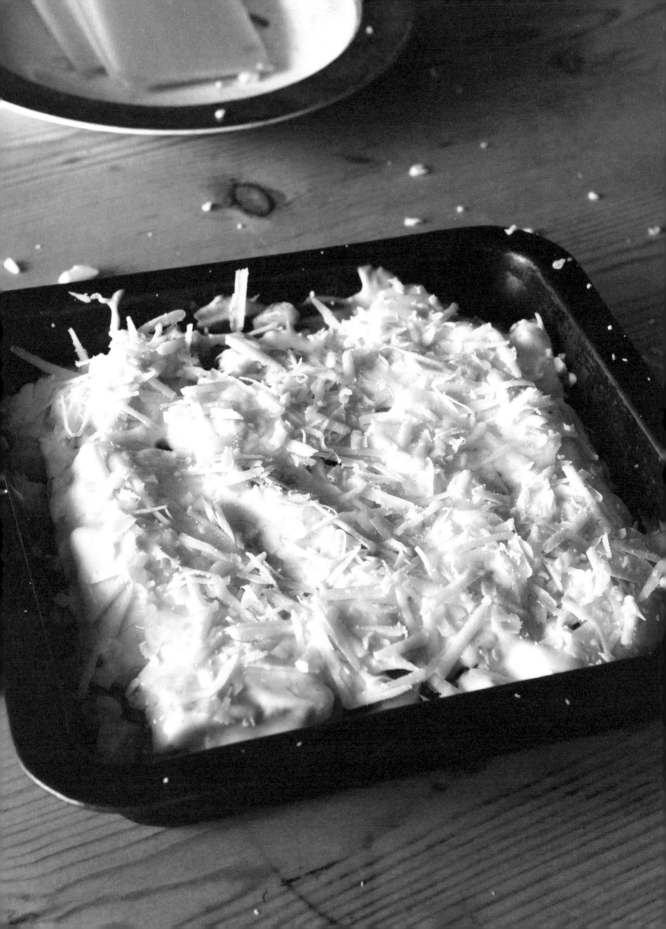

Squash and fennel lasagne

There are endless versions of veg lasagne and many of them are disappointing, being over-reliant on pulses and tomato sauce. I think this unusual recipe is really special, proper comfort food and just what you need on a chilly autumn night: lots of earthy flavours, plenty of creamy béchamel sauce and a good dose of melting cheese.

SERVES 6

1kg squash

6 tablespoons rapeseed or olive oil, plus extra to trickle

1 fat garlic clove, finely chopped

A few sprigs of thyme, leaves only, finely chopped

750g fennel (3 large bulbs)

150g blue cheese or goat's cheese, crumbled

125g lasagne sheets (fresh is best, but dried is fine)

20g Parmesan, Cheddar or other well-flavoured hard cheese, grated

Sea salt and freshly ground black pepper

FOR THE BÉCHAMEL SAUCE

1 litre whole milk

1 bay leaf

1 onion, roughly chopped

1 celery stalk, roughly chopped

A few black peppercorns

50g unsalted butter

50g plain flour

2 teaspoons Dijon mustard

Preheat the oven to 180°C/Gas Mark 4. For the béchamel, heat the milk with the bay leaf, onion, celery and peppercorns until just below simmering. Remove from the heat and set aside to infuse.

Peel and deseed the squash and cut into 2cm cubes. Toss with 4 tablespoons oil in a roasting dish, season well with salt and pepper and roast for 30 minutes, or until tender. Remove from the oven, toss immediately with the garlic and thyme, and set aside.

Trim the fennel, removing the tough outer layer, then cut into roughly 5mm slices. Heat another 2 tablespoons oil in a large frying pan over a medium-low heat. Add the fennel and sauté for 10–15 minutes, or until tender. Set aside.

Gently reheat the infused milk, then strain. Heat the butter in a large saucepan over a medium heat. Stir in the flour to form a smooth roux and cook gently for a minute or two. Take off the heat. Add about a quarter of the hot milk and beat well until smooth. Repeat with the remaining milk, adding it in 2 or 3 lots, until you have a smooth sauce. Return to the heat and cook, stirring often and allowing it to bubble gently for a few minutes, until thickened. Stir in the mustard and season with salt and pepper.

Spread a third of the béchamel sauce over the bottom of a 28 x 22cm (or thereabouts) ovenproof dish. Layer half the lasagne sheets in the dish, then scatter the roasted squash evenly over it. Trickle over another third of the sauce. Add another layer of lasagne, then the fennel. Scatter the crumbled cheese over the fennel, then spoon on the remaining béchamel.

Sprinkle with the grated cheese and add a trickle of oil. Bake for about 30 minutes until golden. Serve at once, with peas or a green salad.

Kale and mushroom lasagne

This is what I call a good weekender: a dish that requires a little bit of preparation, but one you can put together in a relaxed way over an hour or two that results in something truly warming and delicious.

SERVES 6

About 300g curly kale or cavolo nero, tough stalks removed

30g butter

500g mushrooms, sliced

2 garlic cloves, finely chopped

A few sprigs of thyme, leaves only, chopped

175g lasagne sheets (fresh is best, but dried is fine)

20g Parmesan, hard goat's cheese or other well-flavoured hard cheese, grated

A little rapeseed or olive oil

Sea salt and freshly ground black pepper

FOR THE BÉCHAMEL SAUCE

750ml whole milk

1 bay leaf

1 onion, roughly chopped

1 celery stalk, roughly chopped

A few black peppercorns

50g unsalted butter

50g plain flour

2 teaspoons Dijon mustard

Preheat the oven to 180°C/Gas Mark 4. Heat the milk for the béchamel sauce with the bay leaf, onion, celery and peppercorns until just below simmering. Remove from the heat and set aside to infuse.

Roughly shred the kale or cavolo nero. Put into a large saucepan and just cover with cold water. Add salt. Bring to the boil, reduce the heat and simmer for 2–3 minutes, until just tender. Drain well and set aside.

Heat half the butter in a large, wide frying pan over a medium heat. Add half the mushrooms and some salt and pepper. Increase the heat and fry, stirring often, for 5–10 minutes, until the liquid released by the mushrooms has evaporated and they are starting to reduce, concentrate and caramelise. Stir in half the garlic and half the thyme, cook for a minute longer, then remove to a bowl. Repeat to cook the remaining mushrooms and set aside.

Gently reheat the infused milk, then strain. Heat the butter for the béchamel sauce in a large saucepan. Stir in the flour to form a smooth roux and cook gently for a minute or two. Remove from the heat. Add about a quarter of the hot milk and beat vigorously until smooth. Repeat with the remaining milk, adding it in 2 or 3 lots, until you have a smooth sauce. Return to the heat and cook for a few minutes, stirring often, allowing it to bubble gently until thickened. Stir in the mustard, then add some salt and pepper.

Stir about half of the béchamel sauce into the kale; put to one side.

Spread half the remaining béchamel over the bottom of a 28 x 22cm (or thereabouts) ovenproof dish. Layer a third of the lasagne sheets in the dish, then spoon the kale over the top. Add another layer of lasagne, then the mushrooms. Finish with a final layer of pasta and the remaining béchamel.

Scatter over the cheese and add a trickle of oil. Bake for about 30 minutes until golden. Serve straight away.

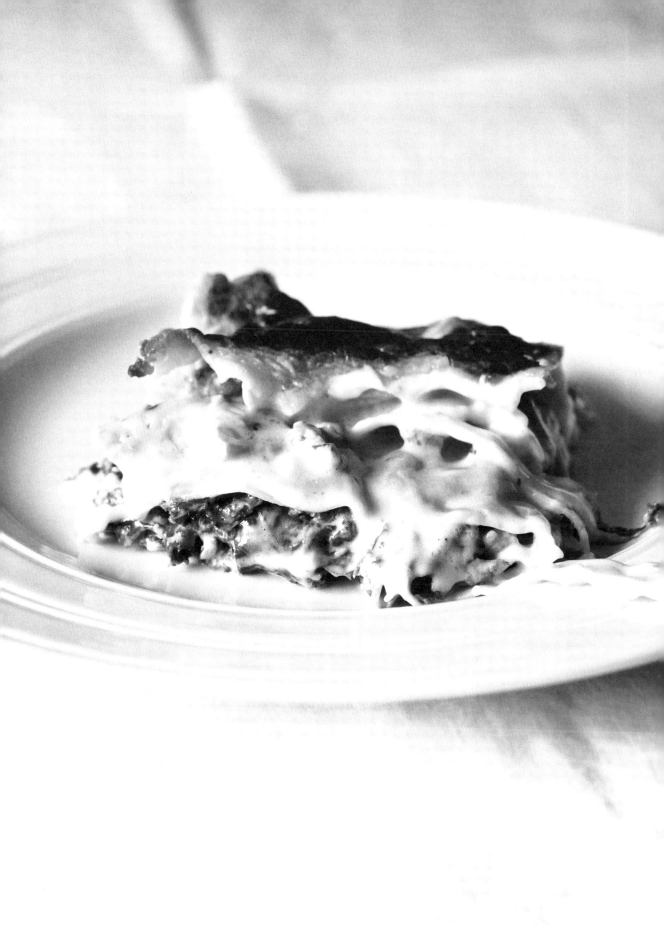

Chillies stuffed with beans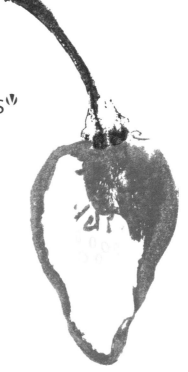

I like to use fat, mildly piquant, poblano chillies for this dish. (You can buy these, as well as chilli seeds and plants, online at www.peppersbypost.biz.) But if you can't get hold of stuffable large chillies, you can use small red or yellow peppers instead.

SERVES 6 AS A STARTER, 2-3 AS A MAIN COURSE

6 large, fresh poblano, Beaver Dam or Hungarian hot wax chillies

1 tablespoon rapeseed or olive oil

2–3 shallots, or 1 medium onion, finely chopped

2 garlic cloves, finely chopped

150–200g tomatoes

400g tin beans, such as borlotti, pinto or butter beans, drained and rinsed

A bunch of coriander, chopped

1 teaspoon ground cumin

1 teaspoon hot smoked paprika

Sea salt and freshly ground black pepper

FOR THE GARLICKY YOGHURT (OPTIONAL)

6 tablespoons plain (full-fat) yoghurt or soured cream

½ garlic clove, crushed

Preheat the grill to high. Lay the chillies on a baking tray and grill, turning from time to time, until the skins begin to char. Leave until cool enough to handle, then carefully peel away the skins, taking care to keep the chillies whole. Cut around and remove the stalks and a flap of flesh to form a 'lid'. Carefully scrape out all the seeds and membranes from inside the chillies and lids, and tip out any juice.

Preheat the oven to 180°C/Gas Mark 4. Heat the oil in a frying pan over a medium-low heat, then gently sauté the shallots or onion and garlic until soft, about 10 minutes. Slice the tomatoes in half and grate their flesh straight into the pan, holding back the skin. Simmer for a minute or two to reduce slightly. Remove from the heat.

Add the drained beans to the pan and roughly mash some of them with a fork, so they break up a little – don't overdo it, you want plenty of them to stay whole. Add the chopped coriander, cumin and paprika, mix well and season with salt and pepper to taste. Stuff the mixture carefully into the chillies and top with the 'lids'. Lay them in a lightly oiled ovenproof dish and bake for 20 minutes.

While the chillies are in the oven, combine the yoghurt with the crushed garlic and some salt and pepper, if serving, and set aside.

Serve the stuffed chillies hot, with a spoonful of garlicky yoghurt if you like, and a crisp, green salad.

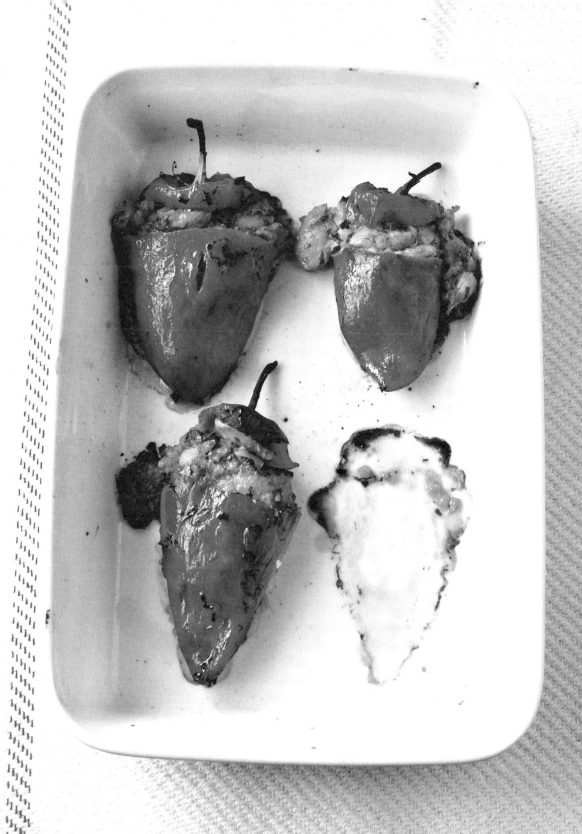

Stuffed cabbage leaves

This is a great dish for a special occasion. It may not be quick, but it's one to prepare when you have a willing accomplice in the kitchen, as in, 'You make the sauce, I'll make the stuffing, and we'll roll the parcels together.'

SERVES 4

12 outer leaves from a large Savoy cabbage

4 tablespoons soured cream, plus extra to serve (optional)

FOR THE TOMATO SAUCE

2 tablespoons olive oil

1 onion, chopped

1 bay leaf

A couple of sprigs of thyme

1 carrot, chopped

1 celery stalk, chopped

2 garlic cloves, finely chopped

600g fresh, ripe tomatoes, skinned and chopped, **OR** a 400g tin plum tomatoes, roughly chopped, any stalky ends and skin removed

A pinch of sugar (optional)

Sea salt and freshly ground black pepper

FOR THE FILLING

120g pearled spelt, rice or pearl barley

1 tablespoon olive oil

1 onion, chopped

1–2 garlic cloves, finely chopped

50g currants

50g walnuts, roughly chopped

Finely grated zest of 1 lemon

A bunch of parsley, chopped

A handful of dill, chopped

¼ teaspoon dried chilli flakes

1 large egg, lightly beaten

First make the tomato sauce. Heat the olive oil in a saucepan over a medium-low heat and sweat the onion, bay leaf and thyme for about 10 minutes until the onion is soft. Add the carrot and celery and sauté for a further 5 minutes, then stir in the garlic and cook for a minute. Add the tomatoes with their juice, some salt and pepper, and a pinch of sugar if you like. Simmer gently until thickened, about 15 minutes.

Preheat the oven to 180°C/Gas Mark 4. If the midribs of the cabbage leaves are thick, pare the thickest part down a bit with a vegetable peeler. Bring a pan of lightly salted water to the boil and blanch the cabbage leaves for 2–3 minutes. Drain and refresh under the cold tap, then pat the leaves dry with a tea towel or kitchen paper.

To make the filling, cook the spelt, rice or barley according to the packet instructions. Heat the olive oil in a small pan, add the onion and sweat over a low heat until soft but not coloured. Add the garlic and stir for a minute. Tip the onion and garlic into a bowl and add the spelt, rice or barley, the currants, walnuts, lemon zest, chopped herbs and chilli flakes. Season very generously with salt and pepper, stir until well mixed, then add the egg and stir again until combined.

Lay the blanched cabbage leaves out on a clean surface. Place a big spoonful of the filling mixture in the centre of each leaf, fold over the sides and roll up from the stalk end, so you have 12 neat packages. Place them in an ovenproof dish, seam side down.

Spoon the tomato sauce over the stuffed leaves, dot some soured cream on top and sprinkle with pepper. Bake for 30–35 minutes until piping hot. Serve with more soured cream, if you like.

VARIATIONS

Instead of cabbage, you can use large fresh or preserved vine leaves, blanching fresh ones for 1 minute only; preserved leaves just need to be rinsed well. Alternatively, you can use the leaves of spring or winter greens: remove coarse stalks and blanch the leaves for a minute or two, to soften.

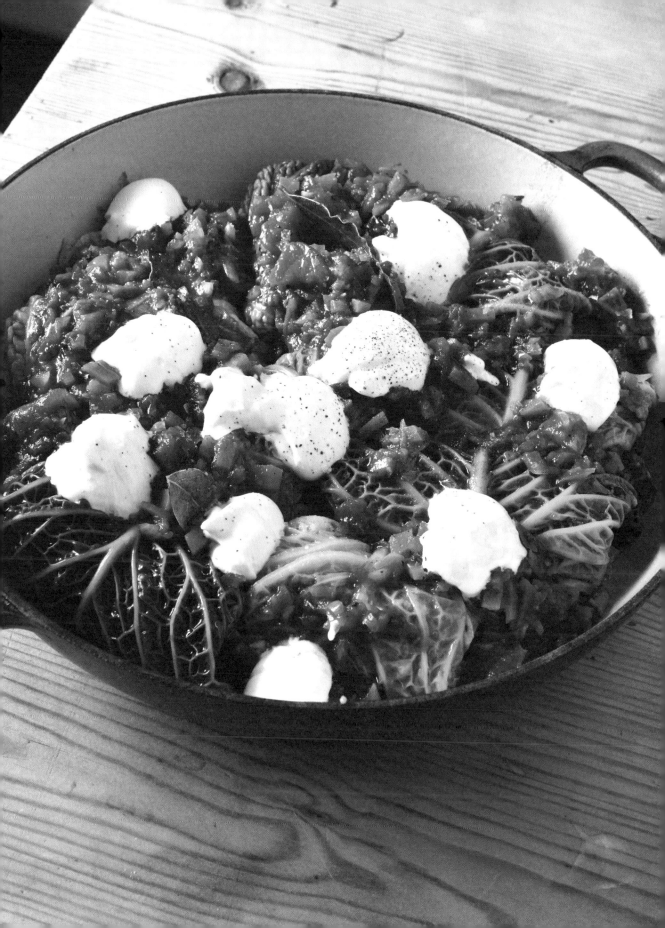

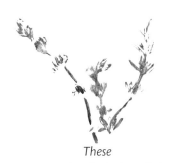

Squash stuffed with leeks

These tempting baked stuffed squash make for an impressive and substantial meal. The scent of thyme, leeks and cheese that wafts up as you lift the lid off is so alluring. Small gem or acorn squash are ideal; you could even use a squat butternut. Those around 400g will serve one; larger squash can be shared.

SERVES 4

35g butter

2 large leeks, trimmed and thinly sliced

1 teaspoon English mustard

4 tablespoons crème fraîche

125g Gruyère or other well-flavoured hard cheese, finely grated

2–4 smallish squash (400–800g each)

A handful of thyme sprigs

Sea salt and freshly ground black pepper

Preheat the oven to 190°C/Gas Mark 5. Heat the butter in a saucepan over a medium heat and add the leeks. As soon as they begin to sizzle, turn the heat right down and cover the pan. Sweat the leeks gently for about 10 minutes, until very soft. Remove from the heat and stir in the mustard, crème fraîche and cheese. Season the mixture well with salt and pepper, as it will be surrounded by a good amount of squash.

Cut a small slice off the base of each squash so it will stand up on a baking tray without wobbling. Carefully slice a 'lid' off the top of each one too and set aside. Now, with a small, sharp knife, cut into the centre of each squash, then use a teaspoon to scoop out all the seeds and fibres.

Fill the squash cavities with the leek mixture – they should be about two-thirds full. Tuck a few thyme sprigs into the centre of each. Put the 'lids' back on top and stand the squash on a large baking tray – there should be plenty of room for hot air to circulate around them.

Bake for 50–60 minutes – possibly longer if the squash are large – until the flesh feels very tender inside. Serve straight away.

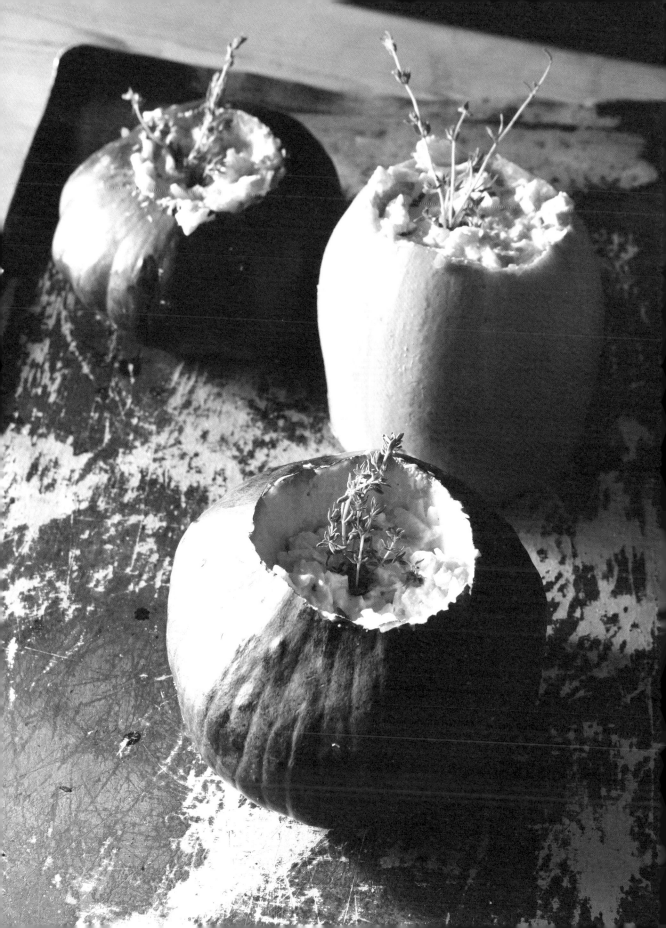

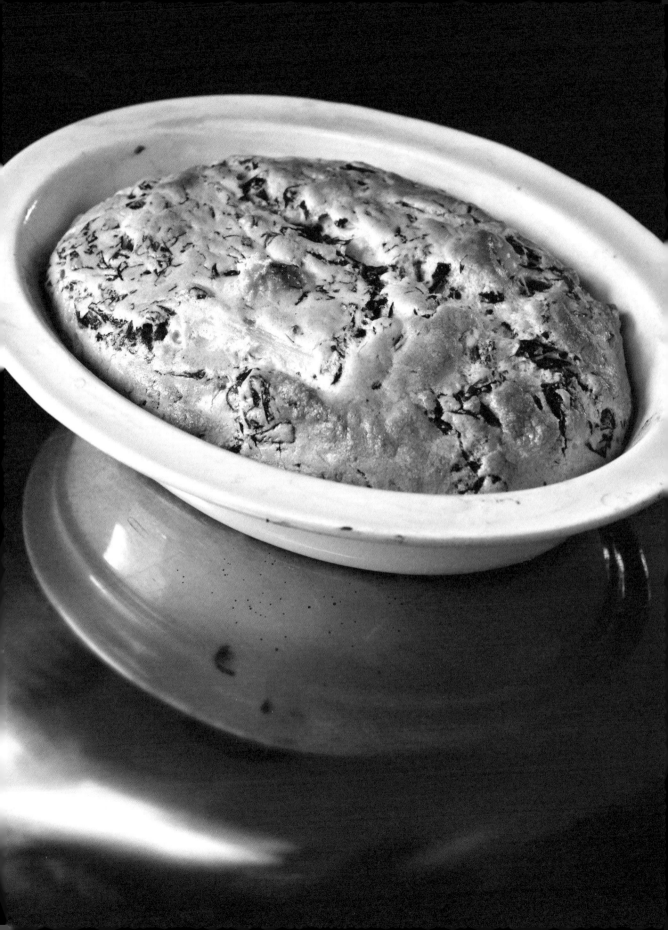

Spinach, penne and cheese spoufflé

I love using pasta to turn a light, puffy spinach soufflé into a sustaining one-pot supper, or 'spoufflé', as I call it. Delicately browned on top, you'll find it's still creamy and soft at the centre. The courgette version (below) is equally good.

SERVES 4

300ml whole milk

1 bay leaf

½ onion

A few black peppercorns

100g penne or similar shaped pasta

A little rapeseed or olive oil

250g spinach, any tough stalks removed

50g unsalted butter, plus extra for greasing

50g plain flour

75g mature Cheddar, finely grated

A little freshly grated nutmeg

3 large eggs, separated, plus 1 extra egg white

Sea salt and freshly ground black pepper

Preheat the oven to 190°C/Gas Mark 5 and put a baking sheet in to heat up. Liberally butter a 1.5 litre soufflé dish or fairly deep ovenproof dish of similar capacity.

Put the milk, bay leaf, onion and peppercorns into a small pan and bring to just below a simmer. Turn off the heat and leave to infuse.

Bring a pan of well-salted water to the boil. Add the penne to the boiling water and cook until *al dente*. Drain well, then toss in a tiny bit of oil to stop it sticking together.

Cook the spinach, with just the water clinging to it after washing, in a large covered pan over a medium heat until wilted – just a few minutes. Drain well. When cool enough to handle, squeeze out the liquid with your hands, then roughly chop the spinach.

Heat the butter in a pan over a medium heat, stir in the flour to form a roux and cook for a few minutes. Reheat the infused milk, then strain. Off the heat, add the milk to the roux, a third at a time, beating well; you will end up with a very thick béchamel sauce. Cook, stirring, for a couple of minutes. Remove from the heat and stir in the cheese, nutmeg, chopped spinach and some salt and pepper – it should be well seasoned. Beat in the egg yolks, then fold in the cooked penne.

In a clean bowl, whisk the egg whites to firm peaks. Stir a spoonful into the béchamel mix to loosen it, then carefully fold in the rest. Tip into the buttered dish and place on the hot baking sheet in the oven. Bake for 25–30 minutes, until well risen and golden. Serve straight away.

VARIATION

Courgette penne spoufflé

Instead of the spinach, use 500g finely sliced courgettes. Heat about 2 tablespoons olive oil in a large frying pan over a medium heat, add the courgettes with a finely sliced garlic clove and a good pinch of salt and fry gently for at least 15 minutes, tossing regularly, without browning. As they soften, break them up a bit with your spatula to form a very rough, creamy purée. Fold into the béchamel along with the cooked penne and continue as above.

Lettuce, spring onion and cheese tart

Cooked lettuce can be absolutely wonderful, combining sweet and slightly bitter flavours. Mixed with fresh-tasting spring onions and a creamy savoury custard, it makes a very lovely tart – perfect for an early summer lunch.

SERVES 4-6

FOR THE PASTRY

250g plain flour

A pinch of sea salt

125g chilled unsalted butter, cut into small cubes

About 75ml cold milk

FOR THE FILLING

1 tablespoon rapeseed or olive oil

4 Little Gem lettuce hearts, trimmed and quartered

15g butter

2 bunches of spring onions (about 250g), trimmed and cut into chunky slices

100g Lancashire, medium Cheddar or hard goat's cheese

2 large eggs, plus 2 extra egg yolks

200ml double cream

200ml whole milk

Sea salt and freshly ground black pepper

To make the pastry, sift the flour and salt together, or give them a quick blitz in a food processor. Add the butter and rub in with your fingertips, or blitz in the food processor, until the mixture resembles fine breadcrumbs. Mix in the cold milk, little by little, until the pastry just comes together, then turn out on to a work surface and knead briefly to bring it into a ball. Wrap and chill for 30 minutes.

Preheat the oven to 180°C/Gas Mark 4. On a lightly floured surface, roll out the pastry quite thinly and use to line a 25cm tart tin. Leave the rough edges of the pastry hanging over the sides of the tin. Line with foil and baking beans and bake blind for 15 minutes. Remove the foil and beans, prick the pastry in a few places with a sharp fork, and bake uncovered for a further 10–15 minutes, or until the pastry is just starting to colour. Using a small, sharp knife, trim away the excess pastry from the edge.

To make the filling, heat the oil in a frying pan over a medium heat. Add the quartered lettuce hearts, sprinkle with salt and pepper and cook for about 5 minutes, turning once or twice, until the cut surfaces are golden brown. Add the butter towards the end of cooking, letting it melt in the pan, then spooning it over the lettuces. Using a slotted spoon, remove the seared, buttery lettuce hearts and arrange in the pastry case.

Reduce the heat under the frying pan a little. Add the spring onions and sauté gently for 5 minutes, then scatter in the tart case over and around the lettuce hearts. Crumble or grate the cheese over the top.

Lightly beat the eggs, egg yolks, cream and milk together in a bowl and season generously with salt and pepper. Carefully pour this mixture over the tart filling (depending on the depth of your tin, you might not need all of it). Bake for about 35 minutes until golden. Serve warm or at room temperature.

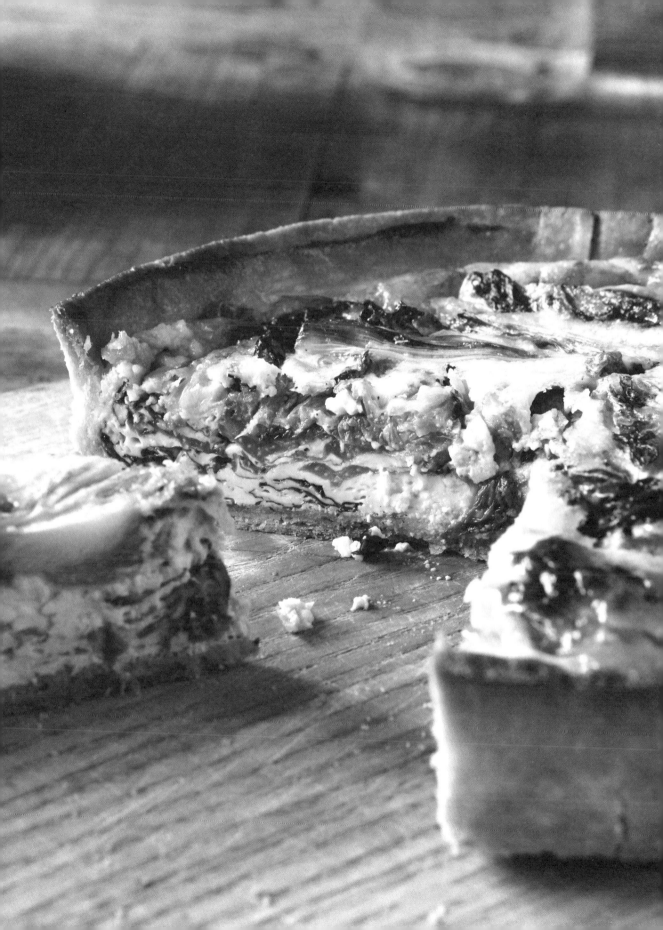

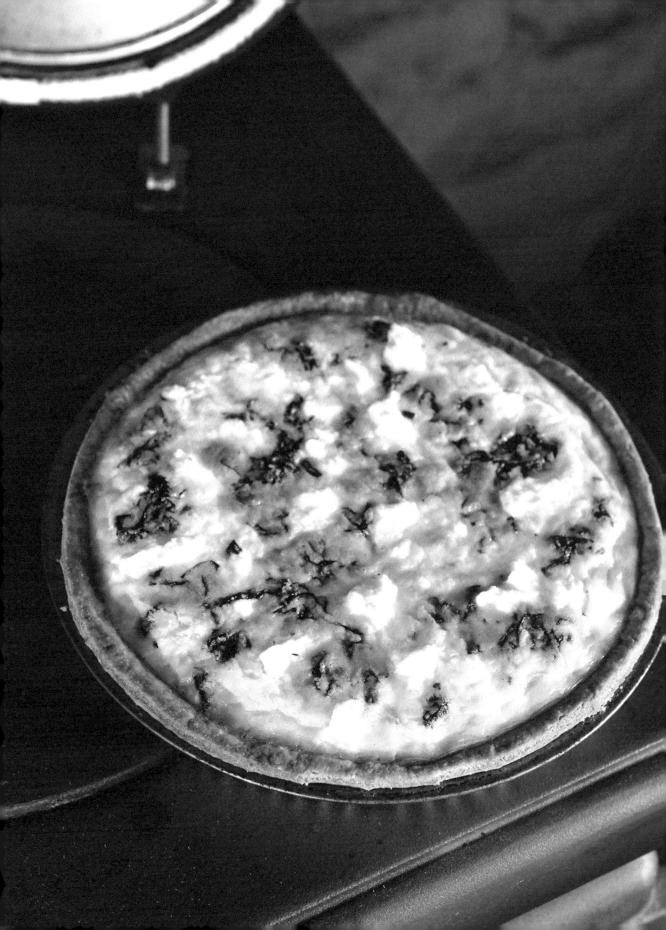

Beet top (or chard) and ricotta tart

If you come by bunched baby beetroot with the leaves and stems still attached, this is a great use for them. Fine-stemmed varieties of chard, such as ruby or rainbow, are ideal too. You can use any ricotta for this, but a delicate, crumbly sheep's milk ricotta is particularly good.

SERVES 4-6

FOR THE PASTRY

250g plain flour

A pinch of sea salt

125g chilled unsalted butter, cut into small cubes

About 75ml cold milk

FOR THE FILLING

Tops from a bunch of beetroot OR a bunch of ruby or rainbow chard (about 300g in all)

1 tablespoon rapeseed or olive oil

1 large onion, sliced

A handful of thyme sprigs, leaves only, chopped

1 garlic clove, finely chopped

100g ricotta, finely crumbled

2 large eggs, plus 2 extra egg yolks

200ml double cream

200ml whole milk

Sea salt and freshly ground black pepper

Make the pastry, rest, then use to line a 25cm tart tin and bake blind, following the method on page 44.

To make the filling, chop the stalks from the beet tops or chard and shred the leaves. Heat the oil in a large frying pan, add the onion with the thyme and sweat gently for about 10 minutes, until softened. Add the garlic and chopped beet or chard stalks. Cook, stirring often, for about 10 minutes, until the stalks are tender. Add the shredded leaves and cook for another 5 minutes or so until the leaves have wilted right down. Season well with salt and pepper.

Spread the leafy mixture in the tart case. Scatter the crumbled ricotta over the top. Lightly beat the eggs, egg yolks, cream and milk together in a bowl and season well with salt and pepper. Carefully pour this mixture over the tart filling. Bake the tart at 180°C/Gas Mark 4 for about 35 minutes until golden. Serve warm or cold.

VARIATION

Samphire and spinach tart
Salty, succulent marsh samphire, which is at its best in June and July, makes an unusual and delicious alternative filling for this tart – it's especially good combined with fresh spinach. Wilt down about 250g spinach, drain well and squeeze out all water, then chop coarsely. Thoroughly wash about 150g marsh samphire and remove any woody ends. Cook the onion as above, adding the thyme and garlic, and seasoning with pepper but no salt as the samphire is already salty. Distribute the onion, chopped spinach and samphire around the tart case, then scatter over the ricotta. Add the custard and bake as above.

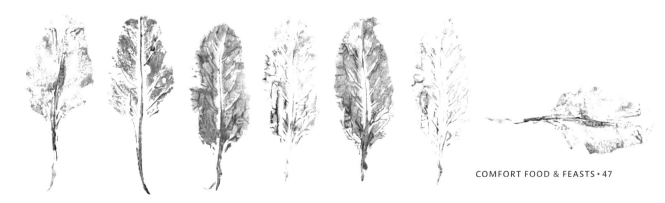

Baby beet tarte tatin

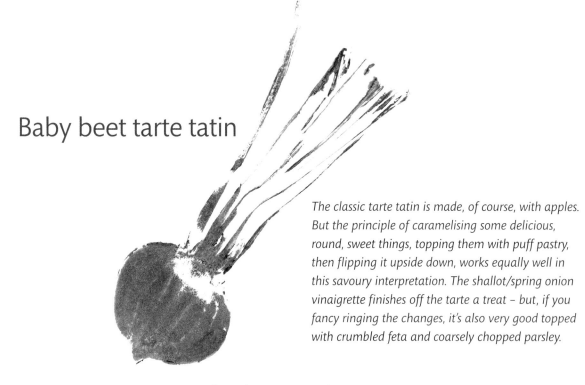

The classic tarte tatin is made, of course, with apples. But the principle of caramelising some delicious, round, sweet things, topping them with puff pastry, then flipping it upside down, works equally well in this savoury interpretation. The shallot/spring onion vinaigrette finishes off the tarte a treat – but, if you fancy ringing the changes, it's also very good topped with crumbled feta and coarsely chopped parsley.

SERVES 4

250g rough puff pastry
(see page 52) or all-butter puff
(ready-made)

A knob of butter

1 tablespoon rapeseed
or olive oil

2 teaspoons cider vinegar

2 teaspoons soft brown sugar

About 300–400g baby beetroot
(the size of a golf ball or no
bigger than a small apple),
scrubbed and halved

Sea salt and freshly ground
black pepper

FOR THE VINAIGRETTE

1 or 2 shallots, or 3 or 4 spring
onions, trimmed and very finely
chopped

1 teaspoon English mustard

1 tablespoon cider vinegar

4 tablespoons rapeseed oil

A pinch of sugar

A handful of parsley leaves,
finely chopped

Preheat the oven to 190°C/Gas Mark 5. Roll out the pastry on a lightly floured surface to a thickness of about 5mm. Take an ovenproof frying pan (or a tarte tatin dish) roughly 20cm in diameter, place it upside down on the pastry and cut around it. Wrap the pastry disc and place it in the fridge.

Melt the butter with the oil in the frying pan (or tatin dish). Add the cider vinegar, sugar and some salt and pepper, stir well, then add the halved beetroot and toss in the juices. You want the beetroot to fill the pan snugly, so add a few more if you need to. Cover the pan with foil, transfer to the oven and roast for 30–40 minutes, until the beetroot are tender.

Take the pan from the oven and rearrange the beetroot halves neatly, placing them cut side up. Lay the pastry disc over the beetroot, patting it down and tucking in the edges down the side of the pan. Return to the oven and bake for 20 minutes, until the pastry is fully puffed up and golden brown.

Leave the tarte to cool in its dish for about 15 minutes, then turn it out by putting a plate over the top and inverting it. Pour any juices left in the pan back over the beetroot.

Put the ingredients for the vinaigrette into a screw-topped jar, season well with salt and pepper and shake to combine. Trickle over the tarte tatin and serve.

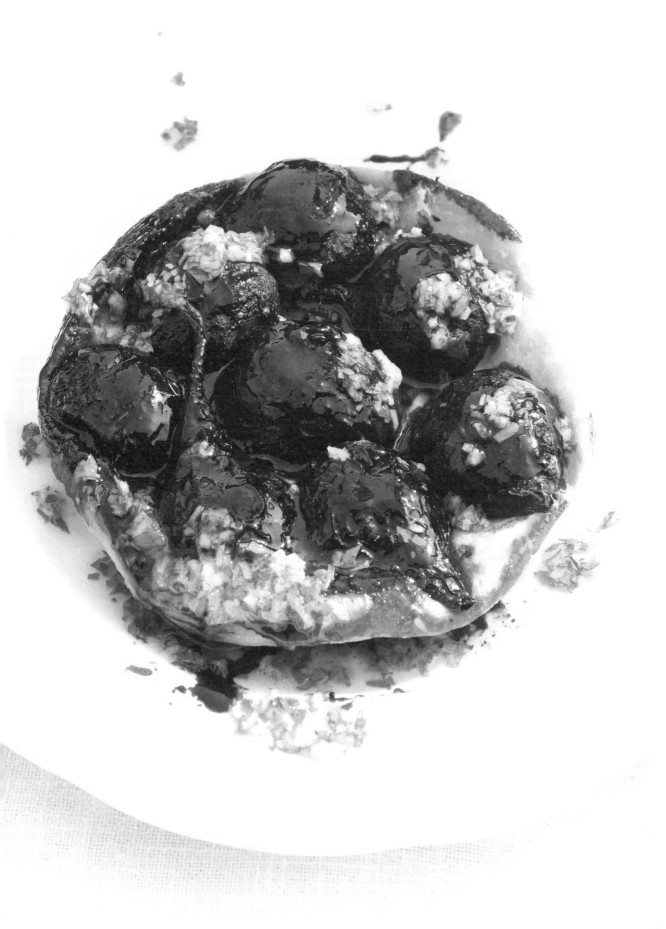

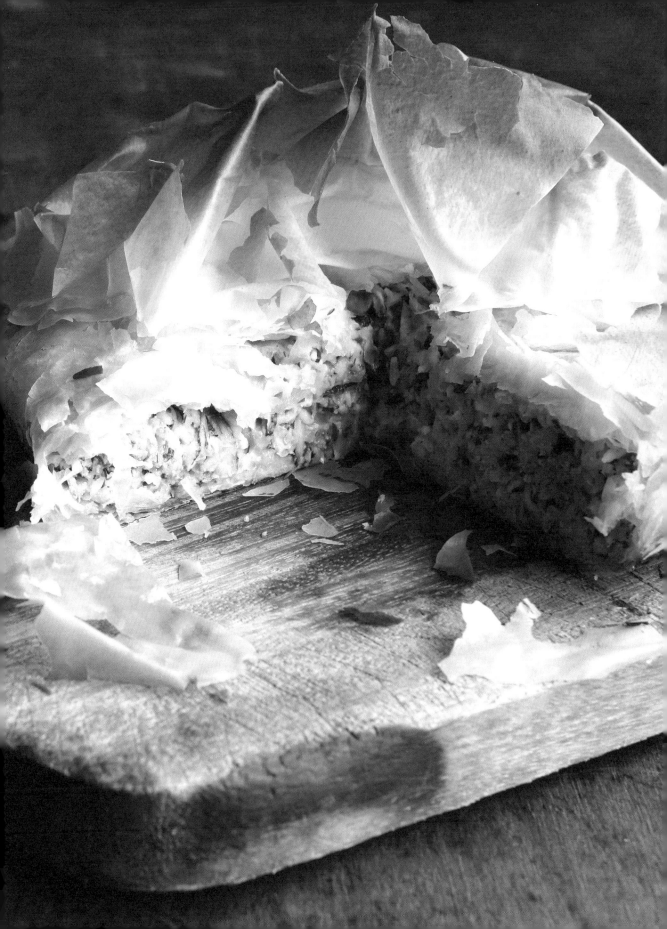

Courgette and rice filo pie

This is based on an intriguing, delicious Greek dish that I came across in a battered old copy of Mediterranean Vegetable Cookery by Rena Salaman. The rice steals the water from the grated courgettes and plumps up as the two cook together inside the pie. It's as tasty as it is cunning.

SERVES 4

500g courgettes, coarsely grated

75g long-grain white rice

½ medium red onion, finely chopped

75g hard goat's cheese or mature Cheddar, grated

2 large eggs, lightly beaten

2 tablespoons olive oil

A handful of dill, chopped

A good handful of flat-leaf parsley, chopped

250g ready-made filo pastry

75g unsalted butter, melted

Sea salt and freshly ground black pepper

Preheat the oven to 190°C/Gas Mark 5. Mix the courgettes, rice, onion, cheese, eggs, olive oil and chopped herbs together in a large bowl. Season with plenty of salt and pepper.

Take a sheet of filo pastry, brush with a little melted butter and use it to line a smallish ovenproof dish, about 1.5 litre capacity, placing the pastry butter side down. Let any excess hang over at the ends. Add another buttered sheet on top and continue until you've used all but one sheet of the pastry.

Tip the filling into the pastry-lined dish. Fold over the pastry ends to enclose the filling, dabbing with a little more melted butter to keep the pastry together. Take the remaining sheet of pastry, crumple it lightly in your hands to give a nicely textured finish and place on top of the pie, tucking in the edges around the side.

Dab a little more butter over the surface and bake for 45 minutes until golden. Serve hot or warm.

Swede and potato pasties

Generously seasoned root vegetables make a hearty pasty filling. These are delicious served hot, but are great cold too – in packed lunches or as a sustaining snack. You can use ordinary shortcrust or a shop-bought puff pastry, but the pasties are particularly good with the easy-to-make rough puff I suggest here. The cheese is optional. Being a bit of a swede purist, I like it without, but it does give an extra dimension of savouriness.

SERVES 4

FOR THE ROUGH PUFF PASTRY

300g plain flour

A pinch of sea salt

150g chilled unsalted butter, cut into small cubes

FOR THE FILLING

225g potato

125g swede

75g carrot

1 small onion, grated

A handful of parsley, finely chopped

A few sprigs of thyme, leaves only, chopped

1 teaspoon vegetable bouillon powder

½ teaspoon freshly ground black pepper

½ teaspoon sea salt

50g strong Cheddar, grated (optional)

30g butter, melted

TO FINISH

1 egg, lightly beaten with 1 teaspoon milk, to glaze

To make the pastry, mix the flour with the salt, then add the cubed butter and toss until the pieces are coated in the flour. Add just enough iced water (about 150ml) to bring the mixture together into a fairly firm dough.

On a well-floured surface, shape the dough into a rectangle with your hands and then roll it out in one direction, away from you, so you end up with a rectangle about 1cm thick. Fold the far third towards you, then fold the nearest third over that (rather like folding a business letter), so that you now have a rectangle made up of 3 equal layers. Give the pastry a quarter turn, then repeat the rolling, folding and turning process 5 more times. Wrap the pastry in cling film and rest in the fridge for about 30 minutes, up to an hour.

Preheat the oven to 190°C/Gas Mark 5. For the filling, peel the potato, swede and carrot and cut into 3–4mm dice. Mix together with all the other ingredients in a bowl, adding the butter last of all to bind.

Roll out the pastry on a lightly floured surface to approximately a 3mm thickness. Using a 19cm plate as a template, cut out 4 circles; you may have to gather up the trimmings then re-roll them to get your fourth circle.

Spoon the vegetable mixture on to one half of each circle. Brush the pastry edges with a little water, fold the other half of the pastry over the filling to form a half-moon shape and crimp the edges well to seal.

Place the pasties on a baking sheet lined with baking parchment and brush with the egg glaze. Bake for about 35–40 minutes, until the pastry is golden brown. Eat hot or cold.

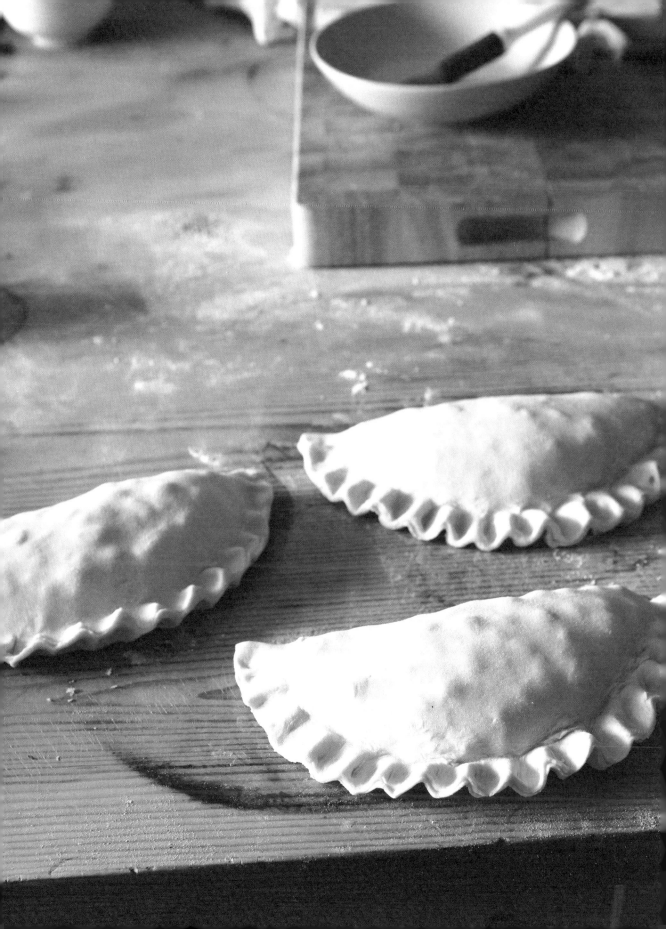

Corner shop spanakopitta

This spinach pie is a pretty loose take on the classic Greek spanakopitta. It came about in response to a challenge laid down by a friend: could I cook up a menu using only ingredients available from the average convenience store? I bit the bullet and this is one of the recipes I came up with. I can't say frozen spinach is an ingredient I use often but you can now get decent frozen whole leaf stuff, and it works well here. Of course, you could use fresh spinach, wilted, drained, squeezed and chopped, if you prefer.

SERVES 4

1kg bag frozen whole-leaf spinach

2 tablespoons olive oil

1 teaspoon cumin, fennel or caraway seeds (whichever is handy)

1 large onion, finely sliced

½ teaspoon dried thyme or a few sprigs of fresh thyme, leaves only, chopped

A squeeze of lemon juice

2 large eggs, lightly beaten

100g soft goat's cheese or feta, broken into small chunks

35g pine nuts, toasted (or roughly chopped cashews)

375g all-butter, ready-made puff pastry (ideally ready-rolled)

Sea salt and freshly ground pepper

Preheat the oven to 200°C/Gas Mark 6. Put the frozen spinach into a saucepan with a splash of water. Cover and heat gently, stirring from time to time, until completely defrosted. Tip into a colander or sieve to drain off all water, pressing with a wooden spoon to help it along.

Meanwhile, heat the olive oil in a frying pan over a medium heat. Add the spice seeds and let them cook for a minute or two, shaking the pan frequently, then add the onion and sauté for 5–10 minutes, or until soft and golden. Add the thyme.

When the spinach has cooled a little, squeeze as much liquid out of it as you can with your hands, then chop it roughly. Combine with the onion, along with a squeeze of lemon juice and plenty of salt and pepper. Set aside 2–3 tablespoons of the beaten egg for glazing and stir the remainder into the spinach and onion mixture.

Spoon half the spinach mixture into a 25 x 20cm (or thereabouts) ovenproof dish. Scatter over the cheese and toasted pine nuts, then top with the remaining spinach. Brush a little of the reserved beaten egg around the rim of the dish.

On a lightly floured surface, roll out the pastry (unless, of course, it's ready-rolled), to a thickness of about 5mm. Lay the pastry over the dish and trim off the excess overhanging the rim. Press the edge of the pastry down so that it sticks to the rim. Brush the pie with the reserved beaten egg and bake for about 25 minutes until the pastry is puffed and golden brown. Serve immediately.

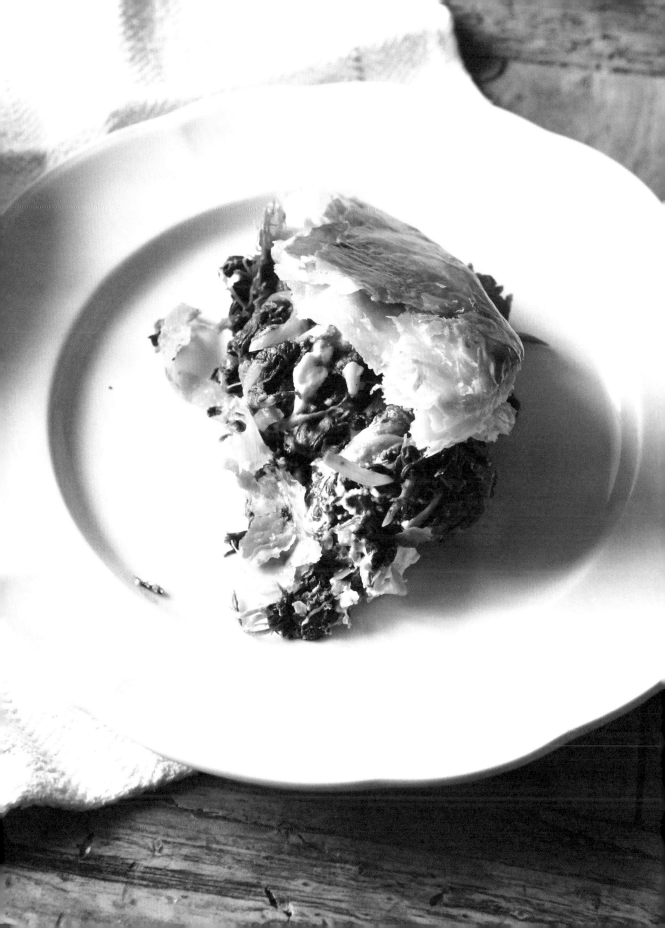

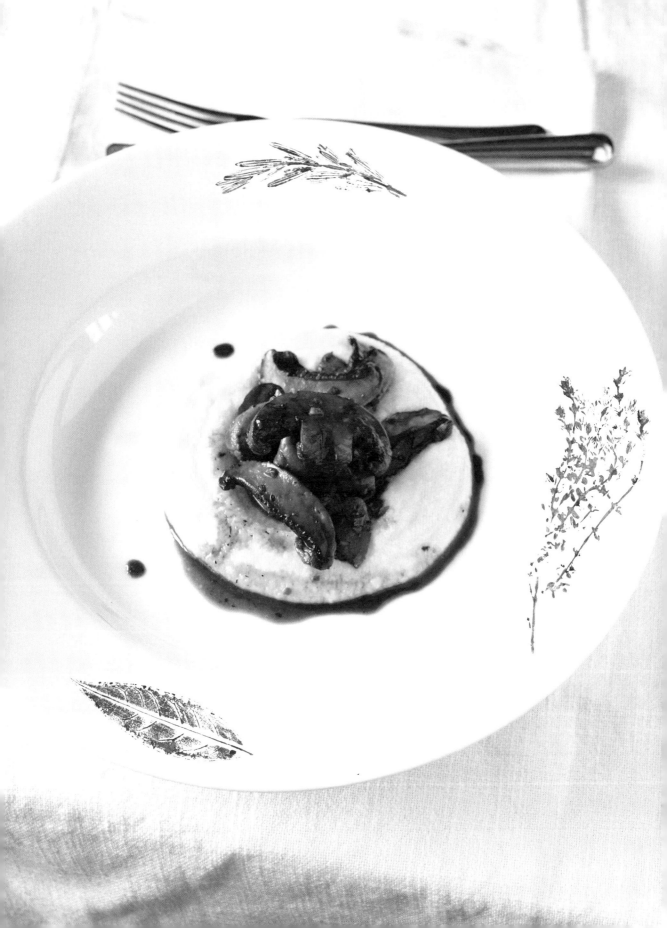

Mushroom ragout with soft polenta

This is very easy to put together, and pretty quick too. Use a mix of well-flavoured mushrooms, such as chestnut, portabellini and big, flat, dark-gilled varieties, adding wild or exotic mushrooms if you have some to hand. If you have any polenta left over, let it go cold, then cut into chunks or cubes and fry it to make polenta 'chips'. In fact, it's worth making more than you need, just so you can do this…

SERVES 4

FOR THE POLENTA

400ml milk

1 bay leaf

A sprig of thyme

A few peppercorns

½ onion and/or 2 garlic cloves, bashed

150g quick-cook polenta

20g butter

1 teaspoon finely chopped rosemary

20g Parmesan, hard goat's cheese or other well-flavoured hard cheese, finely grated

FOR THE RAGOUT

2 tablespoons rapeseed or olive oil

A large knob of butter

650g mushrooms, thickly sliced

1 large garlic clove, finely chopped

A few sprigs of thyme, leaves only, chopped

150ml red wine

150ml vegetable or mushroom stock (see page 130)

Sea salt and freshly ground black pepper

TO SERVE (OPTIONAL)

A trickle of top-notch olive oil

Extra Parmesan or other hard cheese, shaved

For the polenta, put the milk and 400ml water into a saucepan. Add the bay leaf, thyme, peppercorns and onion/garlic. Bring to just below the boil, then set aside to infuse for 20 minutes.

Meanwhile, make the ragout. Heat 1 tablespoon oil and half the butter in a large, wide frying pan over a medium heat. Add half the mushrooms and some salt and pepper and turn the heat up high. Cook, stirring often, to encourage the mushrooms to release their juices. Continue to cook until most of the juices have evaporated and the mushrooms are starting to concentrate and caramelise. Add half the garlic and thyme and cook for a minute more, then tip the contents of the pan out on to a plate and set aside.

Repeat with the remaining mushrooms, using the rest of the garlic and thyme. Return the first batch of mushrooms to the pan. Add the wine and stock, reduce the heat and simmer for about 15 minutes until the liquid has reduced by about half. Check the seasoning.

To cook the polenta, strain the infused milk and water into a clean pan (or just scoop out the flavourings with a slotted spoon, as I do). Bring to a simmer, then pour in the polenta in a thin stream, stirring as you do so. Stir until the mix is smooth and then it let it return to a simmer. Cook for just 1 minute, then remove from the heat. Stir in the butter, rosemary and cheese, then season generously with salt and pepper (adding at least ¼ teaspoon salt).

Immediately scoop the polenta into warmed dishes, top with the juicy mushroom ragout and serve, with an extra trickle of best olive oil and a few slivers of shaved cheese, if you like.

Chilli, cheese and rosemary polenta with tomato sauce

This is a really great way to cook polenta: well flavoured, well seasoned and nicely caramelised. The simple sauce, based on tinned tomatoes, is a mainstay in my kitchen, used in many different ways – with pasta or roasted vegetables, or on a pizza base (see page 180), for example.

SERVES 4

FOR THE POLENTA

4 tablespoons olive oil

1 garlic clove, chopped

1 red chilli, deseeded and finely chopped, or a good pinch of dried chilli flakes

1 tablespoon finely chopped rosemary

150g quick-cook polenta

100g strong Cheddar, hard goat's cheese or other well-flavoured hard cheese, grated

Sea salt and freshly ground black pepper

FOR THE TOMATO SAUCE

2 tablespoons olive oil

2 garlic cloves, finely slivered

2 x 400g tins plum tomatoes, any stalky ends and skin removed

1 bay leaf (optional)

A pinch of sugar

To make the polenta, heat 2 tablespoons of the olive oil in a frying pan over a medium-low heat. Add the garlic and chilli and sweat gently for a couple of minutes – don't let the garlic colour. Add the rosemary and remove from the heat.

Pour 800ml water into a saucepan and bring to the boil. Now pour in the polenta in a thin stream, stirring all the time. When smooth, allow it to return to a simmer. Cook for 4–5 minutes, stirring often, then remove from the heat. Stir in the garlic, chilli and rosemary mixture, then add the grated cheese and a generous amount of salt and pepper. Mix well.

Tip the polenta on to a cold surface, such as a plate or a marble slab, and spread it smoothly into an even disc, about 2cm thick. Leave to cool completely.

To make the tomato sauce, heat the olive oil in a wide frying pan over a medium-low heat. Add the garlic and sweat gently for a couple of minutes; don't let it colour. Put the tomatoes into a large bowl with their juice and crush them with your hands. Tip the lot into the frying pan, adding a bay leaf if you have one handy. Bring to a simmer then cook for 20–30 minutes, stirring often and crushing the tomatoes with a fork until you have a thick, pulpy sauce. Season with salt, pepper and a pinch of sugar.

When the polenta is cool and firm, cut into slices or wedges. Heat 2 tablespoons olive oil in a non-stick pan over a medium-high heat and fry the polenta pieces for 2–3 minutes each side, until they have a light golden brown crust. Serve topped with the hot tomato sauce.

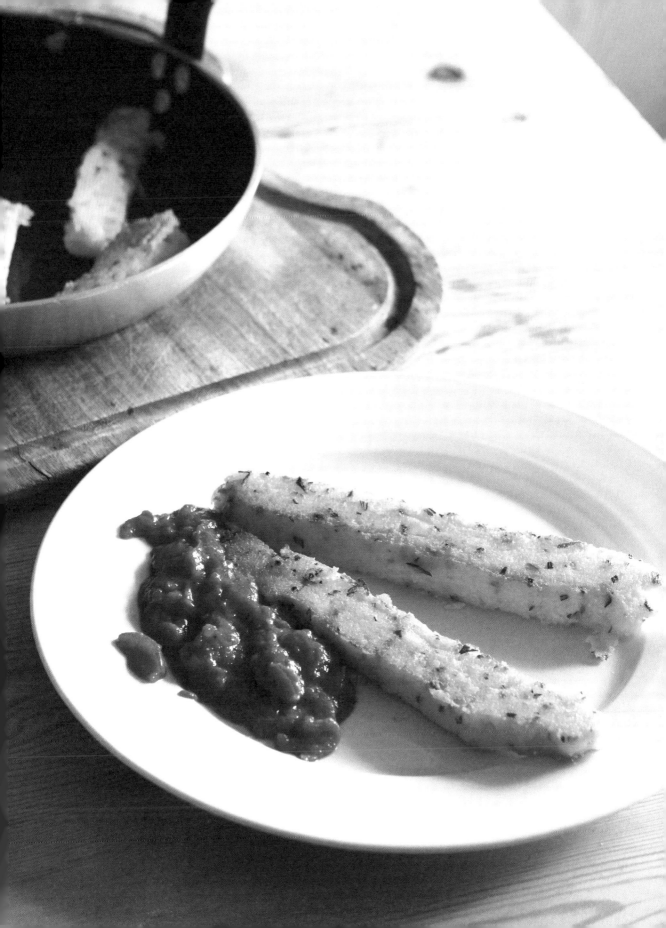

Potato dauphinoise

This classic potato dish with its glorious caramelised top and rich, melting interior will always be one of my favourites. Something magical happens when you bake potatoes, thinly sliced, in garlic-scented cream. I tend to use whichever floury variety I have to hand, but you can also make it with large, new potatoes. The texture is a bit different but still very good. I love a dauphinoise with a green salad and plain-cooked Puy lentils (see page 237).

(see page 237)

SERVES 6

30g butter
1kg floury potatoes
400ml double cream
2 large garlic cloves, crushed
¼ teaspoon freshly grated nutmeg
Sea salt and freshly ground black pepper

Preheat the oven to 160°C/Gas Mark 3. Rub a gratin dish liberally with the butter.

Peel the potatoes and slice them thinly, either with a sharp knife or a mandoline. In a large bowl, whisk together the cream, garlic and nutmeg and season well with salt and pepper. Toss the potatoes in the creamy mixture, then layer them in the gratin dish, spreading them as flat and evenly as you can. Pour over any remaining cream.

Bake for 1¼–1½ hours, pressing down with a spatula every 15 minutes or so to compress the potatoes and stop them drying out. The gratin is ready when the top is golden and bubbling and the potatoes are tender. You may want to turn the oven up to 190–200°C (Gas Mark 5 or 6) for the last 5 minutes to achieve a bit of extra bubbling crispness. Leave to stand for 5 minutes or so before serving.

VARIATIONS

Half-and-half dauphinoise
For something a little more virtuous, you can substitute half the cream for whole milk. That goes for the following variations too.

Celeriac and potato dauphinoise
A wonderful combination. Replace a quarter to half of the potatoes with celeriac, peeled and finely sliced. It's very good with about 30g grated Parmesan or gruyère sprinkled on top before baking, as above.

Potato and turnip dauphinoise
Peel 2 small turnips (about 200g) and slice very thinly, using a mandoline or sharp knife. Use roughly 800g potatoes and toss with the cream as above. Layer half the creamy potato slices in the bottom of the gratin dish, followed by a thin layer of turnips and the rest of the creamy potatoes. Bake as above.

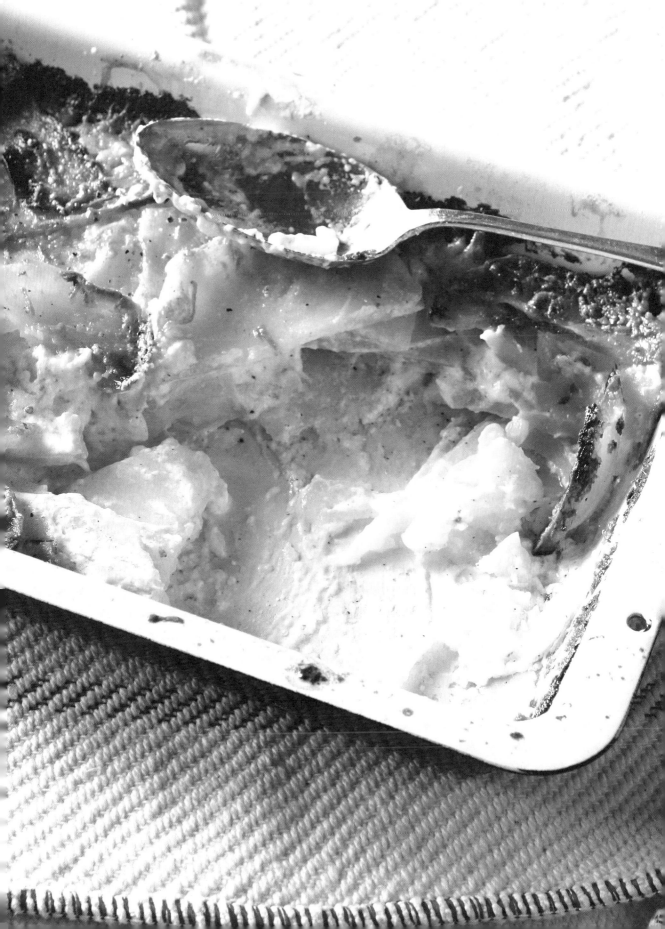

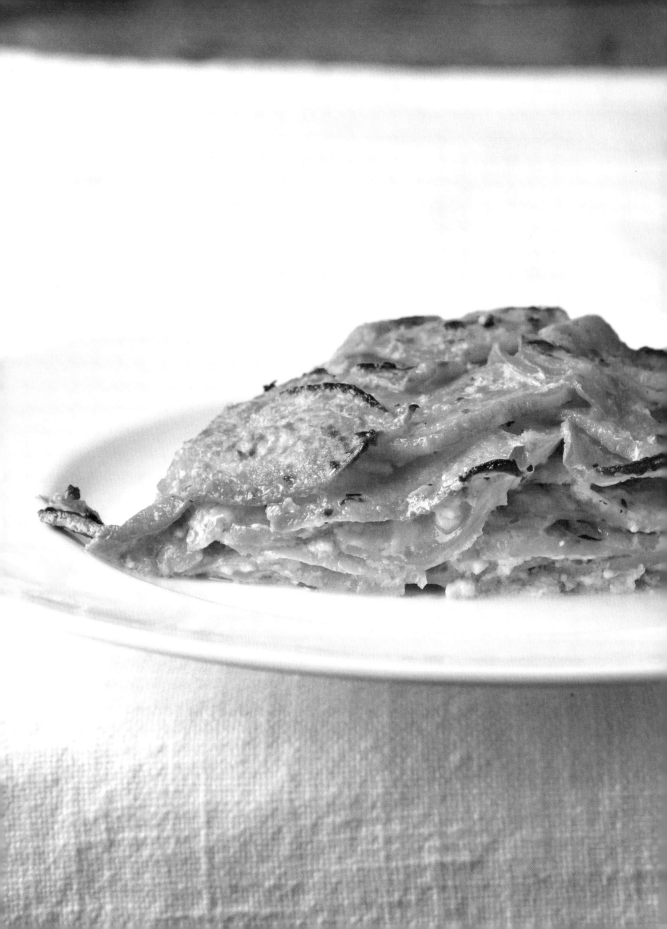

Sweet potato and peanut gratin

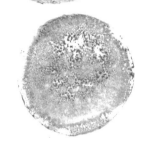

*Although sweet potatoes are not much grown in the UK,
I do enjoy them every now and then. They're extremely good
for you and spiked with a little garlic and chilli to cut their
sweetness, they make a tempting gratin. Here I've added
a seam of slightly salty, crunchy peanut butter with a touch
of lime, which brings a hint of satay-like flavour to the whole
thing, but you can leave this out if you prefer. A bitter-leaved
salad is a good accompaniment here.*

SERVES 4

About 1kg sweet potatoes

2 tablespoons sunflower oil, plus
a little more for greasing

1 red chilli, deseeded and finely
chopped, or 1 teaspoon dried
chilli flakes

3 garlic cloves, finely chopped

250ml double cream

150g crunchy (no-sugar-added)
peanut butter

Finely grated zest of 1 lime, plus
about 2 teaspoons juice

Sea salt and freshly ground
black pepper

Preheat the oven to 190°C/Gas Mark 5 and lightly oil a large gratin dish. Peel the sweet potatoes and cut them into slices, about the thickness of a 10p piece. In a large bowl, toss the sweet potato slices with 1 tablespoon of the oil, the chilli, garlic, cream and some salt and pepper.

Arrange half the sweet potato slices evenly in the gratin dish. You do not have to layer them piece by piece, but try to ensure that the slices are mostly lying flat.

Beat the peanut butter with the remaining 1 tablespoon oil, the lime zest and juice. Spread this mixture in dollops over the sweet potato in the dish. Cover evenly with the remaining sweet potato slices. Pour over any cream remaining from the bowl.

Cover the dish with foil and bake for about 20 minutes, then remove the foil. Bake for a further 30 minutes or so, until the sweet potato is completely tender and the top is browned and crisp. For extra crispness, you can finish under the grill for a couple of minutes, but watch carefully. Serve hot, with a crisp leafy salad to balance the sweet richness of the gratin.

Three-root boulangère

One could hardly call this dish 'light', but it's certainly less rich than a creamy, dauphinoise-style gratin, and a lovely way to enjoy the flavours of some seasonal roots. You don't have to stick to the ones I suggest here: try substituting Jerusalem artichokes, carrots or swede, for example; they all work well. I like to serve this with big flat field mushrooms simply baked with some butter, garlic and cheese (see page 385) and some good bread.

SERVES 4

30g butter

2 onions, halved and thinly sliced

2 garlic cloves, sliced

1 small celeriac

2 large potatoes

3 large parsnips

A couple of sprigs of thyme, leaves only, chopped

3 sage leaves, finely chopped

About 1.2 litres vegetable stock (see page 130)

Sea salt and freshly ground black pepper

Preheat the oven to 180°C/Gas Mark 4. Melt the butter in a heavy-bottomed frying pan and use some of it to grease a large gratin dish. Add the onions to the pan and sauté over a medium heat for about 10 minutes, until nice and soft, then add the garlic and cook gently for a further minute or two.

Meanwhile, peel the celeriac, potatoes and parsnips and cut into slices the thickness of a 10p piece, slicing the parsnips lengthways.

Spread out the celeriac in the gratin dish, season generously with salt and pepper, then sprinkle with half the onions and half the herbs. Layer the parsnips on top, then scatter the remaining onions and herbs on top and finish with a layer of potatoes.

Bring the stock to a simmer and add some salt and pepper, then pour over the vegetables to barely cover them (you may not need all of it). Cover the dish with foil and bake for 30 minutes, then uncover and continue to bake for another 30 minutes or so until the vegetables are cooked.

At this point, if there is still liquid covering the potatoes, spoon off a little and return the dish to the oven for 15 minutes or so, to brown the potatoes on the top. You can use the grill in the oven to get a darker, crisper top if you like. Serve piping hot.

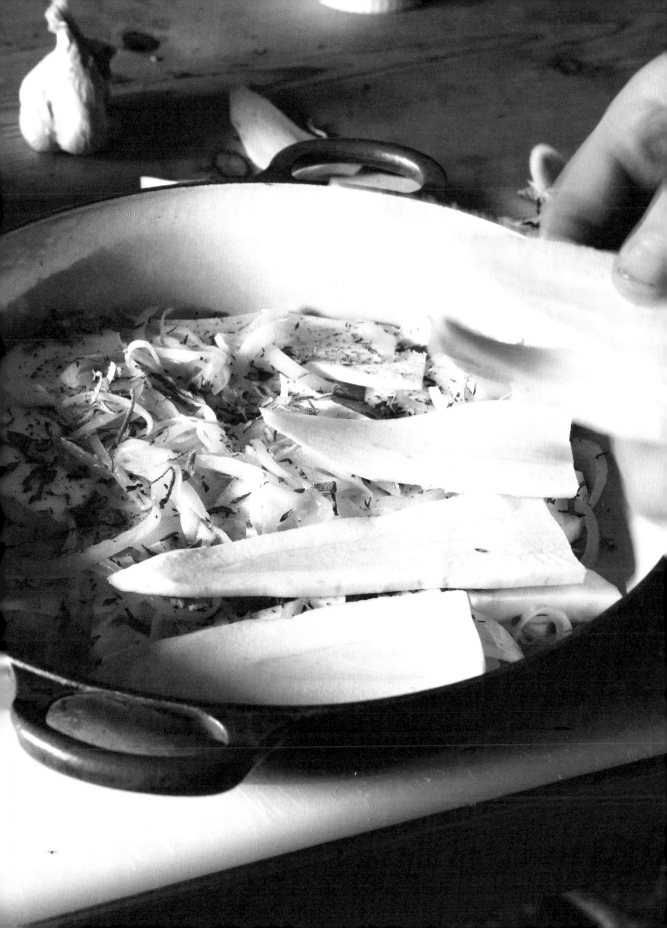

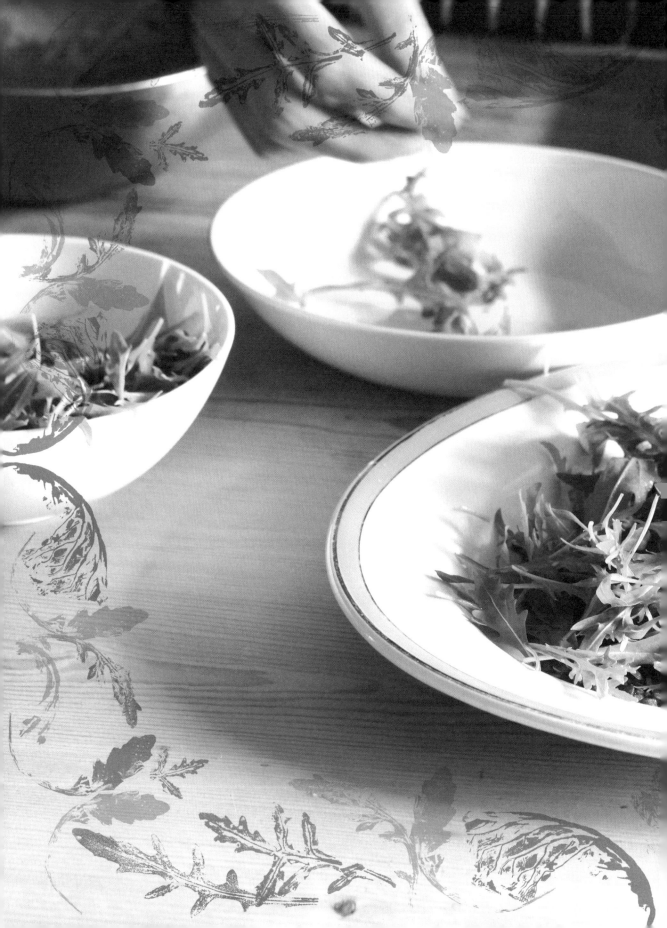

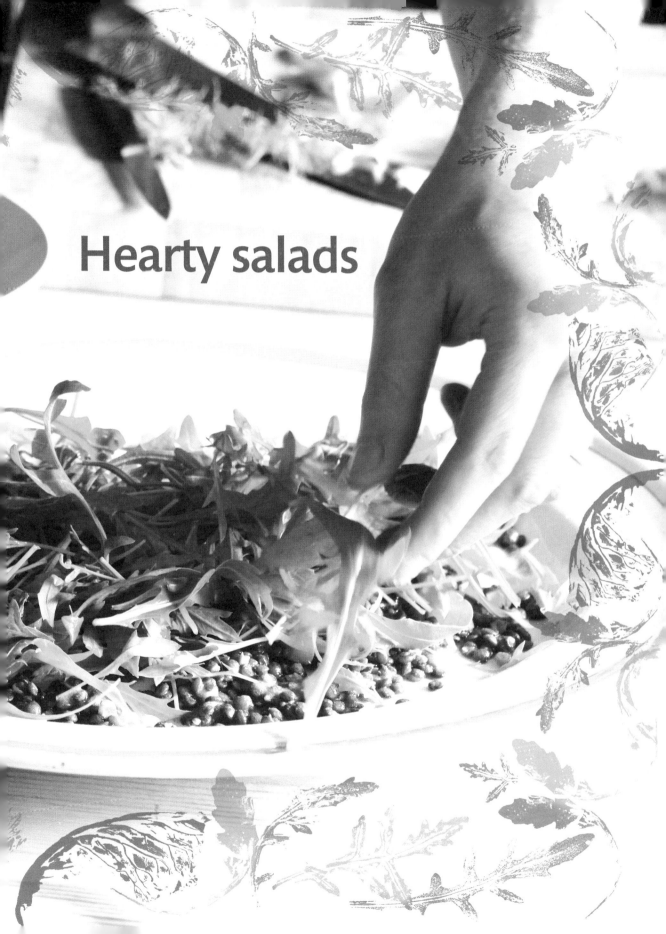

Hearty salads

If you normally think of 'salad' as just a bit of greenery on the side of your plate – more a garnish or afterthought than a meaningful offering to a hearty appetite – then that needs to change. Because the less you are relying on meat and fish, the more you will find that 'salad' is no longer merely a euphemism for limp lettuce, served up to offset the flesh you've just consumed. It's a meal.

In a 'hearty salad', a well-tuned mixture of the raw and the cooked, the chunky and the leafy, perhaps the nutty and the cheesy, creates an enticing, self-contained plateful. Big, gutsy salads like these are fun to eat, full of colour, with lots of different flavours and textures competing for attention. You can taste the ingredients one at a time, or make each forkful an original cocktail. Each mouthful will be different, but all will be good.

These substantial salads need not be bound by any particular conventions – you can play around with all sorts of ingredients, many of which may never have struck you as 'salady' at all. If you're a Yotam Ottolenghi fan – and I certainly am – you may be familiar with this highly eclectic, rule-bending approach to 'salads', in the broadest sense of the word. And if you want to extend your reach into this highly rewarding style of cooking, you should definitely check out his work.

There is, however, a certain logic to the composition of these salads. Generally they are built around a delicious and sustaining trinity of starch, protein and fresh seasonal veg. What makes a salad truly 'hearty' is often a carbohydrate element – most obviously potatoes, pasta, bread or a grain such as rice or spelt. But the addition of some kind of protein – cheese, or eggs, say – can also boost their heft. And pulses such as chickpeas or lentils, being both carb and protein, can do either or both jobs, as well as or instead of another 'hearty' element. The fresh, green, raw, leafy and/or crunchy veg that we more conventionally think of as 'salad' are there too, but often in a supporting role.

What really tickles up many of these salads is the deployment of vegetables that we don't usually eat cold at all – the ones that, all too often, tragically, we boil to oblivion. Here, though, we may emphasise their character, and sweeten and darken their edges, by roasting, grilling or frying them. In particular I like to roast roots from the more colourful and aromatic end of the spectrum – parsnips, beetroot, carrots, Jerusalem artichokes and squashes (which are fruits, I know, but with honorary root status). I also like to fry, grill and barbecue those Mediterranean high summer fruit-vegetables –

aubergines, courgettes, peppers and chillies – along with young leeks and spring onions. What gives them their new-found 'salad' status is a process of gentle assembly, the tumbling or layering together of the still warm, often slightly caramelised pieces with some of the aforementioned items: leaves, pulses, nuts or grains, perhaps some crumblings or shavings of cheese, maybe a final scattering of herbs.

Finally, there are the various 'finishing touches', hinted at already – the dressings and sprinkles that make the salad sing. My dressings often depart from the straight-up vinaigrette, not just with the use of more characterful oils and vinegars, but through the addition of chopped herbs, or a hint of honey, or a spike of chilli. By sprinkles I mostly mean seeds, nuts and (whole) spices, often toasted (dry-fried in a hot pan for a minute or two) to make them more intense and fragrant. They crackle on the tongue or pop between the teeth and add an irresistible snap that puts a real spring into a salad.

The beauty of these hearty salads is that they are endlessly mutable. Almost always, each element can happily be replaced with something else. Don't like blue cheese? Use goat's cheese. No rapeseed oil? Olive will be fine. Or try a dash of walnut oil for a change. And don't think twice about replacing hazelnuts with pumpkin seeds, or basil with parsley. The fact that each combination will inevitably be slightly different each time you make it is a strong part of their appeal.

When it comes to serving these salads, you can relax, too. They are substantial enough to be the main event – perhaps with bread on the side – and that's what I had in mind when putting them together. However, they'll also make a zesty opener to a meal. So, if I've said 'serves 4', you can interpret that as serving 6 or even 8 as a starter or a complement to something else. While I quite often plate them individually – especially as a starter – most work extremely well on a big, generous platter, placed in the centre of the table for everyone to help themselves. Three or four of these lovely combinations are a great way to feed a crowd, or a couple of these and one or two dishes from another chapter, especially Mezze and tapas (pages 290–327) and Side dishes (pages 368–99).

Whether you're entertaining guests with a lavish spread, or just sitting down to a simple family supper, these hearty salads will always bring a riot of seasonal colour and impeccable good taste to your table. This is the kind of food that will make you think, 'I really must do this more often.' And I'm really hoping you will…

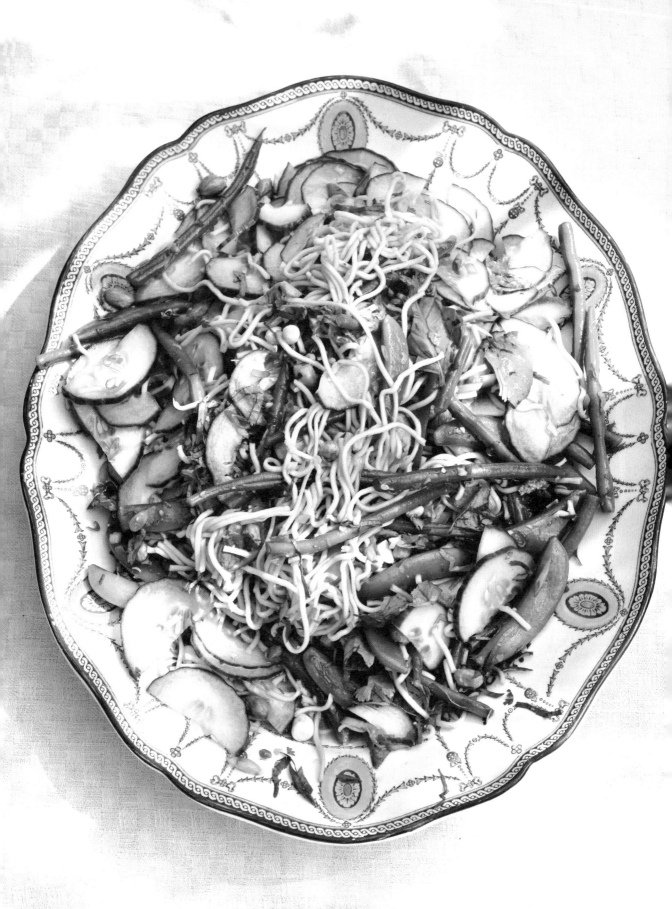

Herby, peanutty, noodly salad ✌

A bright and zingy dressing, handfuls of herbs and crunchy peanuts pack loads of flavour into simple, easy-to-cook noodles. If you can only find salted peanuts, rinse the salt off and pat them dry. When it comes to the fresh herbs, the mint's pretty much a must; the other two are desirable but optional.

SERVES 4

75g raw or roasted unsalted peanuts

200g fine egg noodles or Thai rice noodles

150g French beans or mangetout, or a combination

½ cucumber

6 spring onions, trimmed

About 12 basil leaves (ideally Thai), roughly torn

A small bunch of mint, roughly chopped

A small bunch of coriander, roughly chopped (optional)

FOR THE DRESSING

2 tablespoons rice vinegar

Grated zest and juice of 1 lime, or ½ lemon

½–1 small red chilli, finely chopped

1 garlic clove, finely chopped

1 teaspoon soft brown sugar

1 teaspoon toasted sesame oil

½ teaspoon soy sauce, plus extra to serve

If using raw peanuts, roast on a tray in the oven (at 180°C/Gas Mark 4) for 8–10 minutes, until golden brown. Leave to cool, then bash lightly to break them up a bit.

For the dressing, whisk all the ingredients together in a large bowl.

Cook the noodles according to the instructions on the packet. Drain and rinse under the cold tap. Add to the dressing and toss until well coated. Leave to cool completely in the dressing.

Cook the beans and/or mangetout in a pan of lightly salted boiling water till just tender and still a bit crunchy, 3–5 minutes for beans, 2–3 minutes for mangetout. Drain, refresh in cold water and drain well.

Halve the cucumber lengthways and slice thinly. Finely cut the spring onions on the diagonal.

Toss the cooled noodles with the peanuts, cucumber, spring onions, beans and/or mangetout and herbs. Serve with soy sauce on the side, for everyone to help themselves.

Spelt salad with squash and fennel

This substantial grainy salad makes a lovely autumn/winter lunch or supper. By all means replace the fennel with chunks of leek, or red onion wedges or halved shallots. Indeed you can improvise a spelt salad along these lines for all seasons, and the first baby veg of summer are a great opportunity to play with this idea (see below).

SERVES 4

1 smallish butternut squash (about 600g)

4–5 tablespoons olive oil

2–3 fennel bulbs, trimmed (any feathery fronds chopped and reserved)

1 garlic clove, finely chopped

50g walnuts

200g pearled spelt (or pearl barley), rinsed

Juice of ½ lemon

20g Parmesan, hard goat's cheese or other well-flavoured hard cheese, grated, plus extra to serve

A small handful of parsley, roughly chopped

Sea salt and freshly ground black pepper

Preheat the oven to 190°C/Gas Mark 5. Peel, halve and deseed the squash, then cut into 1.5cm chunks and scatter in a large roasting tin. Trickle over 2 tablespoons of the olive oil and season well with salt and pepper. Toss so that the squash is well coated and put into the oven to roast. Meanwhile, cut the fennel lengthways into 6 or 8 wedges.

After 15 minutes, add the fennel and garlic to the roasting tin and turn with the squash and another tablespoon of olive oil. Roast for a further 20 minutes or so, until the vegetables are soft and starting to caramelise around the edges. Then scatter over the walnuts and cook for another 8–10 minutes. By the end, the veg should be tender and caramelised, and the walnuts lightly toasted and fragrant. If you want to serve this as a cold salad, let the veg cool completely; if you're serving it warm, the veg can go into the spelt straight from the oven.

While the veg are roasting, cook the spelt (or barley) in plenty of well-salted boiling water until tender, but still with just a bit of nutty bite; spelt should take about 20 minutes (allow a bit longer for barley). Drain well and leave to cool a little (or completely, if you're assembling this in advance as a cold salad). Toss with the roasted veg, walnuts and any oil from the roasting tin, the rest of the olive oil, the lemon juice, cheese, parsley and any fennel fronds. Taste and season with salt and pepper. Shave over some more cheese and serve warm or cold.

VARIATION

Summer spelt salad❦

Cook 200g pearled spelt or pearl barley (as above), drain and add 2 tablespoons rapeseed or olive oil and the grated zest and juice of ½ lemon, season with salt and pepper and leave to cool. When cold, toss with about 200g blanched and cooled baby veg, which could include baby broad beans, baby carrots and peas. Add about 300g cubed, cold, cooked new potatoes and a shredded handful of mint. Taste and add more oil, lemon juice, salt and/or pepper as needed. I like to finish this with a scattering of spring onions, gently fried in olive oil for a couple of minutes so they're tender and sweet.

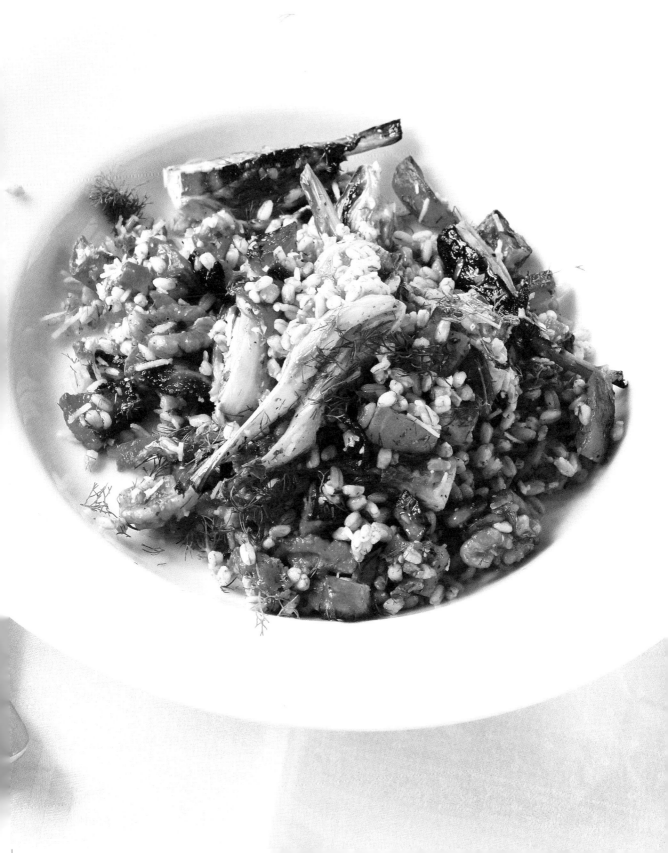

Tahini-dressed courgette and green bean salad

This lovely dish is as much about the dressing as the salad. It's the kind of thick, trickling dressing that Yotam Ottolenghi does so well, and it gives a Middle Eastern edge and a bit of body to all kinds of salads and veg assemblies. It's particularly good whenever courgettes or aubergines – grilled, barbecued or fried – are part of the mix, hence the salad that follows and the serving suggestion for chargrilled summer veg on page 332. It works with lentils, other pulses, spelt and quinoa too. And its coating consistency makes it ideal to use as a dip-cum-dressing for crudités and rolled-up lettuce leaves.

SERVES 4

FOR THE TAHINI DRESSING

½ garlic clove, crushed with a little coarse sea salt

2 tablespoons light tahini (stir the jar well first)

Finely grated zest and juice of ½ lemon

Juice of ½ orange

½ teaspoon clear honey

2 tablespoons olive oil

Sea salt and freshly ground black pepper

FOR THE SALAD

2 tablespoons olive oil

3 medium courgettes (about 400g), sliced into 3mm rounds

Juice of ½ lemon

1 red chilli, deseeded and finely chopped

About 125g French beans, trimmed

4 good handfuls of salad leaves

12-18 oven-dried tomatoes (see page 304) or semi-dried tomatoes (optional)

A handful of mint, finely shredded (optional)

To make the tahini dressing, put the crushed garlic into a small bowl with the tahini, lemon zest and juice, orange juice, honey and a grind of black pepper, and stir together well. The dressing may thicken and go grainy or pastey, but don't worry. Just thin it down by whisking in a little water, 1 tablespoon at a time, until you get a creamy, trickling consistency. Finally, gently stir in the olive oil. Taste and add a little more salt and pepper if needed. The dressing is now ready to use.

For the salad, heat the olive oil in a large non-stick frying pan over a fairly high heat and cook the courgette slices in batches, tossing them occasionally, for a few minutes until tender and browned on both sides, transferring them to a bowl once cooked.

When the courgettes are all cooked, season generously with salt and pepper, add the lemon juice and chilli and toss together well.

Bring a pan of salted water to the boil. Tip in the French beans, return to the boil and blanch for 1 minute. Drain, then dunk in cold water to refresh. Drain again, pat dry with a clean tea towel and toss the beans with the courgettes.

To assemble the salad, spread the salad leaves in a large shallow serving bowl and scatter over the dressed courgettes and beans, tomatoes and shredded mint, if using. Trickle the tahini dressing generously over the whole lot and serve.

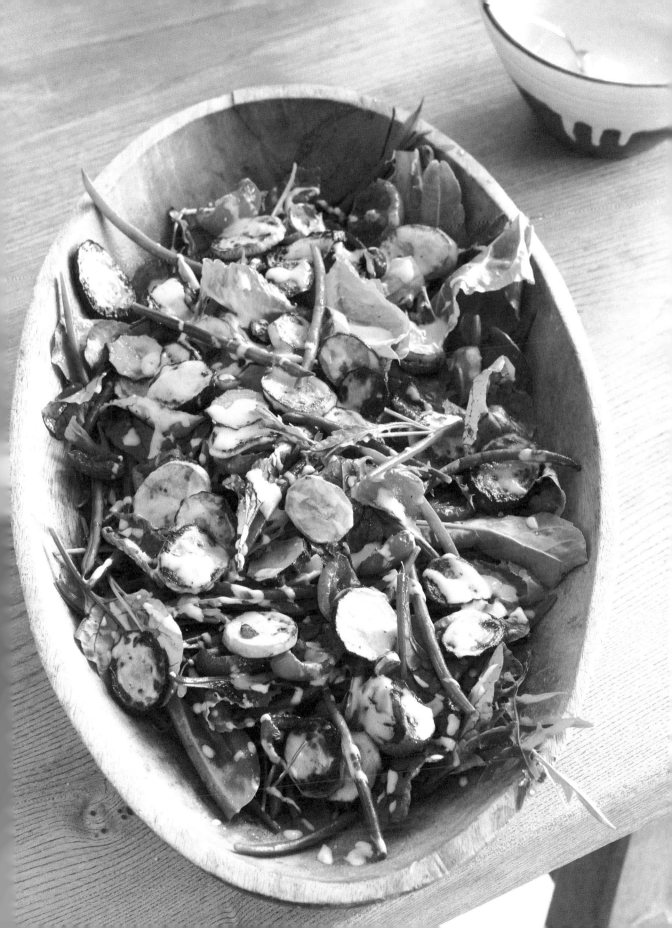

New potato, tomato and boiled egg salad

This rich, yolky dressing, made by combining chopped 'soft, hard-boiled' eggs with a vinaigrette, is one of my favourites. It works brilliantly with new potatoes and sweet, ripe cherry tomatoes.

SERVES 4

About 400g new potatoes

4 large eggs, at room temperature

About 250g cherry tomatoes, halved

A good handful of chives

Sea salt and freshly ground black pepper

FOR THE VINAIGRETTE

6 tablespoons rapeseed or olive oil

4 teaspoons cider vinegar

1 teaspoon English mustard

A pinch of sugar

Cut the potatoes into chunks if they are large. Put in a pan, cover with water, add salt and bring to the boil. Turn down the heat and simmer for 8–12 minutes, or until tender. Drain well and leave to cool.

Meanwhile, to cook the eggs, bring a pan of water to the boil. Add the eggs, return to a simmer, then cook for 7 minutes. Lightly crack the shells of the eggs and run them under cold water for a minute or two to stop the cooking. Leave until cool, then peel the eggs.

For the vinaigrette, put the ingredients into a screw-topped jar with some salt and pepper and shake until emulsified.

Chop the boiled eggs very roughly and put them into a large bowl. Pour on the vinaigrette and mix well, breaking the eggs down a bit as you go. Add the potatoes and cherry tomatoes, and toss together well. Taste and adjust the seasoning if you need to, then snip over the chives and serve.

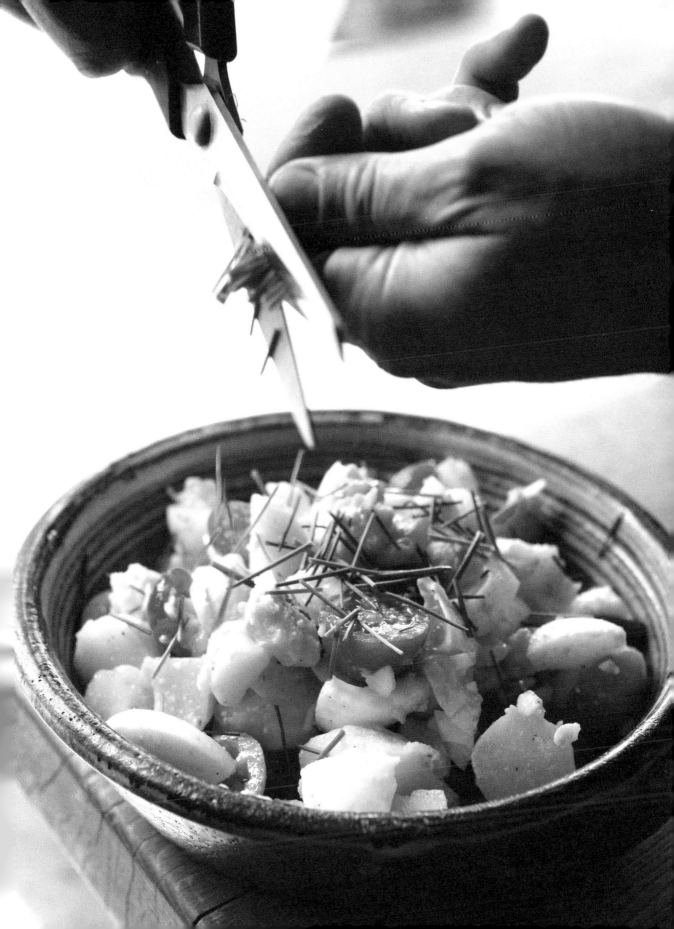

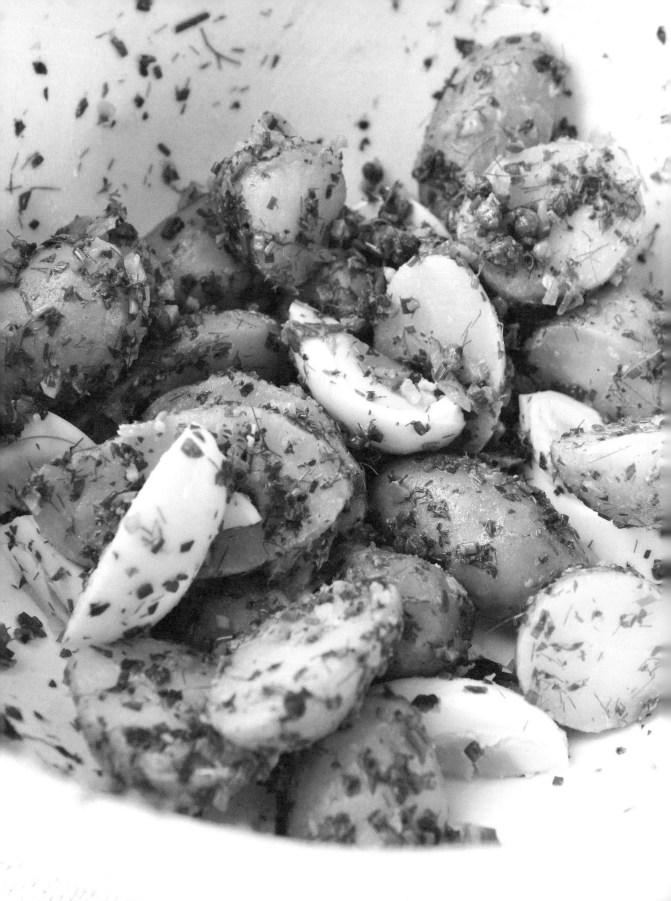

New potato salad 'tartare'

A simple, deconstructed version of good old tartare sauce is used to dress freshly cooked, earthy little new potatoes. Serve as a starter or light lunch.

SERVES 4

1kg small new or waxy potatoes

2 tablespoons capers, rinsed

1 tablespoon chopped gherkins

A handful of chives, finely chopped

A good handful of flat-leaf parsley, finely chopped

A handful of dill, finely chopped

3 soft, hard-boiled large eggs (see page 76)

Sea salt and freshly ground black pepper

FOR THE VINAIGRETTE

1 tablespoon cider vinegar

1½ teaspoons Dijon mustard

3 tablespoons rapeseed or olive oil

Make sure the potatoes are all roughly similar in size (cut up larger ones if necessary). Put the potatoes in a pan, cover with water, add salt and bring to the boil. Lower the heat and simmer for 8–12 minutes until tender.

Meanwhile, for the vinaigrette, put the cider vinegar, mustard, oil and a little salt and pepper in a screw-topped jar and shake to emulsify.

Drain the potatoes and place in a large bowl. While they are still warm, pour on the vinaigrette and toss to mix. Leave until cold.

Add the capers, gherkins, herbs and some salt and pepper and toss again. Quarter the boiled eggs lengthways, gently mix into the salad and serve.

Lettuce, egg and fried bread salad

Many a salad is improved by the addition of croûtons – and what is a croûton if not a big, chunky, golden cube of lovely fried bread? Of course fried bread is fantastic with eggs – and not just in a breakfast fry-up. In this summery salad, the pairing enhances crisp lettuce leaves, while a garlicky dressing brings the whole thing deliciously together. Try it...

SERVES 3–4

4 large eggs, at room temperature

1 Romaine lettuce

2 Little Gem lettuces

1 small butterhead lettuce

A handful of chives

FOR THE CROÛTONS

2 large slices of coarse, robust bread, such as sourdough

3 tablespoons olive or rapeseed oil

FOR THE DRESSING

½ teaspoon Dijon mustard

½ garlic clove, crushed with a little coarse sea salt

1 tablespoon cider vinegar

5 tablespoons rapeseed or olive oil

A pinch of sugar

Sea salt and freshly ground black pepper

Start with the croûtons. Cut the bread into chunky cubes. Heat the oil in a large non-stick pan over a medium heat. Add the bread cubes and fry for a few minutes, turning often, until crisp and golden all over. Set aside to cool.

To cook the eggs, bring a pan of water to the boil. Add the eggs, return to a simmer, then cook for 7 minutes. Lightly crack the shells of the eggs, then run them under cold water for a minute or two to stop the cooking. Leave until cool, then peel the eggs.

Separate the lettuce leaves and put them all into a large bowl.

For the dressing, put all the ingredients into a screw-topped jar, seasoning well with salt and pepper, and shake until emulsified.

Tip about half of the dressing over the lettuce leaves and toss gently to dress. Roughly chop the boiled eggs and combine with the remaining dressing.

Arrange the dressed leaves on a large serving platter and distribute the egg over the top. Scatter the croûtons over the salad, snip over the chives and serve.

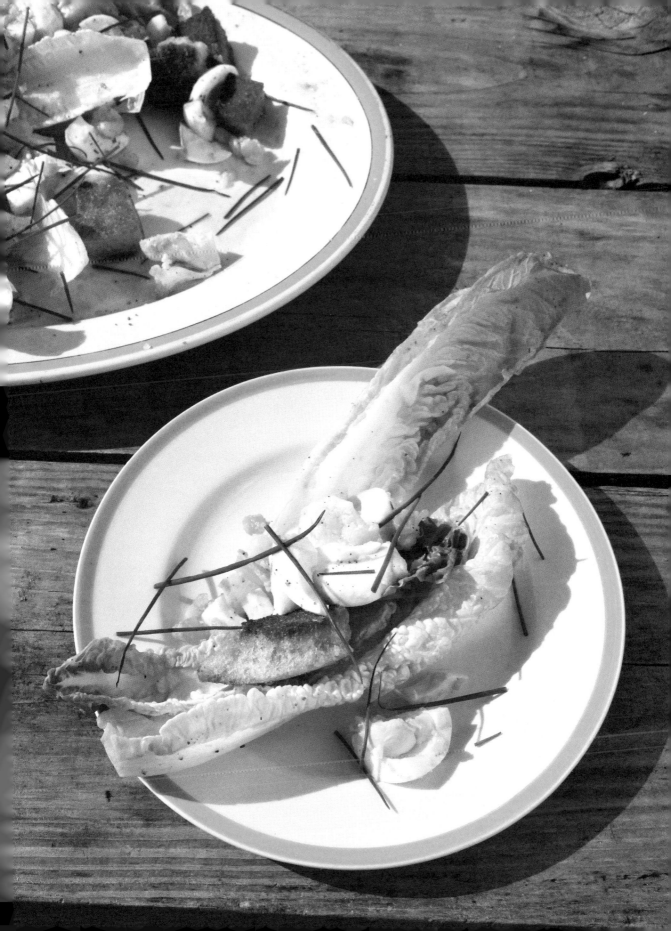

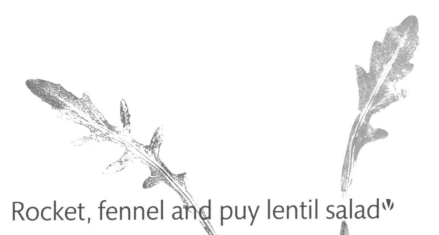

Rocket, fennel and puy lentil salad ✪

Rocket has become such a ubiquitous leaf, so often thrown into generic mixes of salad leaves, that it's easy to forget how well it shines solo, or nearly solo. Combined with the delicate aniseed note of fennel, some earthy lentils and a lemony dressing, it really comes into its own. Adding a few other peppery leaves also works well. With some good bread, this simple assembly is a supper in itself. It also makes a great starter.

SERVES 4

125g Puy lentils

1 bay leaf

½ small onion

A few parsley stalks (optional)

1 large or 2 small fennel bulbs

About 75g rocket, or rocket mixed with a few other peppery leaves such as mizuna

FOR THE DRESSING

2 teaspoons Dijon mustard

Finely grated zest of 1 lemon

2 tablespoons lemon juice

120ml rapeseed or olive oil

A pinch of sugar

Sea salt and freshly ground black pepper

Put the lentils in a saucepan and add plenty of water. Bring to the boil and simmer for a minute only, then drain. Return the lentils to the pan and pour on just enough water to cover them. Add the bay leaf, onion and parsley stalks, if using. Bring back to a very gentle simmer, and cook slowly for about half an hour, until tender but not mushy.

Meanwhile, to make the dressing, shake all the ingredients together in a screw-topped jar until emulsified.

When the lentils are done, drain them well and discard the herbs and onion. While still warm, combine with a good half of the dressing. Leave until cooled, then taste and adjust the seasoning; you could add a little more salt, sugar, pepper or lemon juice if needed.

Trim the fennel, removing the tough outer layer (unless they are young and very fresh). Halve the bulb(s) vertically, then slice as thinly as you can, tip to base.

Pile about two-thirds of the lentils into wide serving bowls. Scatter over the rocket and fennel and trickle over the rest of the dressing. Scatter over the remaining lentils and serve.

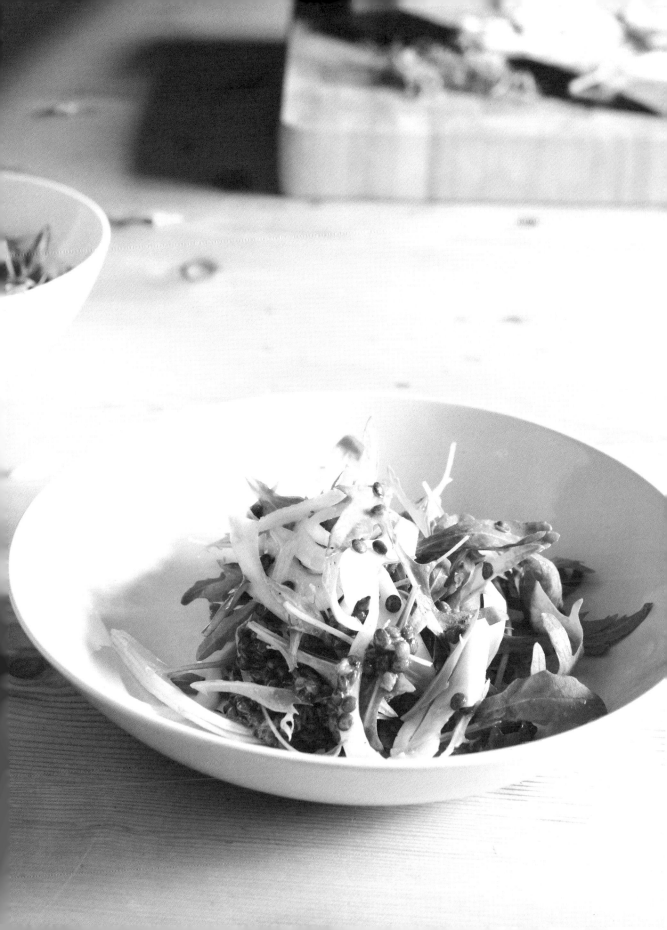

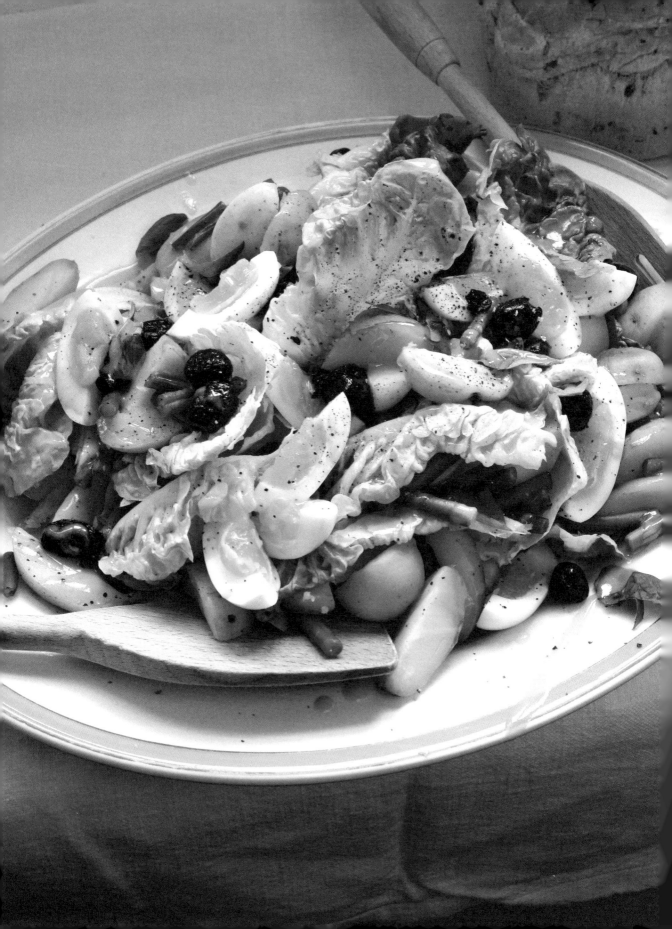

Fish-free salad niçoise

Without any tuna or anchovies, I guess you might upset the good people of Nice a bit with this one, but it is an exceptionally delicious and substantial salad – with plenty going on. I like to cook the eggs so they are hard-boiled but with the yolk still quite soft and sticky.

SERVES 4

500g new potatoes

200g French beans, cut into roughly 3cm lengths

4 large eggs, at room temperature

2–3 Little Gem or similar lettuces

A handful of small black olives

About 12 large basil leaves, torn (or use small ones whole)

Sea salt and freshly ground black pepper

FOR THE DRESSING

½ small garlic clove, crushed with a little coarse sea salt

3 tablespoons olive oil

1 tablespoon cider vinegar

1 teaspoon Dijon mustard

A pinch of sugar

You can cook small new potatoes whole, but cut any larger ones in half or smaller, so they're all roughly the same size. Cover with cold water, add salt and bring to the boil. Reduce the heat and simmer for 8–12 minutes until tender, adding the beans for the last 4 minutes. Drain, tip into a bowl and leave to cool.

To cook the eggs, bring a pan of water to the boil. Add the eggs, return to a simmer, then cook for 7 minutes. Lightly crack the shells and run the eggs under cold water for a minute or two to stop the cooking, then leave to cool. Peel and quarter the eggs.

To make the dressing, put all the ingredients into a screw-topped jar, seasoning with salt and pepper, and shake until emulsified.

Halve, quarter or thickly slice the cooked potatoes. Put them back with the beans, add some of the dressing and toss gently together.

Separate the lettuce leaves and gently toss in a bowl with a little of the dressing. Arrange the lettuce, potatoes and beans on a serving platter and distribute the olives and eggs over the salad. Scatter with torn basil, trickle over the remaining dressing and grind over some pepper. Serve straight away, with bread.

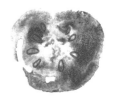

Panzanella ^v

This classic Italian combination of tomatoes and stale bread, pepped up with onion, olives, capers and basil, is hard to beat for a summer lunch. There are various approaches to this dish, but I like to 'sacrifice' about two-thirds of the tomatoes by sieving them into a fresh pulp, to soak into the bread with the rest of the dressing. Then I add more tomatoes, perhaps a different variety, along with the rest of the ingredients. The tomatoes must be sweet and ripe.

SERVES 4

About 700g large,
very ripe tomatoes

4 tablespoons extra virgin
olive oil

2 tablespoons cider vinegar

300–400g (about ½ small loaf)
slightly stale sourdough,
ciabatta or good country bread

About 25 black olives, such as
Kalamata (60g or so)

1 small cucumber, peeled,
deseeded and cut into thick
half-moons

1 small red onion, halved and
finely sliced

About 350g cherry tomatoes,
halved (or a larger variety, cut
into chunks)

1 tablespoon baby capers,
drained and rinsed

A handful of basil leaves, torn

Sea salt and freshly ground
black pepper

Put the 700g larger/riper tomatoes into a large bowl and crush them with your hands. Tip them into a sieve over a bowl and rub through. Discard the skin and pips. Add the olive oil, cider vinegar and plenty of salt and pepper to the tomato juice.

Tear the bread into bite-sized chunks, put into a large bowl and pour over the tomatoey dressing. Add the olives, cucumber, red onion, cherry/other tomatoes, capers and basil and season well with salt and pepper. Toss everything together well with your hands.

If you can, leave the salad to stand for 20 minutes or so to allow the flavours to develop, then toss one more time and leave for a few minutes before serving.

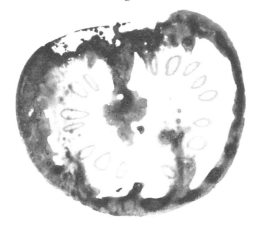

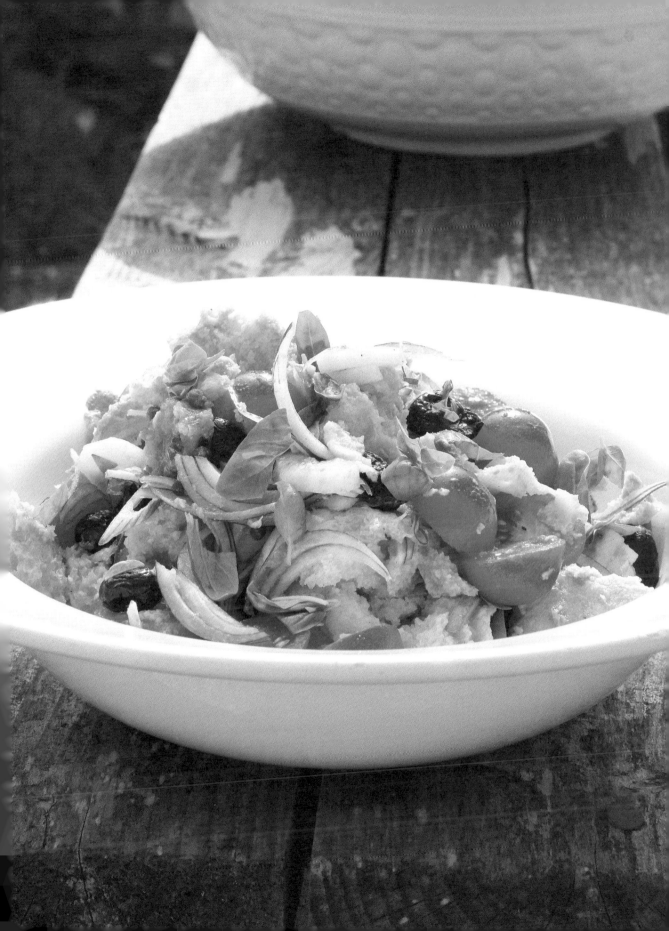

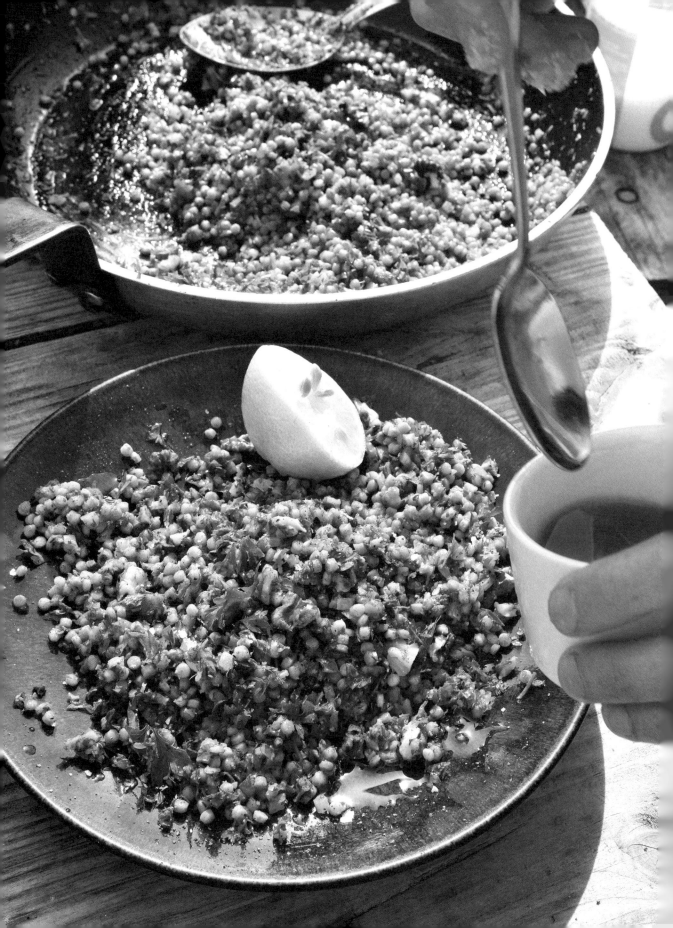

Couscous salad with herbs and walnuts ♥

I like to use a type of 'giant' wholemeal couscous for this salad, which has big, nutty grains. It would also work well with brown rice, quinoa or bulgar wheat instead of the couscous.

SERVES 4

2 teaspoons cumin seeds

1 teaspoon fennel seeds

4–5 tablespoons extra virgin olive oil

1 onion, chopped

2 celery sticks, chopped

1 fennel bulb, chopped

2 garlic cloves, chopped

Finely grated zest and juice of 1 lemon

200g 'giant' wholewheat couscous

A bunch of flat-leaf parsley, chopped

A handful of chives, chopped (optional)

A handful of tarragon, chopped (optional)

75g walnuts, lightly toasted and roughly chopped

Sea salt and freshly ground black pepper

Put the cumin and fennel seeds in a dry frying pan and toast over a medium heat, shaking the pan often, for a few minutes until fragrant. Tip into a mortar and, when cool, grind with the pestle to a powder.

Heat 2 tablespoons olive oil in the frying pan and sauté the onion, celery, fennel and garlic over a medium heat for 5 minutes or so, until softened but still with a bit of bite. Remove from the heat and add the ground spices and lemon zest.

Cook the couscous in plenty of salted water, following the packet instructions, about 9 minutes. Drain well and mix with the onion and spice mixture. Allow to cool.

Stir in the lemon juice, herbs, walnuts and plenty of salt and pepper. Before serving, add more oil to lubricate the couscous to your taste – you might want a little more lemon juice too.

VARIATION

Summer couscous salad ♥

Use a standard, fine-grained couscous instead of the big wholemeal variety and cook in vegetable stock or water, according to the packet instructions. Meanwhile, blanch 100g each peas or petits pois and broad beans in boiling water until just tender. Drain and refresh in iced water. If you have the patience, slip the broad beans from their outer skins. You could also include about 100g small courgettes, cut into 1cm dice and fried in a little olive oil for a few minutes until lightly coloured. For the dressing, whisk the finely grated zest and juice of 1 lemon, 4 tablespoons olive oil, a finely chopped garlic clove and some salt and pepper together. Trickle the dressing over the warm couscous and fork through until fluffy. Cool, then toss with the veg and 200g or so of halved cherry tomatoes, if you like. Add a finely chopped handful each of parsley, basil, mint and coriander. Taste and add more lemon juice and/or salt and pepper if required, then serve.

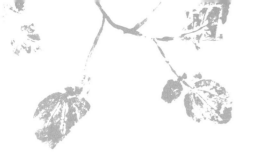
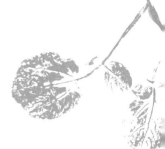

Roasted parsnip, puy lentil and watercress salad

This is a great, if unexpected, three-way combination of lovely flavours and textures, all held together by the nutty rapeseed oil dressing – a perfect autumn salad.

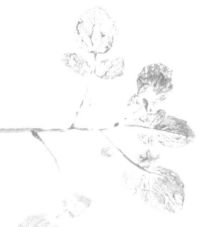

SERVES 4

5 medium parsnips

2 tablespoons rapeseed oil

125g Puy lentils

1 bay leaf

½ onion

A few parsley stalks (optional)

A large bunch of watercress, tough stalks removed

Sea salt and freshly ground black pepper

FOR THE DRESSING

1 garlic clove, crushed with a little coarse sea salt

1 teaspoon English mustard

2 teaspoons clear honey

1 tablespoon lemon juice

4 tablespoons rapeseed oil

TO SERVE (OPTIONAL)

Parmesan, hard goat's cheese or other well-flavoured hard cheese

Preheat the oven to 190°C/Gas Mark 5. Peel the parsnips and halve them lengthways. Cut the wider top parts in half again; the aim is to get chunky pieces roughly all the same size. Put the parsnips into a roasting tin, scatter with some salt and pepper and toss with the oil. Roast for 40 minutes, stirring halfway through, or until tender and starting to caramelise.

Meanwhile, put the lentils in a pan, add plenty of water and bring to the boil. Simmer for a minute only, then drain. Return the lentils to the pan and pour on just enough water to cover them. Add the bay leaf, onion and parsley stalks, if using. Bring back to a very low simmer and cook slowly for about half an hour, until tender but not mushy.

For the dressing, whisk all the ingredients together thoroughly with some salt and pepper.

Drain the lentils and pick out the bay leaf, parsley stalks and onion. While still hot, toss the lentils with the dressing. Taste and make sure they are well seasoned.

Scatter the warm lentils, roasted parsnip chunks and watercress sprigs on serving plates and finish with a few cheese shavings, if you like. Serve warm.

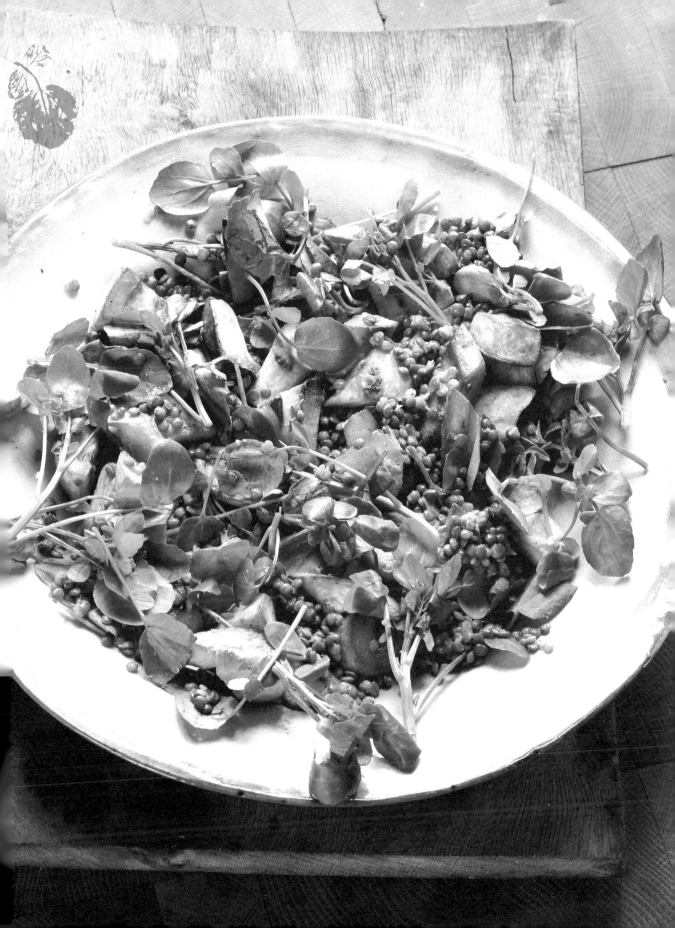

Roasted baby beetroot with walnuts and yoghurt dressing

This salad is lovely to eat and lovely to look at. Fold the beetroot very gently into the dressing to maintain a dramatic marbled look.

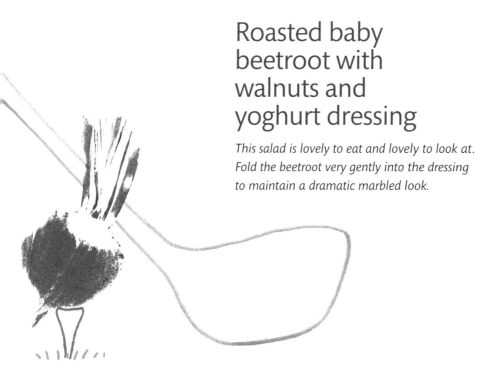

SERVES 4

1kg small beetroot (about the size of golf balls), scrubbed, or halved or quartered larger beetroot

4 garlic cloves (skin on), bashed

4 sprigs of thyme

3 bay leaves

5 tablespoons olive oil

75g walnut halves

Juice of ½ lemon

Sea salt and freshly ground black pepper

FOR THE DRESSING

4 tablespoons plain (full-fat) yoghurt

2 tablespoons soured cream

1 small garlic clove, crushed with a little coarse sea salt

A small handful of chives or dill fronds, roughly chopped

TO FINISH

A couple of handfuls of watercress or rocket

First, roast the beetroot. Preheat the oven to 200°C/Gas Mark 6. Put the beetroot into a baking tin and scatter with the garlic, thyme and bay leaves. Season with salt and pepper and trickle over 3 tablespoons olive oil. Shake the tin so everything is well mingled, then cover with foil, sealing it tightly. Roast until tender – about an hour, though it could take longer, depending on the size of the beetroot. They are cooked when a knife slips easily into the flesh.

Turn the oven down to 180°C/Gas Mark 4. Scatter the walnuts on a baking tray and toast in the oven for 5–7 minutes until just fragrant.

Leave the beetroot until cool enough to handle, then top and tail and remove their skins. Cut the beetroot into halves or quarters and place them in a large bowl. Dress while still warm with the lemon juice, 2 tablespoons olive oil and some black pepper. Allow to cool.

For the dressing, in a small bowl, whisk together the yoghurt and soured cream. Whisk in the garlic and salt and pepper to taste.

Toss the cooled beetroot and about two-thirds of the toasted walnuts lightly in the dressing with most of the chives or dill. Pile the beetroot salad into serving bowls and scatter over the remaining walnuts and chives or dill. Finish with the watercress or rocket.

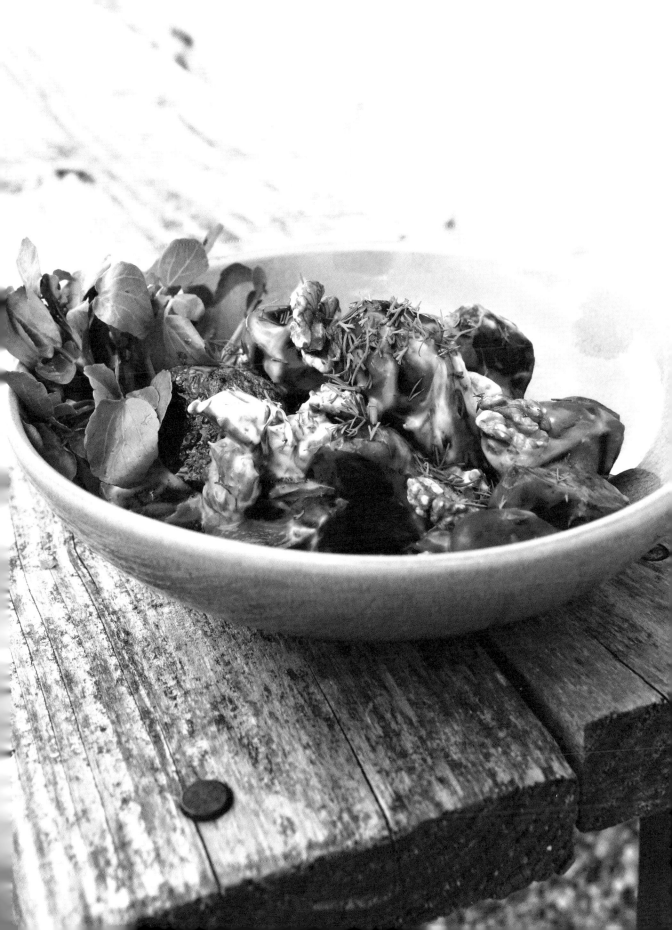

Warm salad of mushrooms and roasted squash

This substantial salad is something of a River Cottage classic, and a great way to bring together two of autumn's finest ingredients: mushrooms and squash. Blue cheese is quite delicious here but you could use other cheeses – shavings of Parmesan, a hard goat's cheese such as Ticklemore, or a firm ewe's milk cheese such as Berkswell would also work well.

SERVES 4

1 small squash, such as butternut, Crown Prince, onion or Harlequin, or ½ larger one (about 1kg)

12 sage leaves, bruised

4 garlic cloves, thickly sliced

100ml rapeseed or olive oil

A large knob of butter

300g open-cap mushrooms, thickly sliced

A small bunch of rocket

150g blue cheese, such as Harbourne blue, Dorset Blue Vinny or Stilton, crumbled

Sea salt and freshly ground black pepper

FOR THE DRESSING

3 tablespoons rapeseed or olive oil

1 tablespoon balsamic vinegar (ideally apple balsamic)

Preheat the oven to 190°C/Gas Mark 5. Peel, halve and deseed the squash. Cut into 2–3cm chunks and put into a roasting tin with the sage leaves, garlic, all but 1 tablespoon of the oil and a generous seasoning of salt and pepper. Roast for about 40 minutes, stirring once, or until soft and coloured at the edges.

Put the remaining 1 tablespoon oil in a frying pan with the butter and place over a medium heat. Throw in the mushrooms along with a little salt and pepper and fry for 4–5 minutes, or until they are cooked through and any liquid they release has evaporated.

For the dressing, in a small bowl, whisk the oil and balsamic vinegar together with some salt and pepper.

In a large bowl, combine the still-warm (but not hot) cooked squash and mushrooms with the rocket and cheese. Add enough dressing to dress them lightly (you may not need it all), toss together and serve.

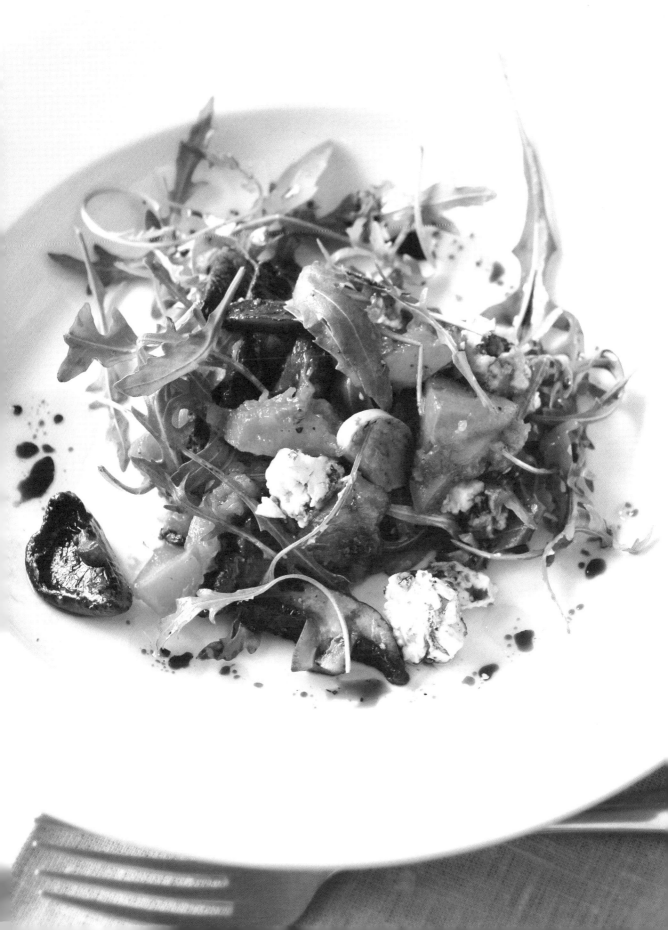

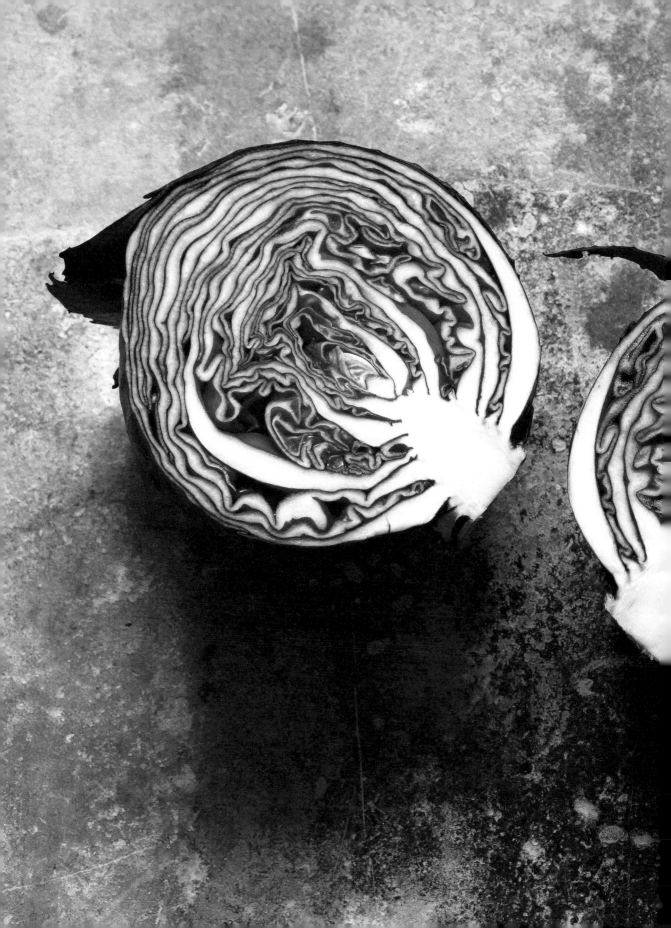

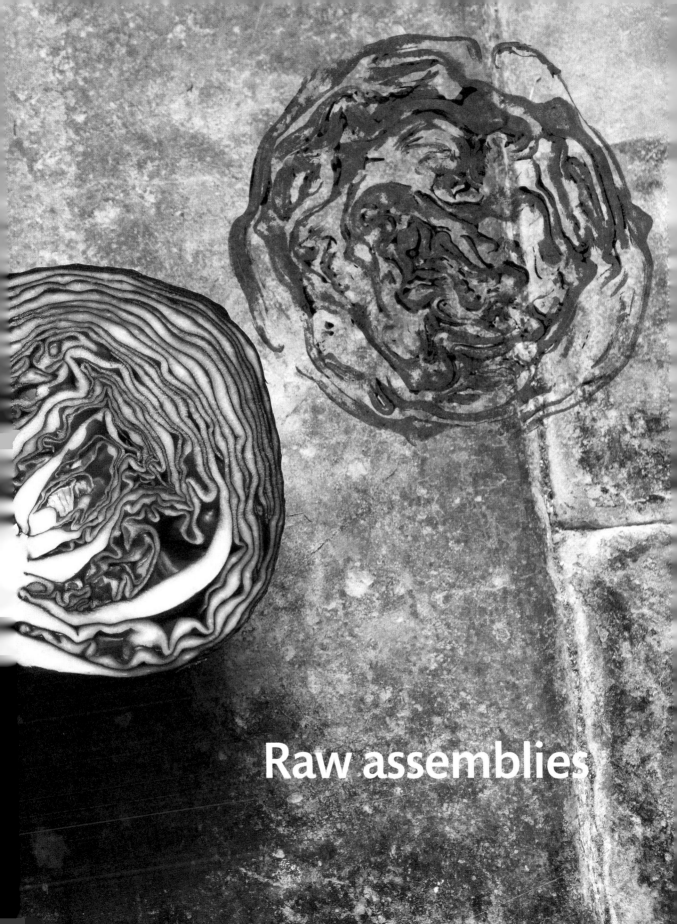

Raw assemblies

There's no question in my mind that most of us don't eat enough raw food. Fond as I am of the art of cooking, the application of heat to vegetables doesn't always do them a favour. And all too often it isn't a great deal for the person dining on them either. School carrots: need I say more? So right now I want to extol those dishes which illustrate that, sometimes, the best thing you can do for the fine, fresh produce in front of you is next to nothing.

The dishes that follow are certainly salads, of a sort, but quite different from the earlier 'hearty salads'. These recipes are for vegetables at their simplest: fresh, raw and barely tinkered with. With the exception of the odd toasted nut or whizzed-up dressing, most of the ingredients require just a little peeling, slicing or grating before bringing together. The result is some really elegant, delicious dishes that will add a resounding crunch of rude health to any meal. If, for instance, you're indulging in one of the greedier, starchier or creamier offerings in the book, stick one of these dishes alongside, and your virtue will be saved. Alternatively, put one at the beginning of a meal, and your dinner party could be made: these are stylish dishes, for the most part, that look lovely on the plate. Serve the kohlrabi 'carpaccio' (on page 116) or the shaved summer veg (on page 100) to your most discerning foodie friends, and you'll see what I mean.

This chapter draws on a lesson I've learned when trying to encourage my kids (and other peoples') to eat more fresh fruit and veg: namely, that preparation and presentation count for a lot. Youngsters, in my experience, are so much more likely to greedily neck that apple, carrot or stick of celery if you cut it into handleable wedges or batons first. I got my kids to eat lettuce by serving the salad dressing as a dip, and encouraging them to roll up their leaves and plunge them in. And I found I could get even more roots and fruits inside them by grating and dressing them.

So a little deft knife-work applied to raw veg, aimed at pleasing the eye and turning on the taste buds, can make all the difference. However, these are not mere tricks of presentation – they change the whole experience of eating the veg in question. The idea of biting into a whole bulb of fennel probably doesn't appeal, but trimmed, finely sliced and dressed with a little peppery oil and fresh lemon juice, it's a vastly more alluring prospect. Cut your vegetables the right way, jumble them up with a dressing or dip, and you have a more unexpected – and tempting – plate of food, but also one that is much more enjoyable to eat. Try offering my cauliflower with toasted seeds (on page 108) to a cauli-phobe or – and this is one of my favourite tests – the Brussels sprouts, apple and cheddar (on page 108) to a sprout-hater, and you could be amazed at the response.

There are dishes here that may raise a few eyebrows. Raw carrots and tomatoes are well embedded in our culinary culture, but raw celeriac, beetroot and parsnip? All I can say is: don't knock them until you've tried them. If you have a fresh, young example of almost any vegetable (potatoes being a rule-proving exception), there's almost always the potential to eat it raw – indeed, to enjoy it raw. This way of preparing veg is another string in the bow of the vegetable cook because it opens up a whole new area of texture and flavour. The difference between a boiled carrot and a raw one (school carrot versus one just pulled from the ground) can be so great as to make them seem two different vegetables. The same goes for cabbage or courgettes. In short, open your mind to the potential of raw veg and you're pretty much doubling your vegetable repertoire.

This leads me on to an important point, which is that the care you take over preparing your lovely veg is never of greater importance than it is here. So have a decent peeler and a sharp knife standing by. You'll also need a sturdy box grater (you'll get most use out of the coarse setting) and you might want to think about acquiring a mandoline – the plastic V-cutter kind with various different slide-in slicing trays are the best, I think, as well as the cheapest. Provided you take care of them, and of yourself while you're using them, they'll last you many years. These tools also exist, of course, as attachments for most modern food processors. Get the hang of them and you can knock up dinner-party quantities of these raw assemblies in very little time.

Such equipment, whether hand-held or automated, is useful because it can give precision to your work, without adding effort, stress or time. I don't like being pedantic about food preparation and, usually, when I say 'chop finely' or 'slice thinly' I'm happy to allow a good margin for error. It rarely matters when veg is going to be cooked. But with these recipes accuracy doesn't go amiss – the dishes will actually taste better for it.

And, finally, though this probably goes without saying, the quality of the vegetables is crucial. Young, tender and snappingly fresh is the order of the day. The rewards for being picky here are, as you're about to find out, really very great. And the best kind of picky, I hardly need tell you, is picking your own.

Shaved summer veg

*Wafer-thin slices of sweet baby root veg and courgettes make
for a deliciously crunchy and gorgeously colourful salad.
The rich dressing ties the lot together nicely – it uses rapeseed
oil, honey and mustard, all of which marry particularly well
with root vegetables. You don't have to stick to these veg –
you can try carrots, fennel or cucumber in the mix as well.*

But always shave or slice as thinly as you possibly can.

SERVES 4

1 medium or 2 small beetroot
(100–150g), any colour you like

1 medium or 2 small kohlrabi
(100–150g)

100–150g radishes

1 medium courgette
(about 150g)

FOR THE DRESSING

1 teaspoon English mustard

2 teaspoons clear honey

1 tablespoon lemon juice

4 tablespoons rapeseed oil

Sea salt and freshly ground
black pepper

Trim all the vegetables, and peel the beetroot and the kohlrabi. Use a mandoline, a vegetable peeler or a very sharp knife to shave/slice them as thinly as you can. (Trying to shave radishes with a potato peeler is quite high risk – take care!) Mix them together and divide between serving plates.

For the dressing, shake all the ingredients together in a screw-topped jar to mix and emulsify. Trickle generously over the salad and serve.

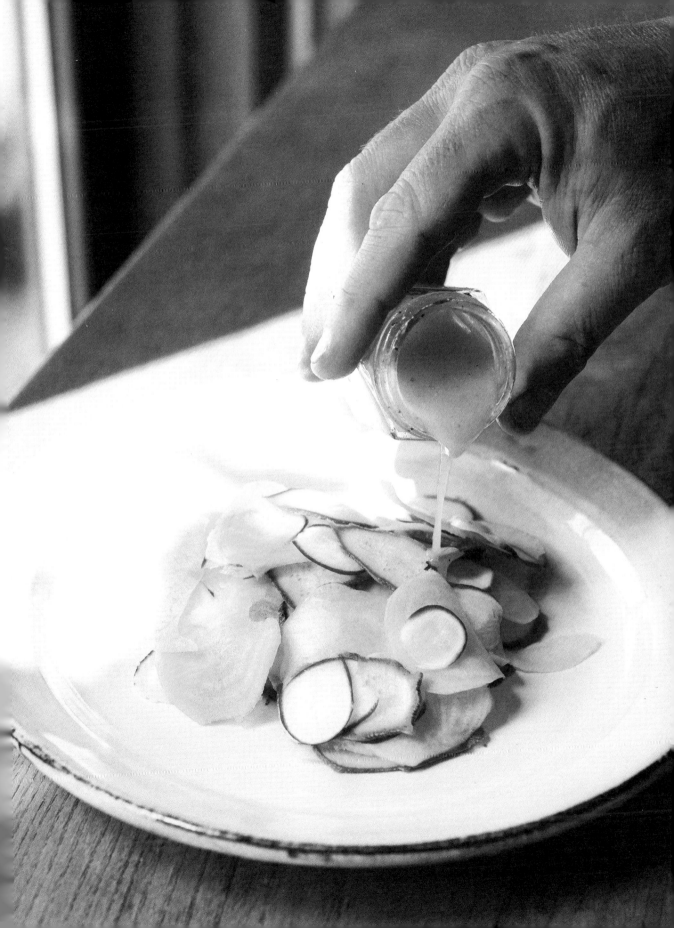

Radishes with butter and salt

This is a simple, time-honoured way of serving radishes, and it is hard to beat. My one caveat, as with all radish recipes, is that it's really only worth doing this with very fresh little roots. Radishes quickly lose their crunch and peppery flavour. It's essential to use a good, sweet sea salt too, such as Maldon, Cornish or Halen Môn.

SERVES 4

About 400g radishes

A pat of unsalted butter, at room temperature but not too soft

A little dish of best quality flaky sea salt

Arrange everything on the table and make sure each diner has a knife. To eat, just smear a little of the butter on the end of a radish then sprinkle with the tiniest pinch of salt before popping into your mouth.

Fennel and goat's cheese

A simple but lovely way to enjoy very fresh, crisp bulb fennel.

SERVES 4

2 large or 3 medium fennel bulbs, trimmed (any feathery fronds chopped and reserved)

1 lemon

2–3 tablespoons rapeseed or extra virgin olive oil

About 30g soft, fresh goat's cheese, rind removed

Sea salt and freshly ground black pepper

Remove and discard the tough outer layer of the fennel bulbs (unless they are young and very fresh). Cut the bulbs in half vertically. Now, using a large sharp knife, slice the fennel as finely as you can, from tip to root.

Put the fennel into a large bowl, squeeze over the juice of ½ lemon, trickle over the oil and add some salt and pepper. Toss everything together with your hands, then cover and set aside for 30 minutes, to allow the fennel to macerate in its dressing. Taste and add a little more lemon, oil and/or salt and pepper if you like.

Transfer to a serving dish, then crumble the cheese over the top. Finish with a scattering of fennel fronds, if you have them, then serve.

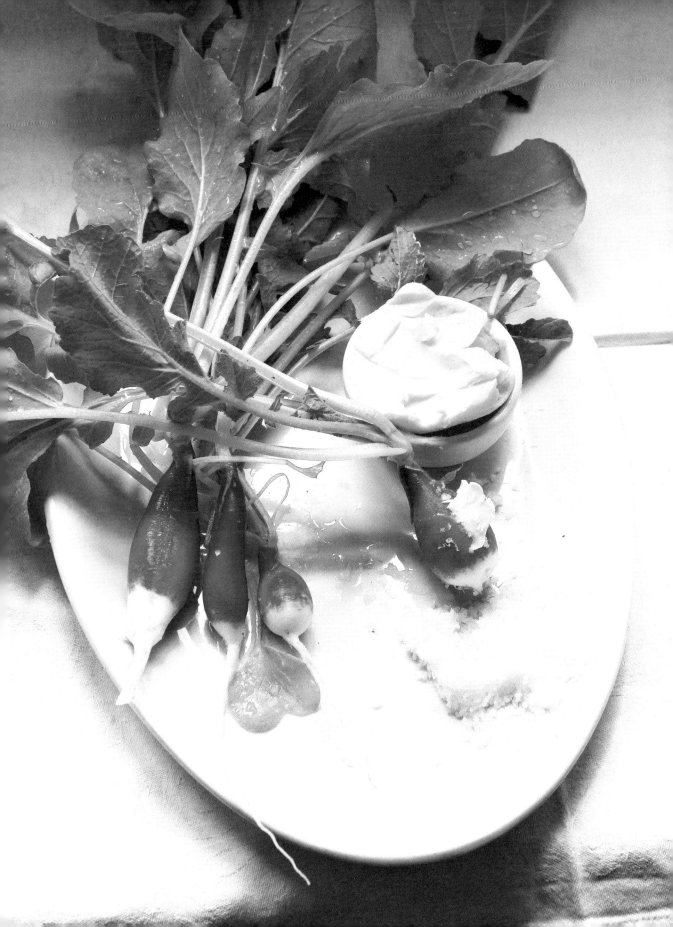

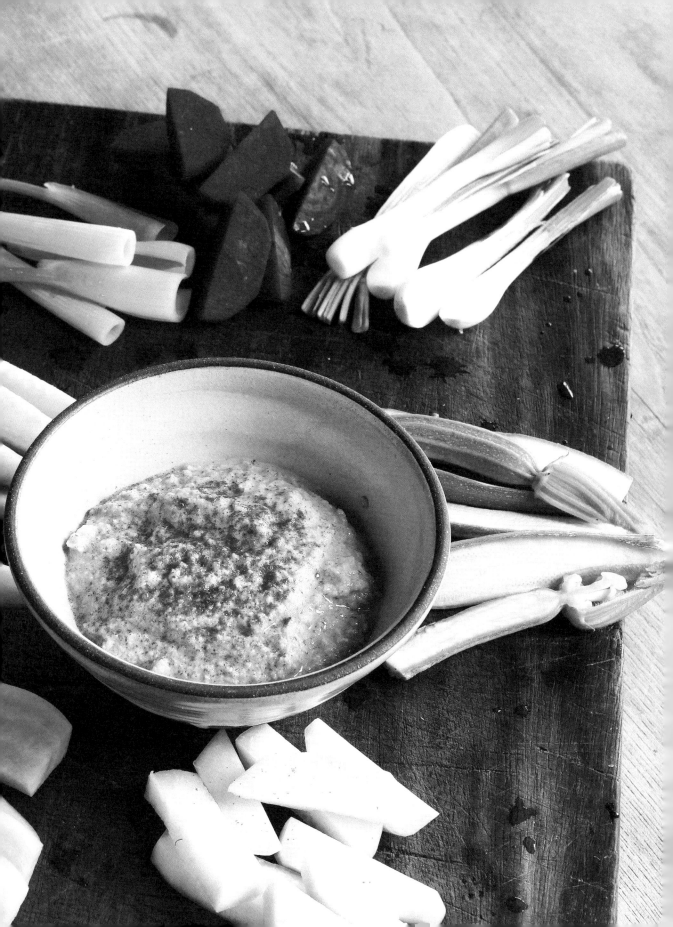

Crudités with tarator sauce

That's really not a misprint for tartare. Tarator is a rich and very garlicky walnut sauce that works brilliantly as a dip for fresh, crunchy crudités. It's lovely summer party food, and a brilliant way to show off the raw harvest from your garden or allotment.

SERVES 6

FOR THE TARATOR SAUCE

100g walnuts or blanched almonds

2 slices of good white bread (about 100g), crusts removed

1 fat garlic clove, crushed

150ml olive oil

Juice of ½ lemon or 2 tablespoons red wine vinegar

Sea salt and freshly ground black pepper

Paprika, to finish

FOR THE CRUDITÉS

A selection from:

Cucumber batons

Firm young courgettes, halved lengthways

Baby carrots, or carrot batons

Small beetroot, peeled and cut into wedges or sticks

Baby fennel

Kohlrabi batons

Spring onions, halved lengthways

Sugarsnap pea pods

Preheat the oven to 180°C/Gas Mark 4. Scatter the nuts on a baking sheet and toast for 5–7 minutes, giving them a shake halfway through. Leave to cool.

Soak the bread in water to cover for a minute or two, then squeeze out most of the water.

Blitz the nuts and garlic in a food processor until quite finely ground. Add the bread and pulse until fairly smooth. With the motor running, add the olive oil in a thin stream, through the feeder tube. Finally, add the lemon juice or vinegar and season to taste with salt and pepper. Dollop into a small bowl and dust with a little paprika.

Arrange a selection of crudités around the tarator sauce to serve.

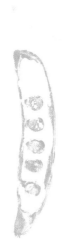

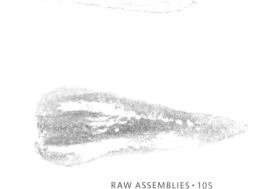

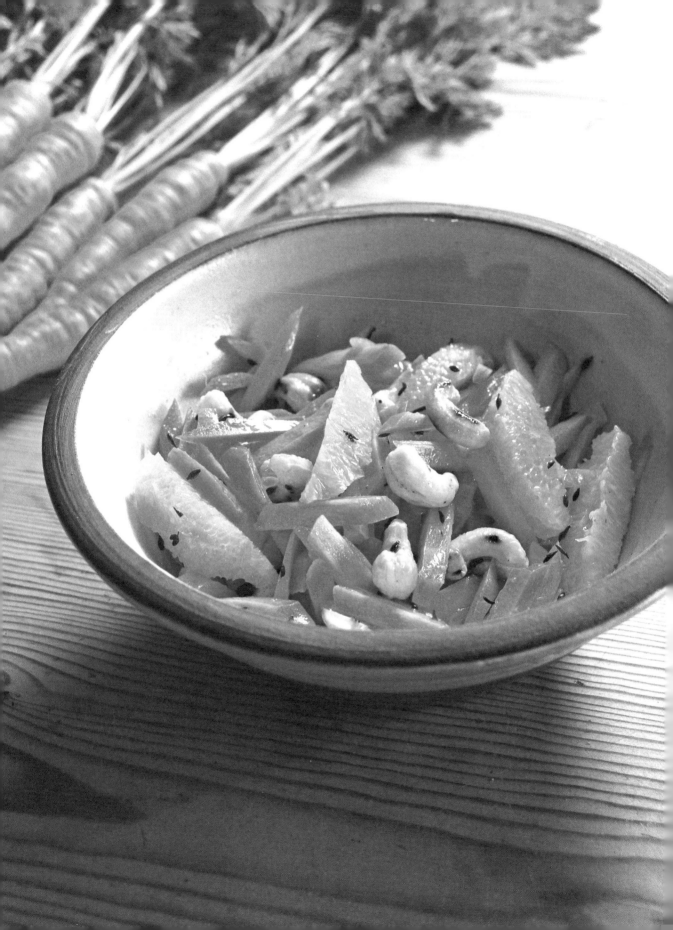

Carrot, orange and cashews ⱽ

*This sweet-nutty combination is an ideal starter before something fairly
substantial, such as my lettuce, spring onion and cheese tart (see page 44).
It's also great with a potato salad, a green salad and some good bread.*

SERVES 2

About 50g cashews

1 teaspoon cumin seeds

2 oranges

2-3 large carrots, peeled

A dash of rapeseed or olive oil

A few drops of cider vinegar

Sea salt and freshly ground
black pepper

Toast the cashews in a hot, dry frying pan over a medium heat for
about 5 minutes until lightly browned, tossing frequently and adding
the cumin seeds for the last minute or so. Tip on to a plate to cool.

Finely grate the zest from one of the oranges and set aside. Using a
small, sharp, serrated knife, slice the peel and pith off both oranges.
Working over a serving bowl, carefully slice each segment out from
between the membranes, letting it fall into the bowl. Squeeze the
remaining membrane to extract all the juice and add the zest too.

Cut the carrots into thick matchsticks, using a mandoline or by hand.
Add to the oranges with the oil, cider vinegar and some salt and
pepper. Toss well together, check the seasoning and scatter over the
cashews and cumin seeds to serve.

Celeriac with apple, raisins and parsley ⱽ

*I like to serve this with Puy lentils – cooked as in the recipe on page 90. It's
important to use a good, fresh, firm celeriac, ideally an early-season one.
Big, old roots can be woody and a bit spongy in the middle.*

SERVES 4

200g celeriac (peeled weight)

1 eating apple

50g raisins

A good handful of flat-leaf
parsley, roughly torn

FOR THE DRESSING

1 teaspoon English mustard

1 teaspoon sugar

1 tablespoon cider vinegar

2 tablespoons sunflower or
rapeseed oil

2 tablespoons olive oil

Sea salt and freshly ground
black pepper

For the dressing, shake all the ingredients together in a screw-topped
jar to emulsify. Tip into a bowl.

Cut the celeriac into matchstick-sized pieces. The easiest way to do
this is with a mandoline, but you can use a large, sharp knife. Transfer
directly to the bowl of dressing and toss them in, so they don't get
a chance to brown.

Peel, quarter, core and thinly slice the apple, and add to the salad with
the raisins. Taste and adjust the seasoning if you need to.

Serve straight away, or leave for an hour or so, which will allow the
celeriac to soften slightly. Toss in the parsley leaves just before serving.

Brussels sprouts, apple and cheddar

Fresh, young Brussels, sliced thinly and served raw, can be a revelation – crisp, earthy and not bitter at all. I love them paired with sweet apple and nutty Cheddar in this raw salad.

SERVES 2

50g shelled hazelnuts, pecans or almonds (optional)

150g very fresh, small Brussels sprouts, trimmed of outer leaves

A good squeeze of lemon juice

2 tablespoons extra virgin olive oil

A few sprigs of thyme, leaves only, roughly chopped

1 tart, crisp eating apple, such as Cox's or Ashmead's Kernel

35g nutty Cheddar

Sea salt and freshly ground black pepper

If using nuts, preheat the oven to 180°C/Gas Mark 4. Scatter the nuts on a baking sheet and toast in the oven until fragrant and browned, 8–10 minutes. If they are skin-on, wrap in a clean tea towel and leave for a minute, then rub vigorously in the tea towel to remove most of the skins. Chop the nuts roughly, or leave whole if you prefer.

Slice the trimmed Brussels sprouts from top to root fairly thinly. Put them into a bowl and add a good squeeze of lemon juice, the olive oil, thyme and plenty of salt and pepper. Toss together well.

Quarter and core the apple, and thinly slice straight into the bowl, then toss together with the sprouts. Crumble in the Cheddar and toss lightly again.

Serve the salad straight away, scattered with the toasted nuts, if using.

Cauliflower with toasted seeds ᵛ

Sumac lends a lovely, lemony-sweet tang to this salad of finely sliced raw cauliflower, but if you can't get hold of this bright red spice, use the finely grated zest of ½ lemon instead.

SERVES 4

1 small, firm cauliflower (about 600g), broken into florets

4 tablespoons pumpkin seeds

2 tablespoons sesame seeds

A small handful of parsley leaves, roughly chopped

3 tablespoons rapeseed oil

2 lemons

½ teaspoon sumac, plus a little more to finish

Flaky sea salt and freshly ground black pepper

Using either a sharp knife or a mandoline, slice the cauliflower florets thinly lengthways, so they are roughly the thickness of a 10p piece.

In a small frying pan, dry-fry the pumpkin seeds over a medium heat until they are fragrant and just beginning to take on some colour. Tip into a bowl and set aside. In the same pan, fry the sesame seeds until they just begin to crackle and turn golden. Tip into the bowl with the pumpkin seeds.

Whisk together the rapeseed oil, the juice of 1 lemon and the sumac. Toss the sliced florets and the seeds in the dressing and season well with salt and pepper. Arrange on serving plates, squeeze over more lemon juice, and scatter a few pinches of sumac over the top to serve.

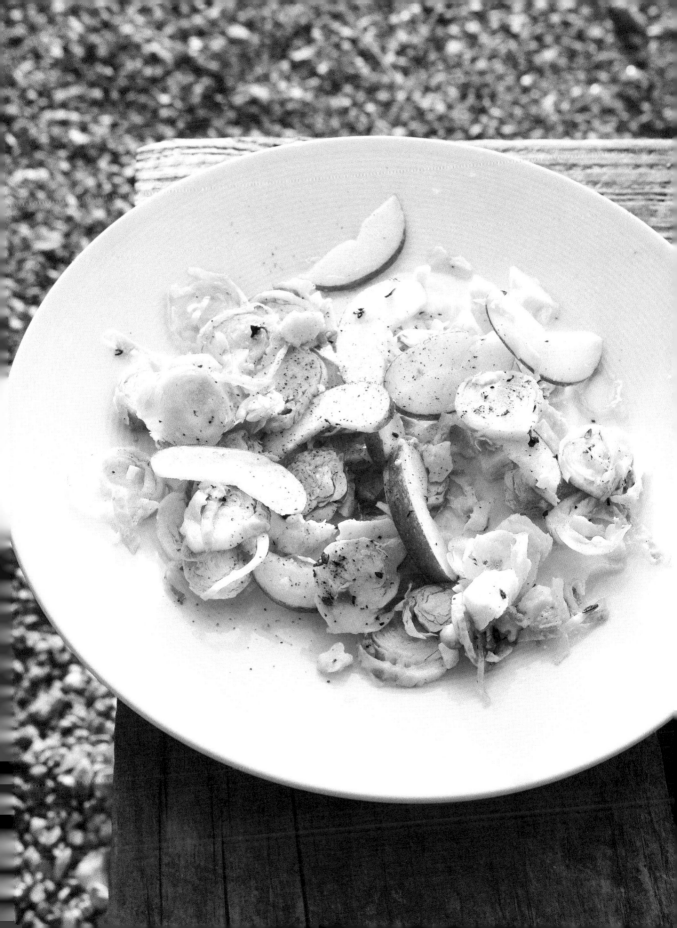

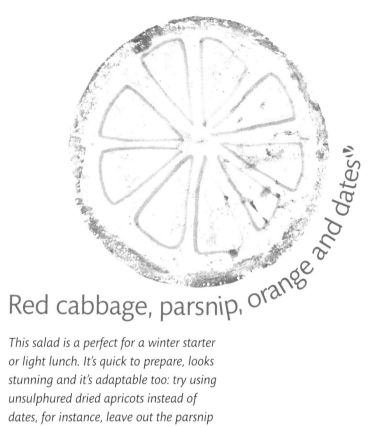

Red cabbage, parsnip, orange and dates"

This salad is a perfect for a winter starter or light lunch. It's quick to prepare, looks stunning and it's adaptable too: try using unsulphured dried apricots instead of dates, for instance, leave out the parsnip for a lighter salad, or substitute a large carrot if you like. Chervil and parsley both work well in place of thyme.

SERVES 2

1 large or 2 small oranges

¼ small red cabbage, core removed, finely shredded

1 small-medium parsnip, peeled and coarsely grated or cut into julienne

2 tablespoons extra virgin olive oil

2 Medjool dates, stones removed, sliced

A couple of sprigs of thyme, leaves only, chopped

Sea salt and freshly ground black pepper

Slice the top and bottom from the orange. Stand it upright on a board and work your way around it with a sharp knife, cutting off the skin and all the pith. Cut out the segments from between the membranes, working over a bowl to save the juice, letting the segments fall into the bowl. When you've finished, squeeze the juice from the remaining membrane into the bowl too.

Put the finely shredded cabbage and grated parsnip into another bowl, add most of the orange juice (not the segments yet) and trickle over the olive oil. Add a little salt and pepper, toss the lot together with your hands, then transfer to serving plates.

Scatter the orange segments and date slices over the red cabbage and parsnip, then finish with a scattering of thyme. Serve straight away.

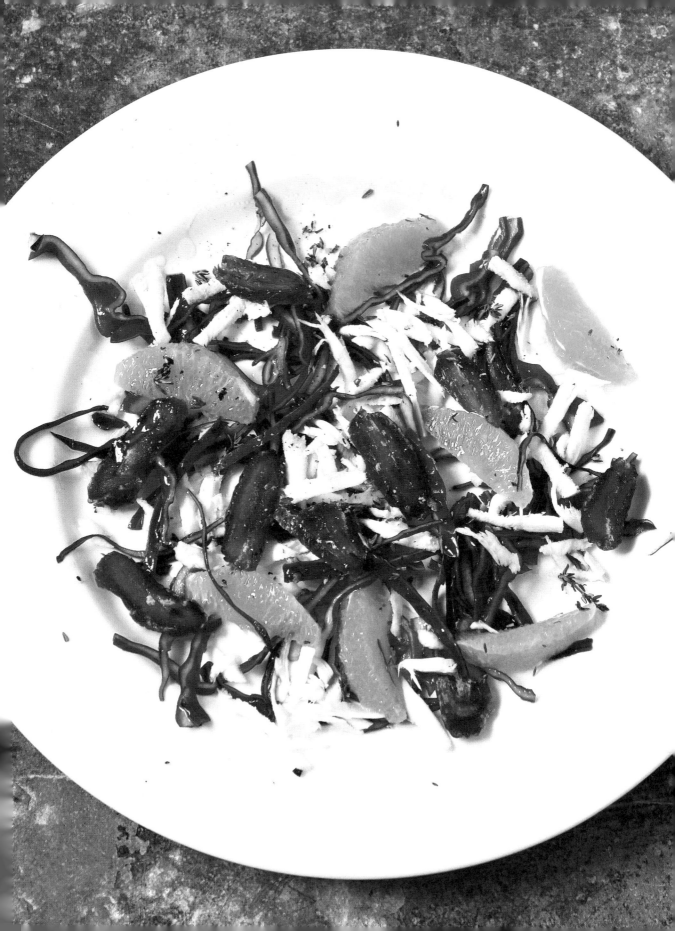

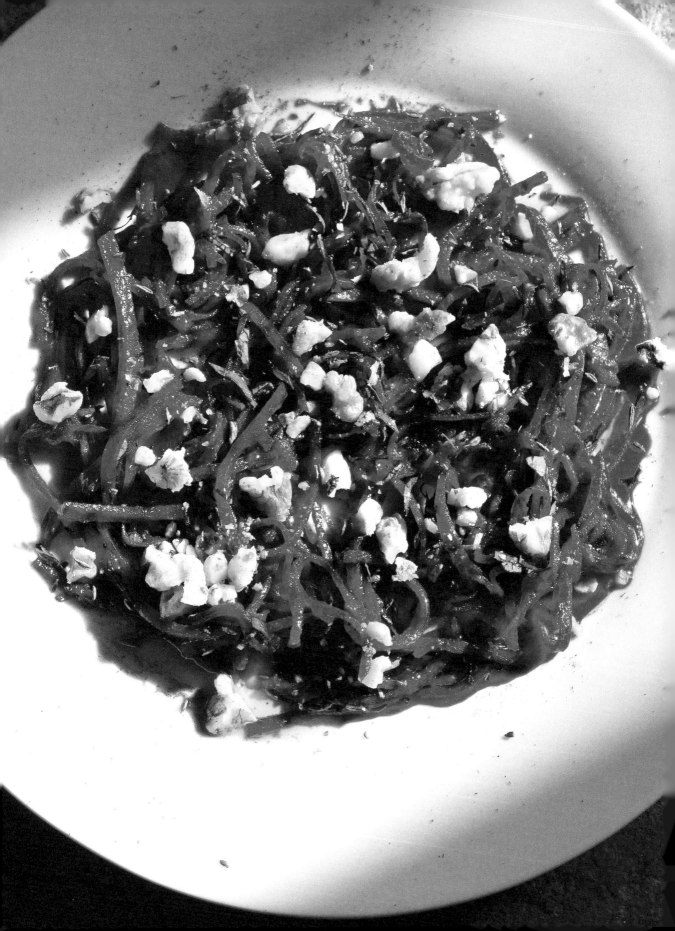

Beetroot with walnuts and cumin ^v

This is a lovely way to use raw beetroot, balancing its rooty sweetness with a touch of bitterness from walnuts and cumin's aromatic warmth. The orange and lemon dressing lightens and brightens the whole thing, and the optional yoghurt finish makes it a little more substantial and indulgent. In the summer, if you can get hold of fresh baby beetroot, just peel and thinly slice, rather than grate them. And do experiment with other nuts – pistachios and pecans work well.

SERVES 4

75g walnuts

1 teaspoon cumin seeds

About 400g beetroot

A good handful of parsley, chopped

Juice of 1 small orange

A squeeze of lemon juice

2 tablespoons rapeseed oil

Sea salt and freshly ground black pepper

TO FINISH (OPTIONAL)

2 tablespoons plain (full-fat) yoghurt

A little more toasted and roughly bashed cumin

A pinch of hot smoked paprika

Heat a dry frying pan over a medium heat and add the walnuts. Toast gently for a few minutes, tossing often, until they smell toasted and are colouring in a few places. Tip into a mortar. Put the cumin seeds into the frying pan and toast gently for 1–2 minutes, tossing a few times, just until they start to release their scent. Tip on to a plate to stop them cooking further.

Peel the beetroot and grate it coarsely (or cut into julienne with a mandoline) into a bowl. Add the parsley, orange juice and a squeeze of lemon juice, 1 tablespoon rapeseed oil and some salt and pepper. Give it a good mix, taste and adjust the seasoning. Ideally leave for 20 minutes or so – the dressing will lightly marinate and tenderise the beetroot.

Spread the beetroot in a dish or on a plate. Bash the walnuts roughly with the pestle and mortar and scatter over the beetroot. Tip the cumin seeds into the mortar and give them a rough bashing too, then scatter over the salad.

Finish with another trickle of rapeseed oil, and, if you like, dot with blobs of yoghurt, sprinkling with more cumin and a pinch of paprika.

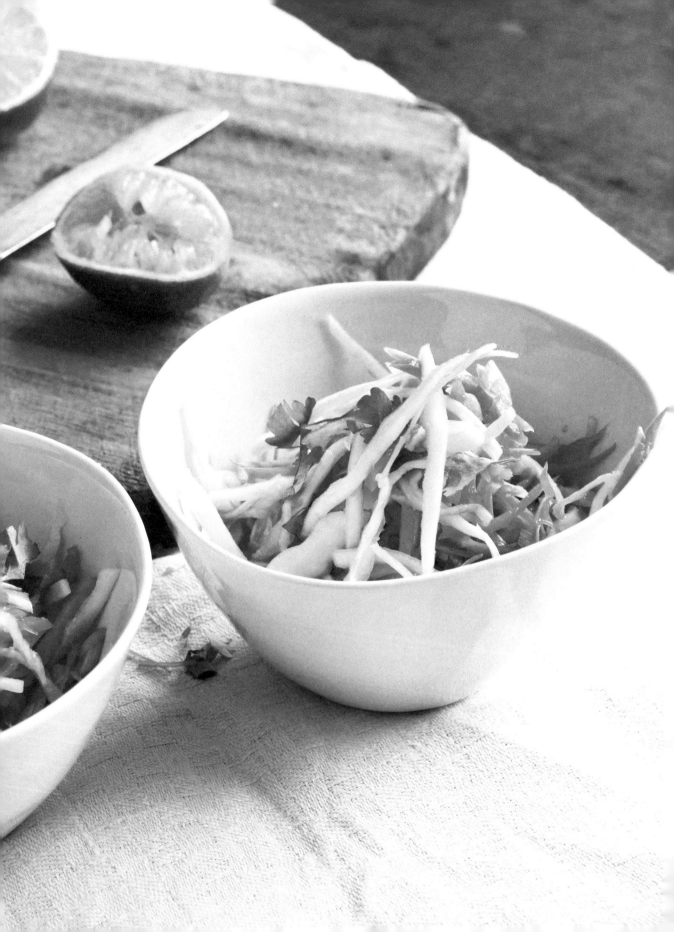

Asian-inspired coleslaw

This is based on a recipe from Taste: A New Way to Cook, by the marvellous Sybil Kapoor. It's wonderfully aromatic, quite unlike any other coleslaw I've ever tried, and I urge you to give it a go.

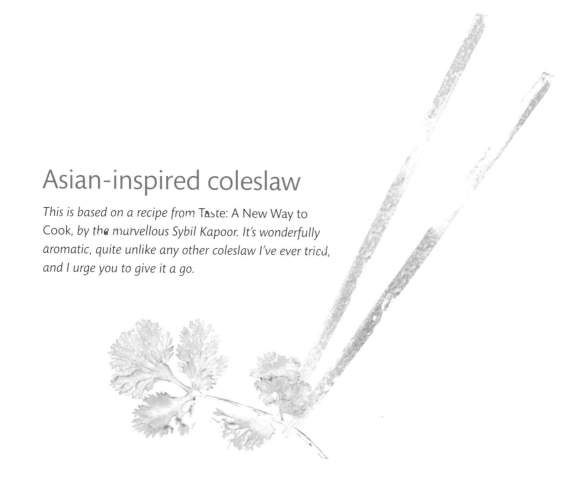

SERVES 6-8

1 bunch of spring onions, trimmed and sliced

4 medium carrots, peeled

1 small white cabbage

FOR THE DRESSING

2 tablespoons soy sauce

1 tablespoon clear honey

1 garlic clove, finely chopped

1 tablespoon finely chopped ginger

2 tablespoons white wine vinegar or rice vinegar

2 tablespoons toasted sesame oil

2 tablespoons olive oil

TO FINISH

A handful of coriander, roughly torn

Lime juice

Put the sliced spring onions into a large bowl. Cut the carrots into fine julienne with a mandoline or grate them coarsely and add to the bowl. Remove any blemished outer leaves from the cabbage, then quarter, cut away the core and shred the leaves as finely as you can. Combine with the spring onions and carrots.

For the dressing, whisk all the ingredients together, making sure the honey is dissolved.

Pour the dressing over the vegetables and toss thoroughly. Leave for 10–20 minutes to soften and 'relax'.

Serve the coleslaw scattered with coriander and sprinkled with a few squeezes of lime juice.

Kohlrabi 'carpaccio'

This elegant salad makes the most of kohlrabi's radishy, water chestnutty crunch. It takes only minutes to make. When I grow kohlrabi, I don't usually let them get any larger than a small eating apple, but they'll probably be a bit bigger than that in the shops. Medium-sized ones are fine but avoid any monsters – they'll be too tough and not sweet enough to serve raw.

SERVES 4

2 medium or 3 small kohlrabi

About 50g hard goat's cheese

A few sprigs of thyme, leaves only, bruised or roughly chopped

Juice of ½ lemon

2 tablespoons rapeseed or extra virgin olive oil

Sea salt and freshly ground black pepper

Peel the kohlrabi and slice them into thin slivers with a vegetable peeler. Divide the slivers between four plates or arrange on a large plate, spreading them out and overlapping – to almost cover the plate.

Shave over some goat's cheese – again, using the vegetable peeler. There's no need to cover the kohlrabi with the cheese, 4 or 5 good shavings per plate is fine.

Sprinkle on the thyme, squeeze over a few drops of lemon juice and trickle on a little oil. Season with salt and pepper and serve.

Celery, orange and pecans ❥

I love the bitter-sweet-sharp combination of celery and orange. Use the sweeter, less fibrous stems from the inside of the celery for this fruity salad. The rich nuts are the perfect foil to the zesty orange and crunchy celery.

SERVES 2

2 oranges

3–4 inner celery stalks, plus a few of the leaves

40g pecans or cashew nuts, lightly toasted

Sea salt and freshly ground black pepper

Finely grate the zest from one of the oranges and set aside. Slice the top and bottom from both oranges, stand upright on a board and work your way around with a sharp knife, cutting off the skin and all the pith. Cut out the segments from between the membranes, working over a large bowl to save the juice, letting the segments fall into the bowl. When you've finished, squeeze the juice from the remaining membrane into the bowl and add the zest too.

Remove any obvious fibres from the outside of the celery stems with a peeler and slice the stems fairly thinly. Add to the oranges, along with the nuts and some salt and pepper.

Transfer the salad to a serving bowl, scatter over a few little roughly chopped celery leaves and serve.

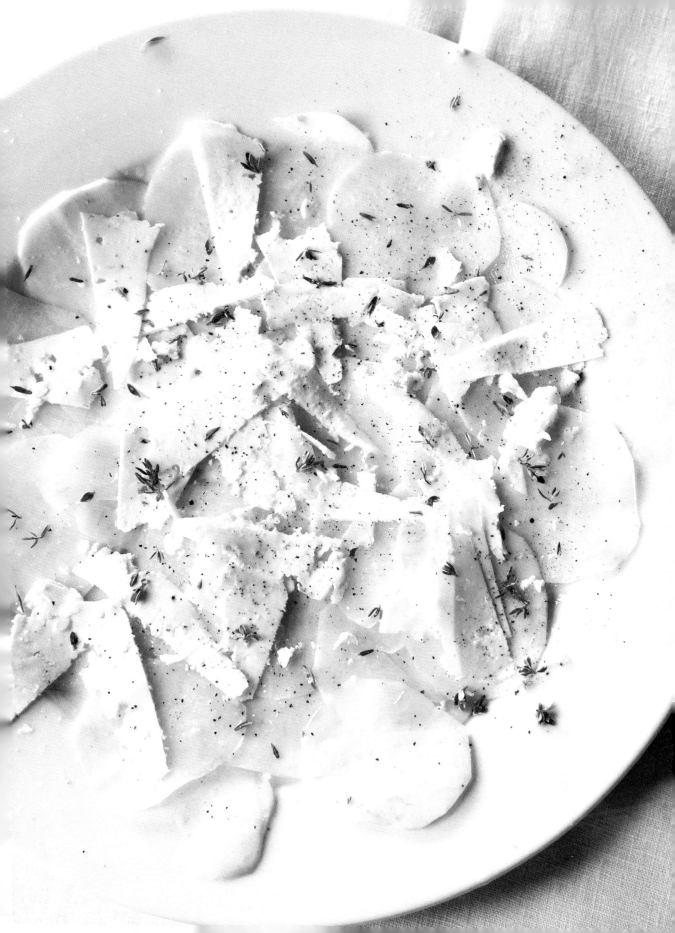

Chicory, pears and salty-sweet roasted almonds

Marcona almonds, if you can get them, are particularly tasty here. The nuts can be prepared well ahead and stored in an airtight container.

SERVES 4

2 heads of white or red chicory

2 ripe pears

FOR THE SALTY-SWEET ALMONDS

½ teaspoon unsalted butter

½ teaspoon sugar

A good pinch of sea salt

50g blanched almonds

FOR THE DRESSING

3 tablespoons rapeseed or olive oil

¼ teaspoon English mustard

A squeeze of lemon juice

Sea salt and freshly ground black pepper

To prepare the almonds, put the butter, sugar, salt and almonds into a small pan and heat gently. Watch the mixture like a hawk, stirring often, as the sugar starts to caramelise. After a few minutes, the nuts will take on some colour and the sugar-butter-salt mix will be nicely caramelised. Remove from the heat and immediately tip out on to a non-stick silicone liner or a sheet of baking parchment. Leave to cool.

To make the dressing, whisk the oil and mustard together in a small cup or jug. Add just enough lemon juice to create a nicely sharp dressing and season with some salt and pepper.

Separate the chicory leaves. Peel, quarter and core the pears, then cut each quarter lengthways in half again. Arrange the chicory and pears on serving plates, add a scattering of salty-sweet nuts, trickle over the dressing and serve.

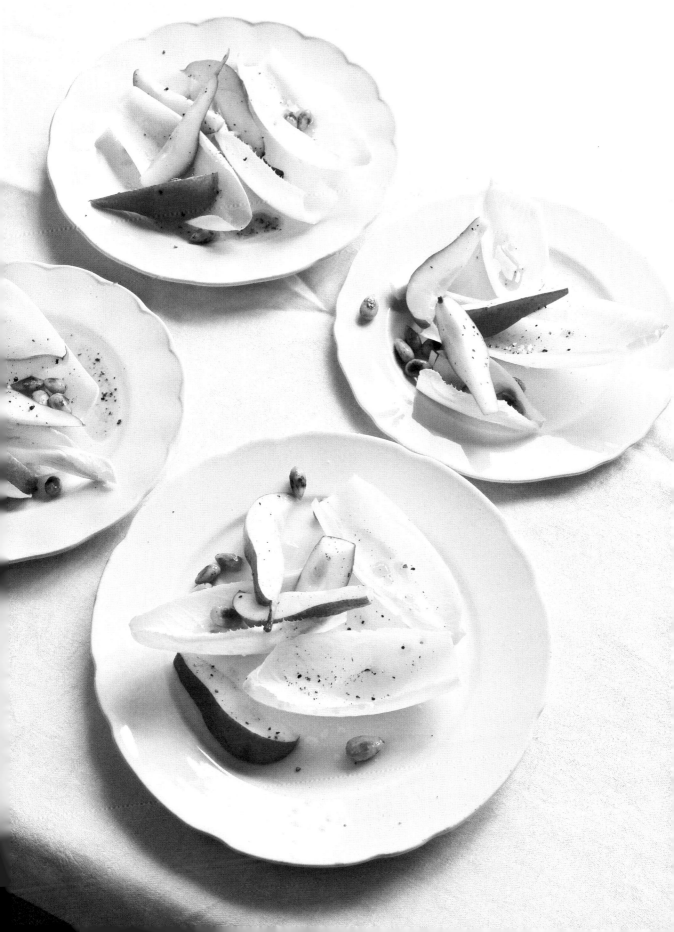

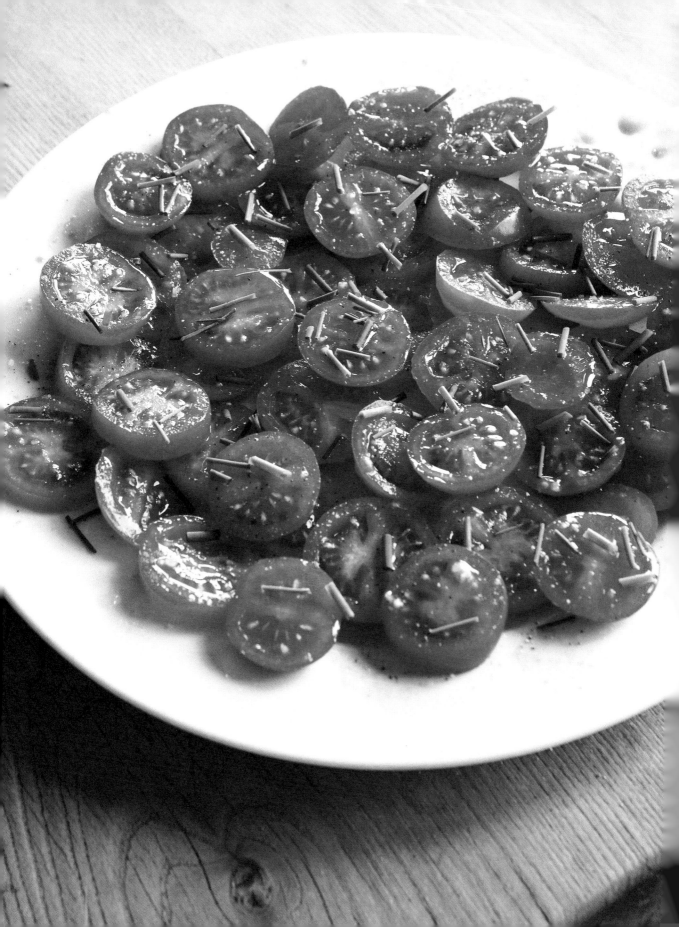

Tomatoes with herbs 🌱

This classic assembly remains one of my favourite ways to serve really good,
ripe, sun-warmed tomatoes, and I like to use two or three varieties if possible.
Vary the herbs as you please – chives, basil and parsley all work well.

SERVES 4

1kg ripe, full-flavoured tomatoes

3–4 tablespoons extra virgin olive oil

1–2 tablespoons balsamic vinegar (ideally apple balsamic)

A small handful of chives, snipped, or torn basil leaves, or chopped parsley

Sea salt and freshly ground black pepper

Thickly slice the tomatoes and arrange on a serving platter, so the slices are only slightly overlapping to ensure each one will receive some of the dressing.

First trickle over the olive oil, then the balsamic vinegar. Scatter over the herbs, season with a little salt and pepper and then serve.

VARIATION

Tomatoes and goat's cheese
I sometimes scatter a thinly sliced firm goat's cheese over the sliced tomatoes before dressing this salad (as shown on page 7).

Tomatoes with thai dressing

This is another simple and delicious way to serve up a tomato salad – with
an unusual Thai-inspired dressing, which goes brilliantly with the mint.
Again, I like to use a few different types of tomatoes.

SERVES 4

1kg ripe, full-flavoured tomatoes

6–8 mint leaves, shredded

Sea salt and freshly ground black pepper

FOR THE DRESSING

½–1 small red chilli or a good pinch of dried chilli flakes

½ garlic clove, crushed with a little coarse sea salt

1 tablespoon balsamic vinegar (ideally apple balsamic)

2 teaspoons rice vinegar or cider vinegar

2 teaspoons sesame oil

1 teaspoon clear honey

For the dressing, halve, deseed and very finely chop the fresh chilli, if using, almost to a paste. Whisk together all the rest of the ingredients for the dressing until the honey has dissolved into the mixture, adding the chilli by degrees to achieve the heat you want.

Thickly slice the tomatoes and arrange them on a large platter, or on individual plates. Season with salt and pepper, trickle over the dressing and sprinkle over the mint. Serve immediately.

Avocado and ruby grapefruit with chilli ᵛ

A lovely, fresh zesty salad, spiked with a little chilli. When available,
I like to use organic small, dark, knobbly Hass avocados.

SERVES 2

1 ruby or pink grapefruit

1 avocado

½ small or medium red chilli, deseeded and finely chopped

A small handful of coriander leaves

Extra virgin olive oil

Sea salt and freshly ground black pepper

Slice the top and bottom from the grapefruit. Stand it upright on a board and work your way around the fruit with a sharp knife, cutting off the skin and all the pith. Now hold it in your hand over a bowl to catch the juice and slice carefully down between each segment to release from the membrane, letting the segments fall into the bowl. Squeeze the juice from the remaining membrane in too.

Halve, peel and stone the avocado, then cut lengthways into thin slices. Arrange on a large plate with the grapefruit segments and trickle over the saved juice.

Sprinkle a little salt and the chopped chilli over the salad. Finish with the coriander and a generous trickle of olive oil. Serve straight away.

Marinated cucumber with mint ᵛ

We don't always get excited about cucumber, because it isn't always served to its best advantage.
This refreshing salad takes just a few minutes to put together, but does a cucumber full justice.
Resting the salad allows the mint to infuse and takes the chilly edge off the cucumber.

SERVES 3–4

1 medium-large cucumber

1 teaspoon cider vinegar

1 tablespoon olive or rapeseed oil

A good handful of mint, finely chopped

A pinch of sugar

Sea salt and freshly ground black pepper

Peel the cucumber, halve it lengthways and scoop out the seeds. Slice into thick half-moons. Place in a dish with the cider vinegar, oil, mint and a pinch each of salt, sugar and pepper. Toss together thoroughly. Leave for 15–30 minutes, toss again and then serve.

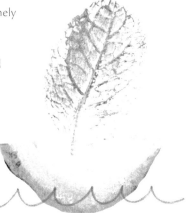

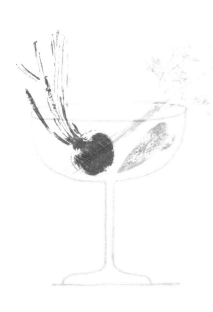

Vegetable juice mixology

Once in a while it's good to get to know your veg intimately, from the inside out, as it were. That's where the juicer comes in handy. And a glass of freshly juiced veg can be very delicious as well as feeling very virtuous. I've been experimenting with lots of juices – in one session I juiced ten different types of veg, and tried out all sorts of blends. One of the revelations was rhubarb (which is of course a vegetable, not a fruit). It's too tart and astringent on its own, but a great way to add zing to sweeter juices like carrot and beetroot. It can be quite tough on the juicer though, with its fibrous stems, so don't force it.

The whole point of owning a juicer, as I see it, is to experiment, play around and come up with your own favourite veg/fruit combinations. But, of course, I'm delighted to share some of my favourites with you. All quantities are approximate. Feel free to adjust the balance to your taste, or what's to hand. Veg juiced cold from the fridge will always make for a more refreshing drink. I prefer not to add ice, though, as it dilutes the flavours.

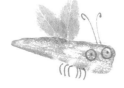

Beetroot bazaar ᴠ
I've always liked the combination of cumin with root veg; you could also try coriander seeds, or a pinch of cayenne.
Lightly toast ½ teaspoon cumin seeds in a dry frying pan for a couple of minutes until fragrant, then pulverise using a pestle and mortar. Juice 2 medium beetroot, 2 large carrots and 2 celery stalks. Add the toasted cumin with a pinch of salt and a grinding of black pepper, then taste and adjust, sharpening the juice with a few drops of lemon or orange if you like.

Bugs' surprise ᴠ
This a great way to give a tart edge to sweet, creamy carrot juice.
Juice 3 large carrots and ½–1 medium rhubarb stalk and mix well. Serve cold, finished with a bruised sprig of mint if you like.

Cuke and tom cooler ᴠ
Freshly juiced ripe tomatoes are quite different from tomato juice in a carton or bottle, which has effectively been cooked to preserve it. The cucumber is a lovely companion.
Juice 250g ripe tomatoes (any kind) and ½ large cucumber, finely chop a few mint leaves and mix all well together.

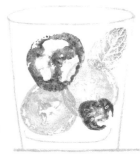

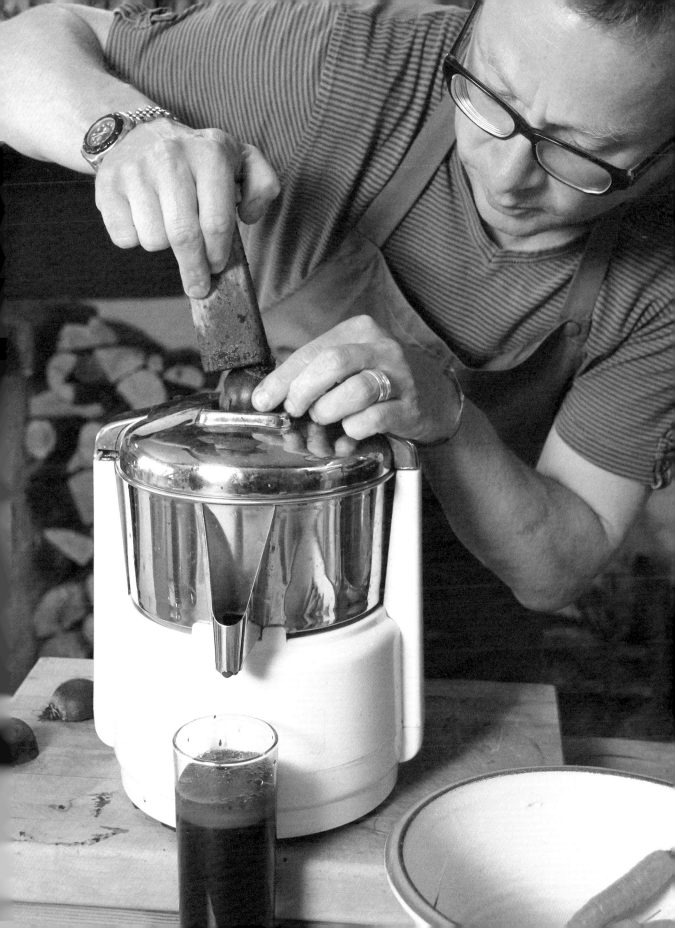

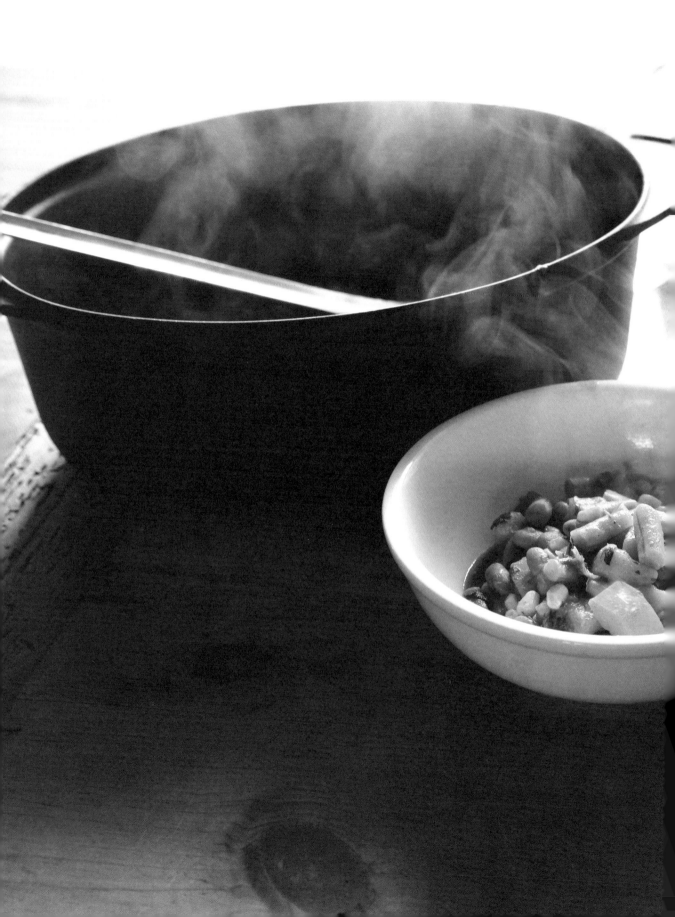

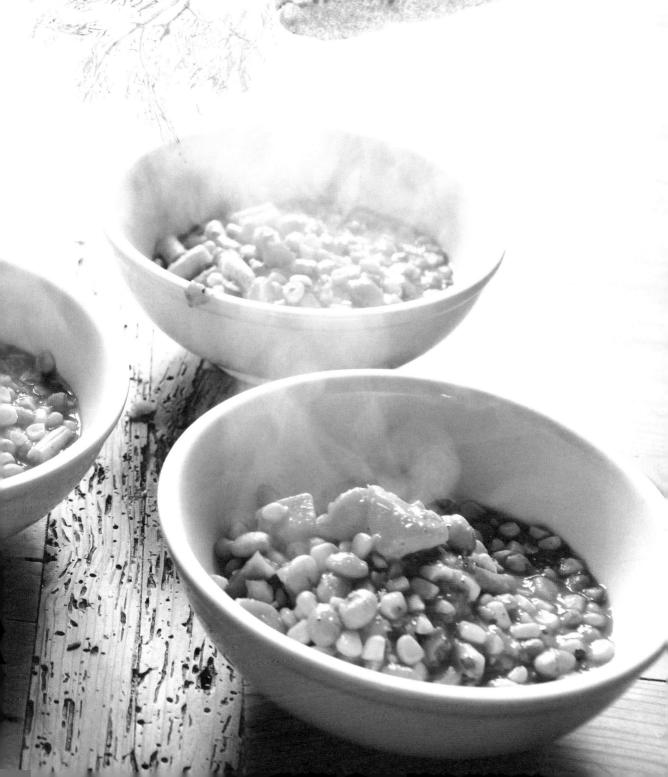

Hefty soups

I hope you're not tempted to skim over this chapter because the idea of 'vegetable soup' doesn't entice you. If you are, I urge you to think again, because these soups are as varied, textured and flavour-packed as any of the other dishes in the book. The only thing that really marks them out is that they generally need to be eaten with a spoon. Although in a couple of cases – the ribollita (see page 151) springs to mind – they're so packed with goodness and goodies that you'd probably get away with a fork.

There's certainly nothing samey about them. There are some broth-based soups, with a whole veg patch of produce to be chased around the bowl, while some are smooth, thick and creamy, others chunky, rich and hearty. And many hover tantalisingly between these poles. Some are almost stews: after all, the point at which a soup turns into a stew is pretty arbitrary. With many 'big' soups, you're simply building up a really hearty mix of vegetables, grains and pulses that happens to sit best in a bowl, on account of the lovely liquor in which they sit.

The purpose of almost all of these soups is to be satisfyingly substantial. A few would be perfect in small portions, as starters – the cucumber and lettuce vichyssoise (see page 134) is particularly elegant. However, for the most part, they have it in them to be main meals. They are the sort of soups I would expect you to have seconds of: not just half a ladleful, but a whole second bowl. Add some bread and you've got supper.

The lovely loose, liquid consistency of soup makes for relaxed eating but also for relaxed cooking. There are no delicate emulsions or veloutés here, just marvellous mixtures of good tasty things. There's no need to get bogged down with precise measurements and long lists of fancy ingredients. The fact is that most of the soups I make at home – and I make soup at least once a week – are not pre-planned or taken from recipe books. They are improvised from ingredients I have to hand – sometimes fresh, sometimes leftovers, sometimes from the store cupboard, often a combination of all three.

Only yesterday I put together a soup that bore little resemblance to one I had ever made before. In the fridge I happened to have a few leftover wedges of roast squash (similar to the recipe on page 346). I also had a meagre portion of the lovely cauliflower and chickpea curry (on page 27). I put them together in the blender, with half a litre of stock from an organic veg stock cube, and a dash of coconut milk from a tin off the shelf. The result, finished with a swirl of yoghurt from the fridge, was a genuinely fine soup – from a combination of ingredients that would never have been premeditated.

Even – especially – when cooking from scratch with garden-fresh ingredients, I'm still often cooking on the hoof, and many of the recipes that follow are the results of impromptu soup sessions. I like to knock out chunky-textured soups that showcase fresh veg in their greatest glory – either whole, or in bite-sized pieces for the eye to see and the mouth to savour. Often they'll feature a composite of creamy beans, leafy greens, cubed roots and cubed fruits (generally in the savoury, courgettey, squashy sense of the 'f' word). They tend to be put together with gay abandon after raiding the garden – and certainly don't require a session in a white lab coat with the digital scales. So, please feel free to cut loose with these recipes in a similar spirit of improvisation. Add less of this, more of that, or throw in something completely different that you have a hunch about. With soups, there are so few rules and so many good outcomes.

Almost all the soups that follow are based on a light vegetable stock; having said that, they could equally well be made with a light chicken stock if you have one to hand. When I have time, I love to make a fresh vegetable stock, and the recipe on page 130 can be done and dusted in half an hour. But frankly, that's half an hour I often don't have, so I am no stranger to the stock cube. My favourite is an organic, yeast-free one by Kallo, which seems to be available these days in most delis and wholefood shops, and some supermarkets. I'll often make a slightly weaker broth, half to two-thirds strength, than that suggested on the pack, as a soup already crammed full of fresh veg shouldn't need much help from a stock.

I'm a great fan of the 'finishing touch' for soups. I flinch from the word 'garnish' – so often an addition you don't actually want to eat – but something on top, or swirled in, that adds an extra dimension of contrasting taste or texture, is usually very welcome. It also makes the lucky person who's supping on that soup feel well looked after. Don't underestimate the pleasing effect on the palate of a trickle of a herb or spice oil, a swirl of yoghurt, a few gratings of cheese, a dab of pesto, or the crunch of croûtons. Again, don't feel my ideas for the final flourish in these recipes are strictly prescriptive either. Mix and match. Knock yourself out. It's all part of bigging up a good soup to give it the billing it deserves, a way of saying: 'I love my soup. And you're going to love it too.'

Vegetable stock

A good vegetable stock, built around the deep savoury notes of bay and celery and the delicate sweetness of onion and carrot, is invaluable for giving body to many soups. You'll also find it indispensable for stews, risottos, gratins and curries. I always try to keep some of this in the freezer – though it can be rustled up in no time if you have the ingredients to hand.

MAKES ABOUT 1.5 LITRES

2 large or 3 medium onions

3 large or 4 medium carrots

3–4 celery stalks

1 garlic clove

1 tablespoon rapeseed oil

1 or 2 bay leaves, roughly torn

A sprig of thyme and/or some parsley stalks, if you have them

A few black peppercorns

½ small glass dry white wine (optional)

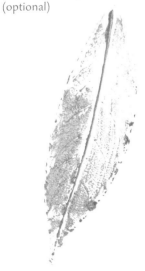

Coarsely grate the onions, carrots, celery and garlic – or chop them, if you prefer, but in fairly small pieces. Heat the oil in a large pan over a medium heat and tip in the vegetables, garlic, herbs and peppercorns. Sauté, stirring from time to time, for about 5 minutes or until the veg have softened slightly (you're largely doing this to mellow the raw onion).

Add the wine, if you are using it, then 1.75 litres boiling water from the kettle. Bring back to the boil and simmer, uncovered. If all your veg were grated, the stock will be ready in about 10 minutes. If they were in larger chunks, give it 20–30 minutes. Either way, strain the stock and use straight away, or cool, then refrigerate or freeze.

VARIATION

Mushroom stock

This stock has an extra kick of 'shroomy flavour. It's ideal for a mushroom soup (see pages 152 and 154), or in a mushroom risotto. However, you can use it in almost any veg soup to give a good deep, earthy base. Make the stock as above but add about 200g fresh, sliced mushrooms to the other veg – use well-flavoured types such as chestnut, shitake or big open-cap varieties. In addition, if you're including any dried mushrooms in the dish the stock is to be used in, be sure to add the soaking liquid to the stock, first straining it through muslin (to remove any grit).

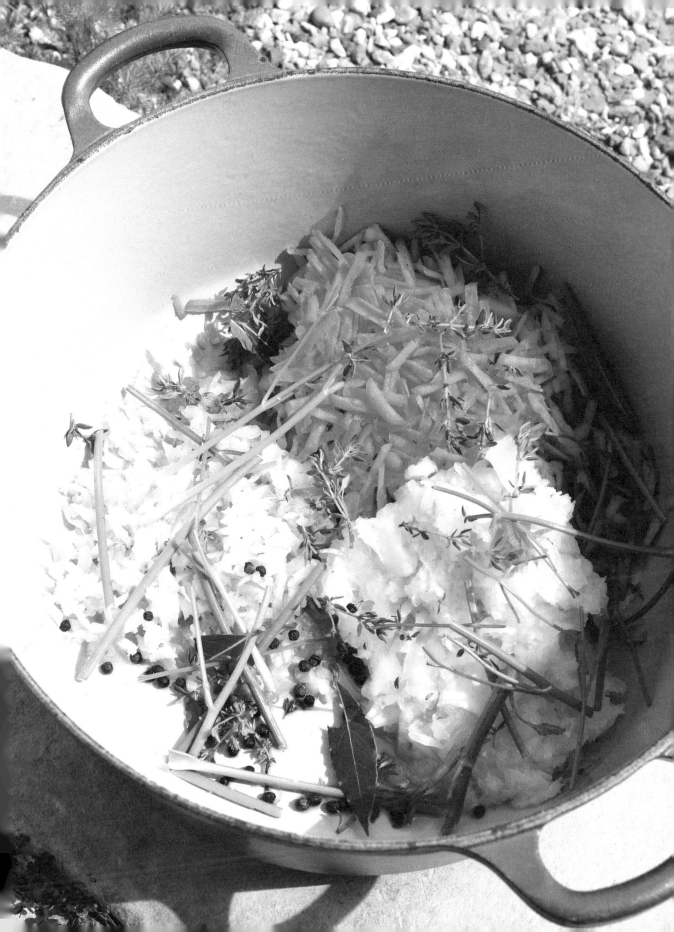

River Cottage summer garden soup

We often prepare this recipe to showcase some of our early summer produce from the River Cottage garden. You may not have access to the same range of just-picked veg, but gather some good, fresh stuff from a farm shop, market or greengrocers and you will get a similar result. Vary the veg according to what is available. Just chop it all into small, similar-sized pieces, and 'build' the soup, cooking the harder, denser veg for slightly longer, and you'll end up with a vibrant, fresh-tasting bowlful.

SERVES 6

2 small fennel bulbs, trimmed (any feathery fronds chopped and reserved)

2 celery stalks

A small bunch of spring onions, trimmed

About 500g small courgettes

A bunch of ruby or rainbow chard

30g butter

1 tablespoon rapeseed or olive oil

1 litre vegetable stock (see page 130)

100–150g freshly podded peas

100–150g freshly podded broad beans, blanched and peeled if large

2 small lettuces, such as Little Gem, shredded

2 tablespoons finely chopped mixed herbs, such as mint, lemon balm, parsley, basil, fennel tops and/or chives

A few fresh pea shoots (optional)

Sea salt and freshly ground black pepper

Chop the fennel, celery, spring onions and courgettes into small dice, keeping them separate. Tear the leaves from the chard stalks and shred them; cut the stalks into small pieces.

Heat a medium saucepan over a medium heat and add the butter and oil. Add the fennel, celery, spring onions and chard stalks and cook gently for about 10 minutes, until soft but not coloured. Add the stock and bring to a simmer. Season with salt and pepper.

Making sure your broth is simmering well, add the courgettes. Once returned to a simmer, cook for 1 minute, then add the peas and broad beans. Simmer these for another 2 minutes. Check the peas and beans are just tender, then add the lettuce and the shredded chard leaves. Simmer for another minute.

Add the chopped herbs along with any feathery fennel fronds and, if you have them, the pea shoots, then immediately remove from the heat. Check the seasoning, then ladle into warmed bowls and serve.

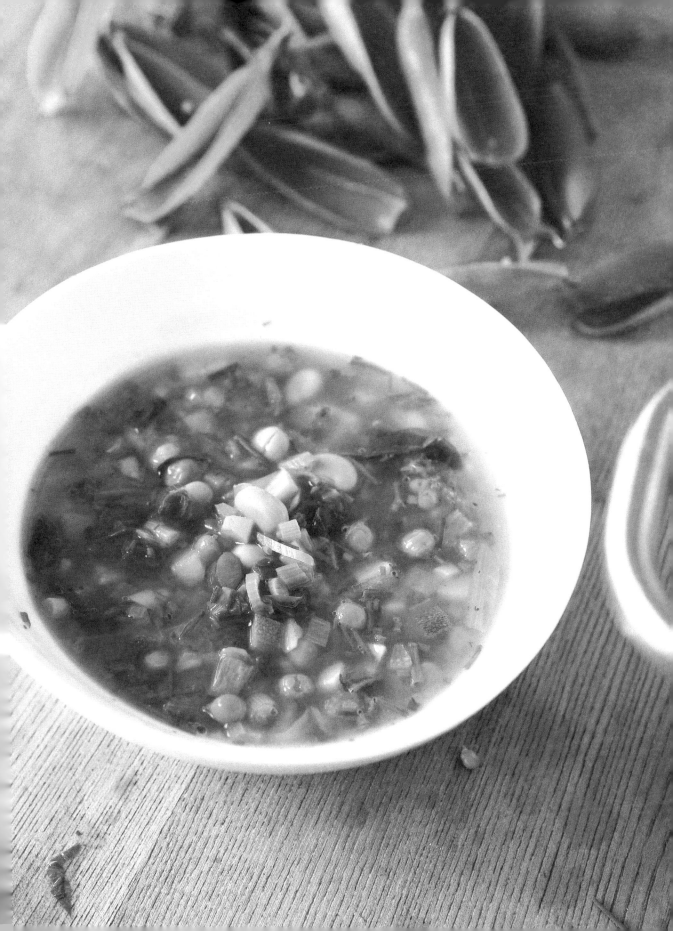

Cucumber and lettuce vichyssoise

Light, delicate and pretty, this chilled soup – a take on the classic vichyssoise – is a great way to start a summer meal. You can also make a deep green version with spinach instead of the lettuce.

SERVES 6

50g butter

2 leeks, trimmed (white and pale green part only), washed and sliced, OR 1 large onion, sliced

1 large, floury potato (about 250g), peeled and cut into large chunks

1 litre vegetable stock (see page 130)

2 cucumbers, peeled and cubed

2 Little Gem or butterhead lettuces, washed and shredded

3 tablespoons double cream or crème fraîche, plus a little extra to finish

Sea salt and freshly ground black pepper

FOR THE CROÛTONS

4 tablespoons rapeseed or olive oil

4 slices of bread, crusts removed, cut into cubes

TO FINISH

Chopped chives

Melt the butter in a large pan over a medium-low heat. Add the leeks or onion, cover and sweat gently for about 10 minutes, until soft. Add the potato and stock. Bring to the boil, then simmer for about 10 minutes, until the potato is almost cooked. Add the cubed cucumbers and shredded lettuce, return to the boil and simmer for a further 4 minutes.

Fish out the potato chunks and rub them through a sieve, mouli or potato ricer into a large bowl (whizzing them in a blender would make the soup gluey). Purée everything else in a blender, add to the sieved potato and stir well. Stir in the cream or crème fraîche and season with salt and pepper. Leave to cool completely, then chill for a couple of hours.

Meanwhile, make the croûtons. Heat the oil in a frying pan over a medium-high heat. Add the bread and fry, turning often, for a few minutes, until golden brown. Leave to cool.

Serve the chilled soup topped with a swirl of cream or crème fraîche, chopped chives and the croûtons.

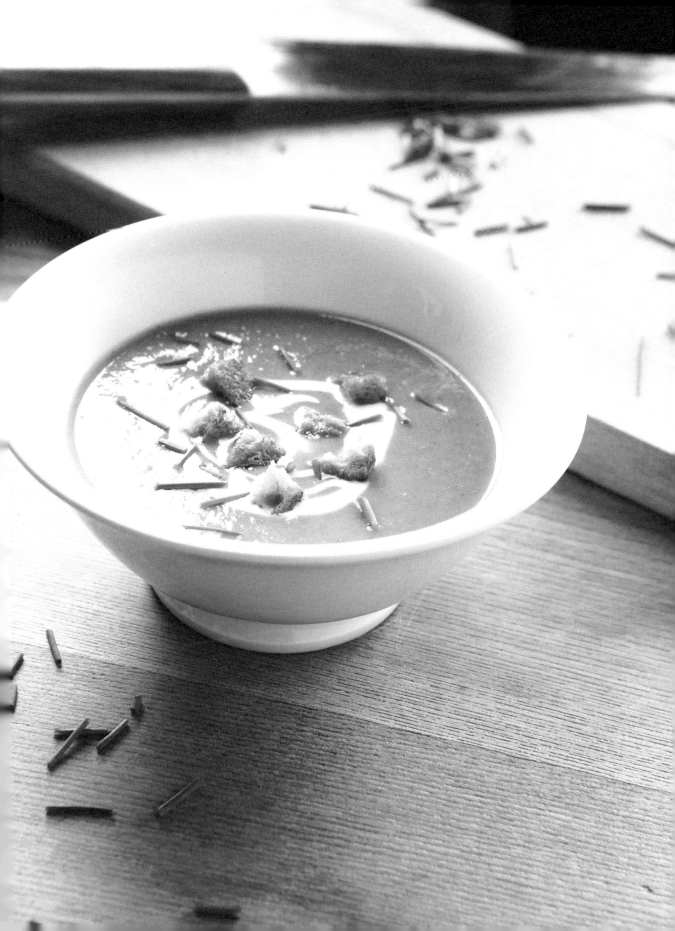

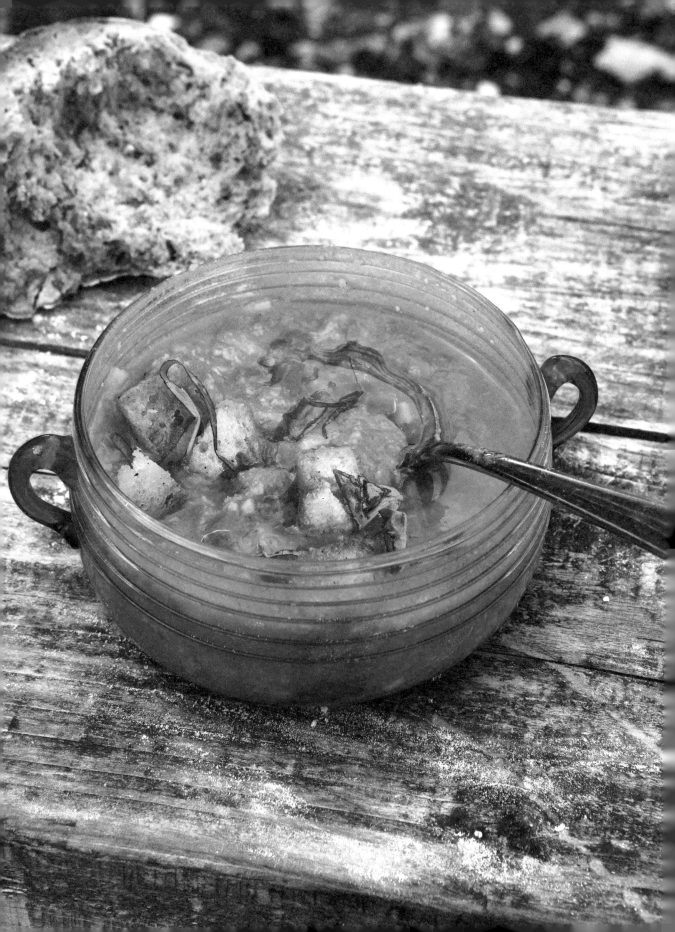

Gazpacho ♥

This traditional, chilled Spanish soup is as cooling as they come: the perfect thing to serve on a hot summer's day or a sultry evening. You can, if you like, press the puréed soup through a sieve to get a really smooth finish – but bear in mind you'll lose some of the volume if you do this. In any case, I like my gazpacho a little bit chunky. It goes without saying that the tomatoes need to be full of flavour or you'll be selling your soup short.

SERVES 4

2 thick slices of stale white bread (about 100g), crusts removed

1 garlic clove, crushed

1–1.5kg large, ripe tomatoes

½ cucumber, peeled and sliced

1 red pepper, deseeded and chopped

½ small red onion, chopped

50ml extra virgin olive oil

1 tablespoon balsamic vinegar (ideally apple balsamic)

1 teaspoon sugar

Sea salt and freshly ground black pepper

TO FINISH

Croûtons (see page 134)

Shredded basil or chopped flat-leaf parsley

Tear the bread into pieces and put into a bowl with the crushed garlic. Pour on 200ml cold water and leave to soak while you prepare the remaining ingredients.

Cover the tomatoes with boiling water, leave for a couple of minutes, then scoop out and peel off their skins. Quarter and deseed the tomatoes, putting all the seeds and clinging juicy bits into a sieve over a bowl. Put the skinned flesh into a separate bowl. When all the tomatoes are done, press the seedy bits in the sieve to extract as much juice as possible, adding it to the tomato flesh.

Put the soaked bread and garlic, tomatoes, cucumber, red pepper, onion, olive oil, balsamic vinegar and sugar in a food processor (you should just about be able to do it in one batch). Process to a coarse purée and season with salt and pepper to taste. You can leave it chunky, or whiz a bit longer then press through a sieve, if you prefer.

Cover and chill for 2–3 hours, then taste and adjust the seasoning. Serve the gazpacho topped with croûtons and shredded basil or chopped parsley.

Mexican tomato and bean soup

This fresh, piquant summer soup combines many of the ingredients you might find in a feisty salsa, but in this case they're all 'souped up'. Add more chillies if you like it hot, and a handful of fresh sweetcorn kernels, sliced straight from the cob, is a good addition if you have them. A scattering of diced avocado can replace the soured cream, if you prefer.

SERVES 4-6

2 tablespoons olive oil

2 red onions, finely chopped

3 garlic cloves, finely chopped

1–2 medium-hot green chillies, such as jalapeño, deseeded and finely chopped

½ teaspoon ground cumin

600ml vegetable stock (see page 130)

200ml roasted tomato sauce (see page 366) or passata

400g ripe tomatoes, cored, deseeded and finely chopped

400g tin black beans or black eyed beans, drained and rinsed

A handful of oregano, chopped

A pinch of sugar

Juice of 1 lime

A small handful of coriander, roughly chopped

Sea salt and freshly ground black pepper

TO FINISH

4–6 tablespoons soured cream (optional)

A small handful of coriander, roughly chopped

Heat the olive oil in a saucepan over a medium-low heat, add most of the onions (reserving a little to finish the soup) and sauté for about 5 minutes, or until softened. Add the garlic, chillies and cumin and stir for a minute.

Add the stock, roasted tomato sauce or passata, tomatoes, beans, oregano and sugar. Season with salt and pepper, bring to the boil and simmer gently for 10 minutes. Remove from the heat and add the lime juice and coriander. Taste and adjust the seasoning if necessary.

Serve the soup topped with dollops of soured cream, if you like, and scattered with the reserved red onion, chopped coriander and freshly ground pepper.

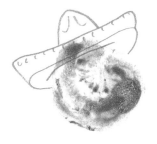

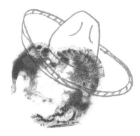

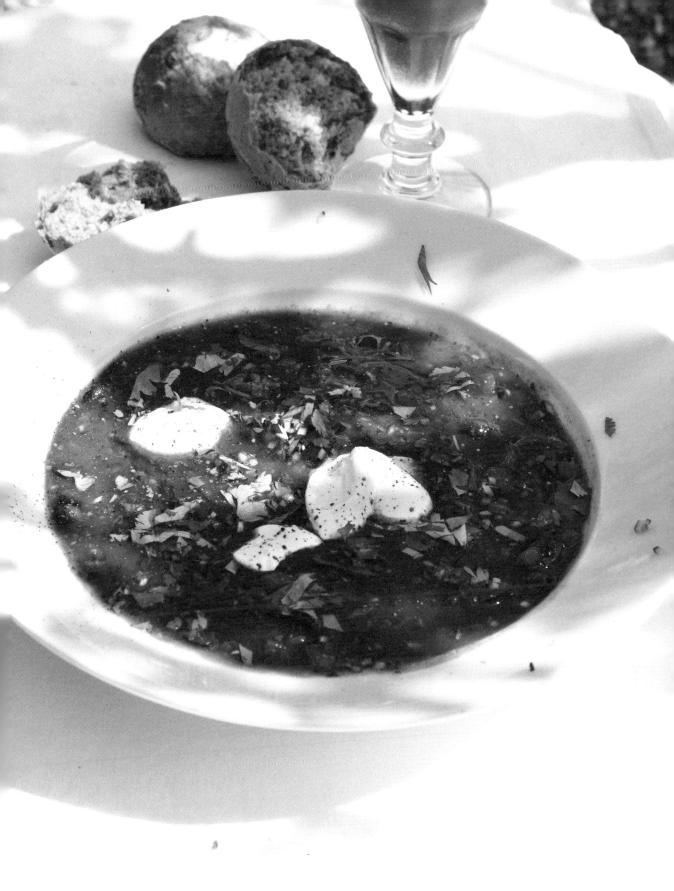

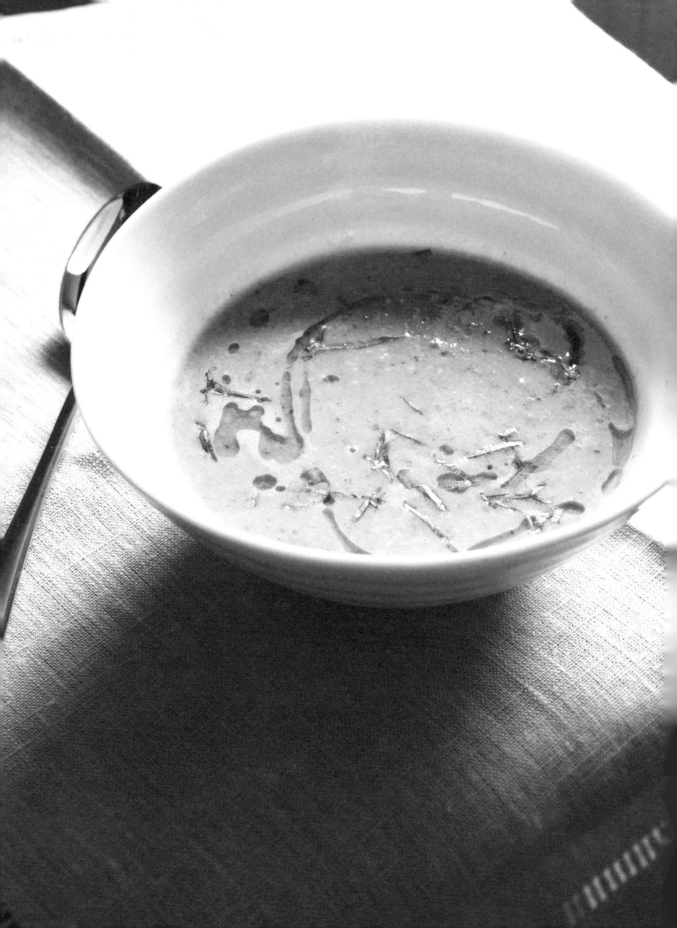

Pea and parsley soup

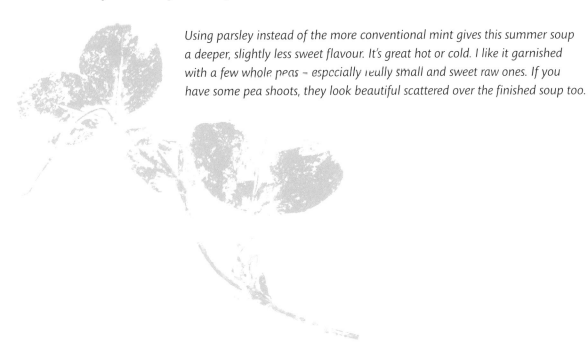

Using parsley instead of the more conventional mint gives this summer soup a deeper, slightly less sweet flavour. It's great hot or cold. I like it garnished with a few whole peas – especially really small and sweet raw ones. If you have some pea shoots, they look beautiful scattered over the finished soup too.

SERVES 4

1 tablespoon olive or rapeseed oil, plus extra to trickle

20g butter

1 medium onion, finely chopped

A few sprigs of thyme, leaves only, chopped

1 litre vegetable stock (see page 130)

500g fresh shelled peas, or frozen peas

20g flat-leaf parsley, chopped

Sea salt and freshly ground pepper, to taste

A few mint leaves, shredded, to finish (optional)

Heat the oil and butter in a large saucepan over a medium-low heat and sweat the onion with the thyme until soft and translucent, about 10 minutes.

Add the stock, peas (reserving a handful to finish the soup if you like) and parsley. Season with salt and pepper, bring to a simmer and cook for 5–10 minutes, or until the peas are very tender.

Cool slightly, then purée the soup in a food processor or blender, or with a stick blender, until very smooth – you may need to do this in two batches if you are using a processor or free-standing blender. Return the soup to the pan, adjust the seasoning and heat through.

Ladle the soup into warmed bowls. If you have some fresh, raw peas, scatter a few on top (or you could use blanched frozen peas). Add the mint, if using, trickle over a little olive or rapeseed oil and serve.

Alternatively, you can let the soup go cold, then chill it lightly before serving – add the scattering of peas and mint, if using, and trickle of oil at the last minute.

Fennel and celeriac soup with orange zest

This velvety, gently aniseedy soup is given warmth and definition with a touch of orange zest. The rich-but-sharp crème fraîche added at the end balances it all out nicely.

SERVES 4

30g butter

1 tablespoon rapeseed or olive oil

4 shallots, or 1 medium onion, sliced

3 large fennel bulbs (about 750g), trimmed and sliced (any feathery fronds reserved)

¼ large celeriac (about 250g, untrimmed), peeled and cubed

Finely grated zest of 1 orange

About 500ml vegetable stock (see page 130)

Sea salt and freshly ground black pepper

4–6 tablespoons crème fraîche, to finish

Heat the butter and oil in a large saucepan over a medium heat. Add the shallots or onion and sweat gently for a few minutes. Add the fennel and celeriac, stir well, then cover and sweat for about 10 minutes.

Add the orange zest, stock and some salt and pepper. Bring to the boil, then simmer for about 15 minutes until all the veg is tender.

Purée the soup in a blender until completely smooth, adding a touch more stock or water to loosen the consistency if necessary. (You may have to blend longer than usual to blitz out all the fibres from the fennel, but it shouldn't be necessary to pass the soup through a sieve.)

Reheat the soup if necessary, check the seasoning and serve, with a good blob of crème fraîche on top, a few fennel fronds if you have them, and plenty of freshly ground black pepper.

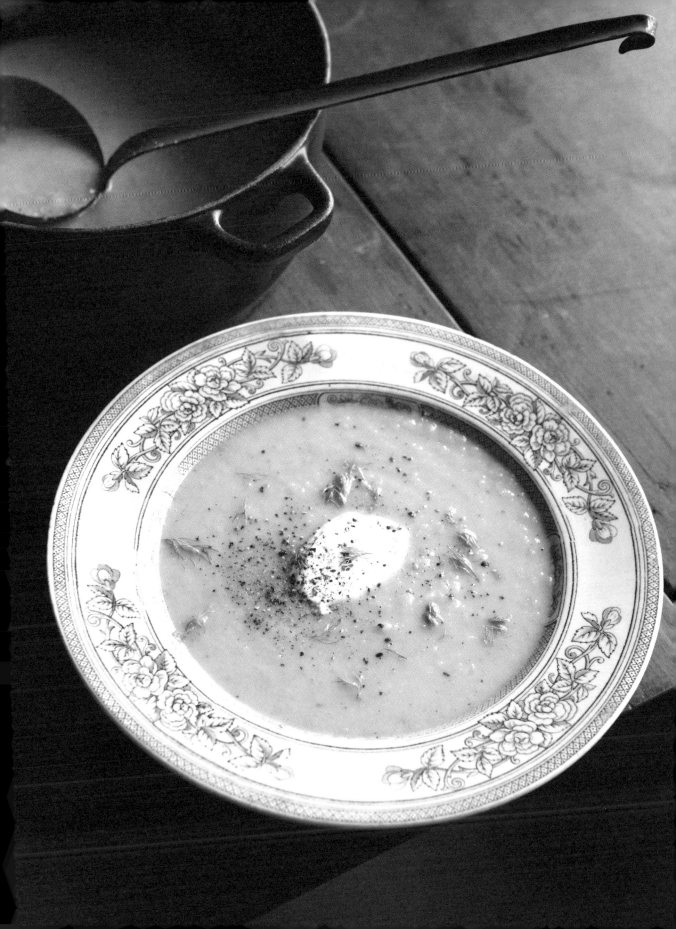

Roasted beetroot soup with horseradish cream

Two fantastic roots take centre stage here: the sharp, hot tang of horseradish is the best foil I know to beetroot's earthy sweetness. The resulting soup, though easy to make, is really very elegant.

SERVES 4–6

1kg beetroot

4 garlic cloves (unpeeled), bashed

2–3 sprigs of thyme

1 bay leaf

3 tablespoons olive or rapeseed oil

1 litre vegetable stock (see page 130)

Sea salt and freshly ground black pepper

FOR THE HORSERADISH CREAM

3–4cm piece of fresh horseradish, peeled and freshly grated (or 1 tablespoon creamed horseradish)

200ml soured cream, crème fraîche or thick, plain (full-fat) yoghurt

TO FINISH

Dill fronds

Preheat the oven to 200°C/Gas Mark 6. Scrub the beetroot well but leave them whole. Place them in a roasting tin and scatter around the garlic, thyme and bay leaf. Trickle on the oil and season well with salt and pepper. Mix everything together with your hands so that it is well coated. Pour a wine glass of water into the tin and cover tightly with foil. Roast until the beetroot are tender when pierced with a knife – about an hour depending on the size of the beetroot.

While the beetroot are roasting, make the horseradish cream: in a bowl, mix the grated (or creamed) horseradish with the soured cream, crème fraîche or yoghurt.

Remove the foil from the roasting tin and leave the beetroot until they are cool enough to handle. Top and tail them and peel or rub off the skins – they should slip off easily. Roughly chop the beetroot.

Squeeze the soft garlic from the skins and place in a blender with the beetroot. Process with enough of the stock to make a smooth purée, then transfer to a saucepan and thin further with stock to get the texture you like.

Heat through, over a medium heat, till thoroughly hot but not boiling. Adjust the seasoning to taste. Serve the soup in warmed bowls with a dollop of the horseradish cream and the dill scattered on top.

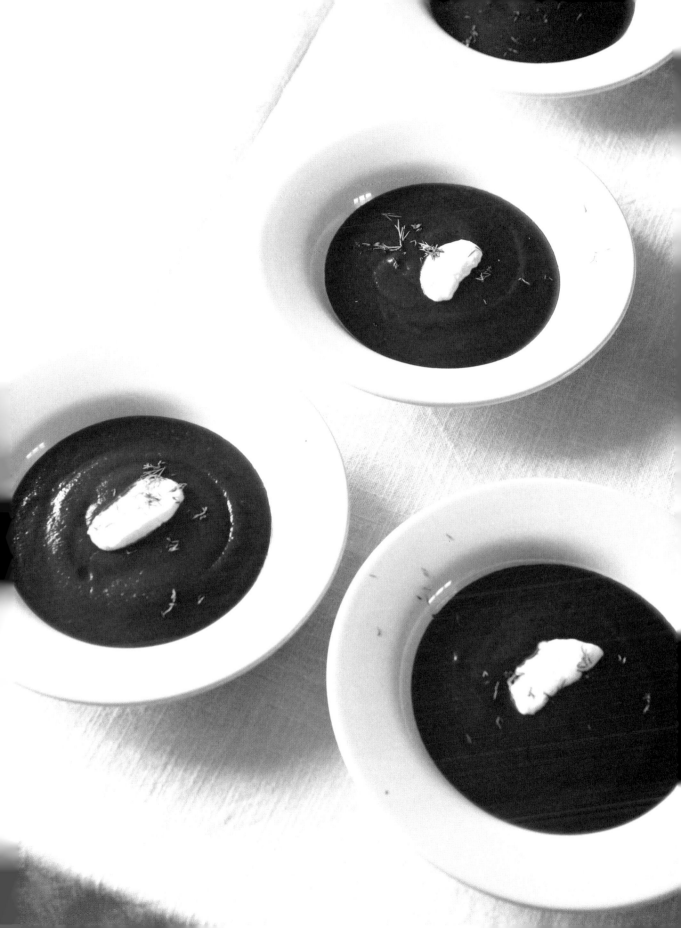

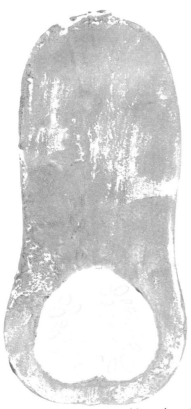

Porotos granados

This is my version of the traditional Chilean squash and bean stew. It's wonderfully hearty and warming and, like so many such dishes, even better if you leave it for 24 hours and reheat gently before serving.

SERVES 6

2 tablespoons rapeseed or olive oil

1 medium onion, chopped

2 garlic cloves, finely chopped

1 teaspoon sweet smoked paprika

A handful of oregano or marjoram, chopped

100g small dried beans, such as pinto, navy or cannellini beans, soaked overnight in cold water, OR 400g tin beans, drained and well rinsed

1 litre vegetable stock (see page 130)

1 bay leaf

750g squash, such as butternut, Crown Prince or onion, peeled, deseeded and cut into 2cm chunks

200g French beans, trimmed and cut into 2cm pieces

Kernels cut from 2 cobs of corn

Sea salt and freshly ground black pepper

Heat the oil in a large saucepan or casserole over a medium heat. Add the onion and garlic and sauté gently for about 10 minutes. Add the paprika and 1 tablespoon of the oregano. Cook for another minute.

If using dried beans, drain them after soaking and add to the pan, with the stock and bay leaf. Bring to the boil, then reduce the heat and simmer for about 45 minutes, or until the beans are completely tender (dried beans vary, and sometimes this may take over an hour). Add the squash, stir well and simmer for 10–15 minutes until the squash is just tender, then add the French beans and corn kernels and simmer for another 5 minutes.

If using tinned beans, add the drained, rinsed beans, the squash, bay leaf and stock at the same time, and simmer until the squash is just tender, 10–15 minutes. Then add the French beans and corn kernels and simmer for a further 5 minutes.

To finish, season well – I use about 1 teaspoon salt and plenty of pepper. Stir in the remaining oregano, leave to settle for a couple of minutes, then serve.

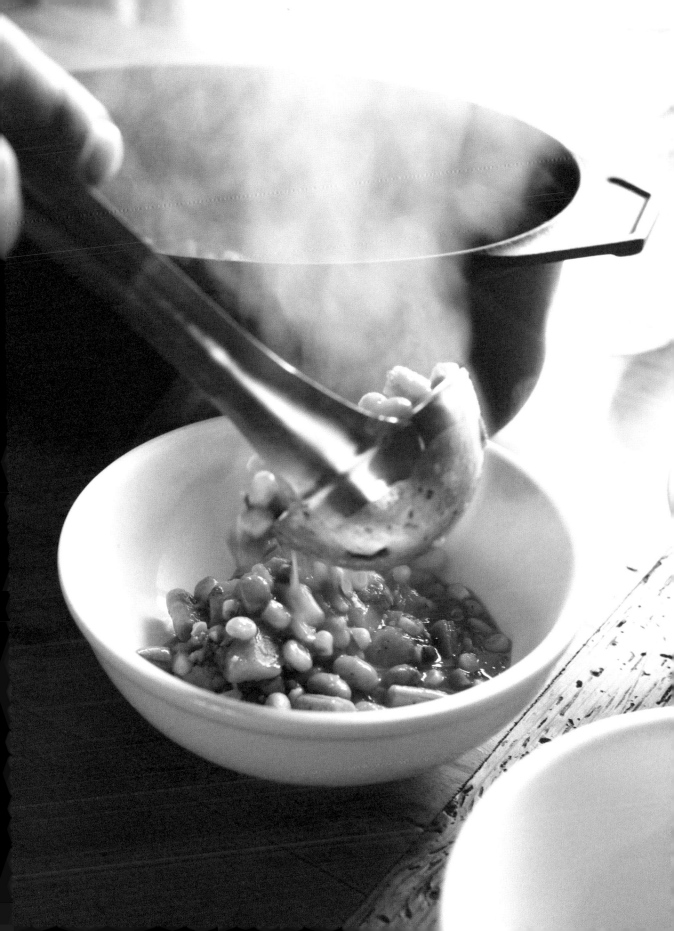

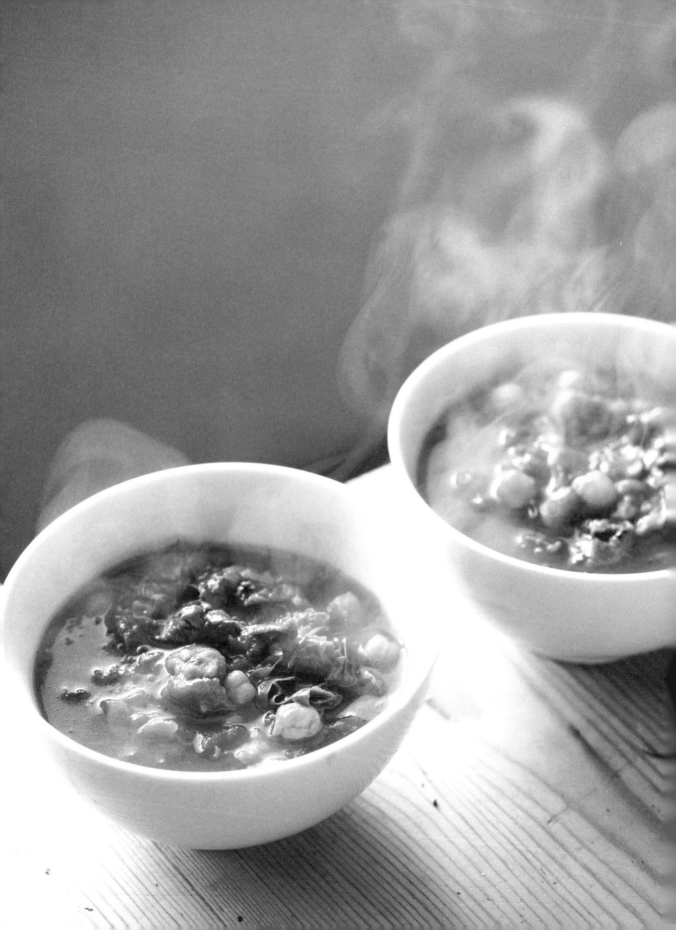

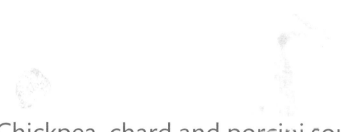

Chickpea, chard and porcini soup

This is a really lovely, hearty, big-flavoured soup, underpinned by the earthiness of porcini mushrooms. You could use tinned white beans, such as cannellini, in place of the chickpeas, and kale or spring greens instead of the chard or spinach.

SERVES 4

30g dried porcini mushrooms

30g butter

3 tablespoons olive oil

1 small onion, diced

2 garlic cloves, finely chopped

400g passata OR a 400g tin plum tomatoes, chopped, any stalky ends and skin removed

400g tin chickpeas, drained and rinsed

1 sprig of rosemary

300g chard or spinach, shredded

Sea salt and freshly ground black pepper

TO SERVE

Extra virgin olive oil

Parmesan, hard goat's cheese or other well-flavoured hard cheese (optional)

Soak the porcini in about 750ml warm water for 30 minutes. Remove the mushrooms with a slotted spoon, reserving the soaking water. Rinse the mushrooms briefly under the cold tap (they can be gritty) and pat dry with kitchen paper. Roughly chop them.

Strain the mushroom soaking liquid through a sieve lined with muslin or kitchen paper into a bowl.

Heat the butter and olive oil in a saucepan over a medium-low heat and sweat the onion, stirring from time to time, for about 15 minutes, until soft and translucent. Add the garlic and stir for a minute, then add the mushrooms and cook, stirring, for another couple of minutes.

Add the passata or the tomatoes with their juice, chickpeas, rosemary, reserved mushroom soaking liquid and a few grinds of black pepper. Bring to the boil, turn down the heat and simmer gently for about 45 minutes. Add the shredded chard or spinach and cook for a further 8–10 minutes for chard, just 2–3 minutes for spinach.

If the soup seems too thick, thin it slightly with a little water. Discard the rosemary. Taste and add salt and pepper if needed.

Ladle into warm bowls, trickle over some olive oil and use a vegetable peeler to shave a few slivers of Parmesan or hard goat's cheese over the top, if you like. Serve at once.

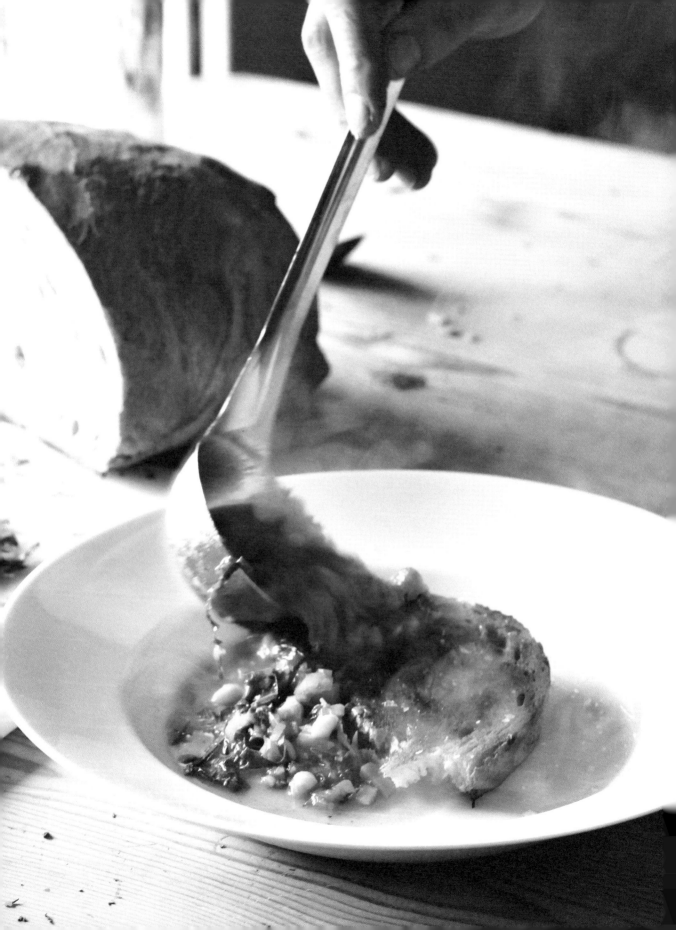

Ribollita ♥

Ribollita literally means 'reboiled': traditionally this Italian soup was made in large quantities so it could be reheated on subsequent days. It's fantastic, economical peasant food and proves how humble ingredients – in this case, a few inexpensive veg and some stale bread – can yield truly delicious results. By all means use a couple of tins of cannellini beans rather than dried beans.

SERVES 6

FOR THE BEANS

200g dried cannellini beans, soaked in cold water overnight

1 onion, quartered

1 bay leaf

1 garlic clove, bashed

1 sprig of rosemary

OR

2 x 400g tins cannellini beans

FOR THE SOUP

4 tablespoons olive oil

1 onion, finely chopped

1–2 carrots, finely chopped

1 celery stalk, finely chopped

1 leek, trimmed, washed and finely sliced

5–6 tomatoes, skinned, deseeded and chopped, OR a 400g tin plum tomatoes, roughly chopped, any stalky ends and skin removed

800ml vegetable stock (see page 130)

1 sprig of rosemary and 1 sprig of thyme, tied together with string

300g kale, cavolo nero or Savoy cabbage, tough stalks removed

Sea salt and freshly ground black pepper

TO FINISH

6 slices of slightly stale country-style or sourdough bread

1 garlic clove, halved

3–4 tablespoons extra virgin olive oil

If you are using dried beans, drain them after soaking, rinse and then put into a large saucepan with the onion, bay leaf, garlic clove and rosemary. Add enough water to cover the beans by about 5cm, bring to the boil, lower the heat to a bare simmer, partially cover and cook until the beans are tender, about 1–1½ hours. Drain, reserving the liquid. Pulse half of the beans with some of the cooking liquid in a blender or processor until you have a rough purée.

If you are using tinned beans, drain and rinse them well, then mash or blend half of them with a little cold water.

In a large saucepan, heat the olive oil and sauté the onion over a medium-low heat for about 15 minutes, until softened. Add the carrots, celery and leek and sauté for 5 minutes, stirring. Now add the tomatoes with their juice, the puréed and whole beans, stock, rosemary and thyme, and simmer gently for about 1 hour.

Shred the kale, cavolo nero or cabbage leaves. Add to the soup and cook for 10 minutes more. Remove the sprigs of thyme and rosemary and add some salt and pepper.

To serve, toast the slices of bread until golden, then rub with the garlic and brush with olive oil. Put a slice of bread in the base of each bowl, ladle over the soup and trickle some olive oil on top before serving.

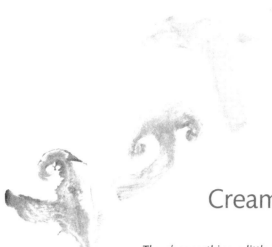

Creamy mushroom soup

There's something a little bit retro about a sherry-spiked cream of mushroom soup but, as a child of the seventies, I have no problem with that. With its beautiful dun colour and rich, earthy flavour, this is a dish I'm happy to revisit regularly. To get the best flavour, I use dark-gilled flat-cap and/or chestnut mushrooms.

SERVES 4–6

30g butter

2 leeks, trimmed (white and pale green part only), washed and finely sliced

A sprig of thyme

750g mushrooms, roughly chopped

1 small garlic clove, chopped

1 tablespoon plain flour

1.2 litres hot mushroom or vegetable stock (see page 130)

100ml double cream, plus extra to finish

A few gratings of nutmeg

2 tablespoons dry sherry (optional)

Sea salt and freshly ground black pepper

A handful of chives, tarragon or parsley, finely chopped, to finish

Melt the butter in a large saucepan over a medium-low heat and sweat the leeks with the thyme, stirring from time to time, until soft – about 10 minutes.

Turn the heat up to medium-high and add the mushrooms with a pinch of salt (this will help the juices to run). Sauté for a few minutes until they soften and lose some of their moisture.

Add the garlic and stir for a minute, then sprinkle over the flour and stir for a couple of minutes. Pour over the hot stock. Bring to the boil and simmer gently, uncovered, for 20 minutes.

Remove the thyme. Whiz the soup in a blender until smooth (or blend three-quarters of it and leave a quarter unblended if you prefer a soup with more texture). Return it to the pan.

Add the cream to the soup, along with the nutmeg, and reheat gently, stirring. Add the sherry, if using, then taste and adjust the seasoning, adding more salt, pepper and/or nutmeg as needed.

Spoon the soup into warmed bowls and add a swirl of cream and a sprinkling of chopped herbs before serving.

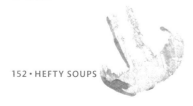

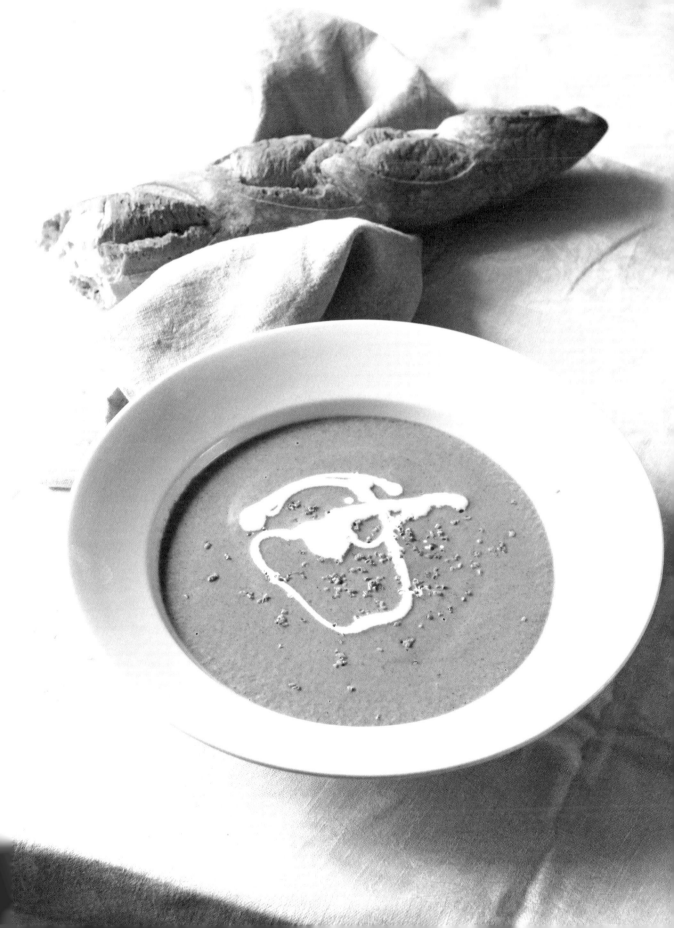

Mushroom stoup

Somewhere between a soup and a stew – hence the name – this is full of lovely earthy mushroom flavour, and can be made even more generous with the addition of some little herby dumplings. Another good way to make it a bit more substantial or suppery would be to throw in a handful of cooked pearl barley or pasta. And if you want to posh it up for a dinner party, a swirl of soured cream or thick yoghurt and a sprinkling of dill is an ideal finishing touch.

SERVES 4

50–60g dried porcini mushrooms

30g butter

1 tablespoon rapeseed or olive oil

2 medium onions, finely chopped

2 medium carrots, finely chopped

1 celery stalk, finely chopped

500g mushrooms, sliced

4 garlic cloves, finely chopped

1 litre mushroom or vegetable stock (see page 130)

A bunch of flat-leaf parsley, finely chopped

A good handful of dill, finely chopped

Sea salt and freshly ground black pepper

FOR THE DUMPLINGS (OPTIONAL)

100g self-raising flour, plus extra for dusting

½ teaspoon English mustard powder (optional)

50g vegetable suet

1–2 tablespoons finely chopped herbs (dill, thyme, parsley, chives or chervil, or a combination)

Soak the dried porcini in 500ml hot water for 30 minutes.

Melt the butter with the oil in a large saucepan over a medium-low heat. Add the onions and let them sweat, stirring occasionally, until they begin to turn golden – 15–20 minutes. Add the carrots and celery and cook, stirring occasionally, for about 5 minutes until softened.

Meanwhile, use a slotted spoon to remove the porcini from the soaking water, rinse them briefly and pat dry on kitchen paper. Strain the soaking liquid through a sieve lined with muslin or kitchen paper (to remove any fine, sandy grit) into a bowl.

Increase the heat under the pan to medium-high and add the fresh mushrooms, stirring until they release some of their moisture. Add the porcini and garlic and fry, stirring, for a minute. Stir in the strained soaking liquid and stock. Add some salt and pepper, then simmer, uncovered, for 15 minutes.

Meanwhile, make the dumplings. Sift the flour together with the mustard, if using, then mix in the suet and chopped herbs, using a whisk. Season well with salt and pepper. Use a knife to mix in just enough cold water – about 5–6 tablespoons should do – to form a soft, but not too sticky, dough. The secret of light dumplings is not to work the mixture too hard. Dust your hands with flour and gently form the dough into 12–14 dumplings.

Check if the soup needs more salt and pepper, then add the parsley and dill. Add the dumplings, and simmer, covered, for a further 12–15 minutes until they are fluffy and cooked through. If you are not using dumplings, continue to simmer the soup, uncovered, for a further 10 minutes. Ladle into warmed bowls and serve.

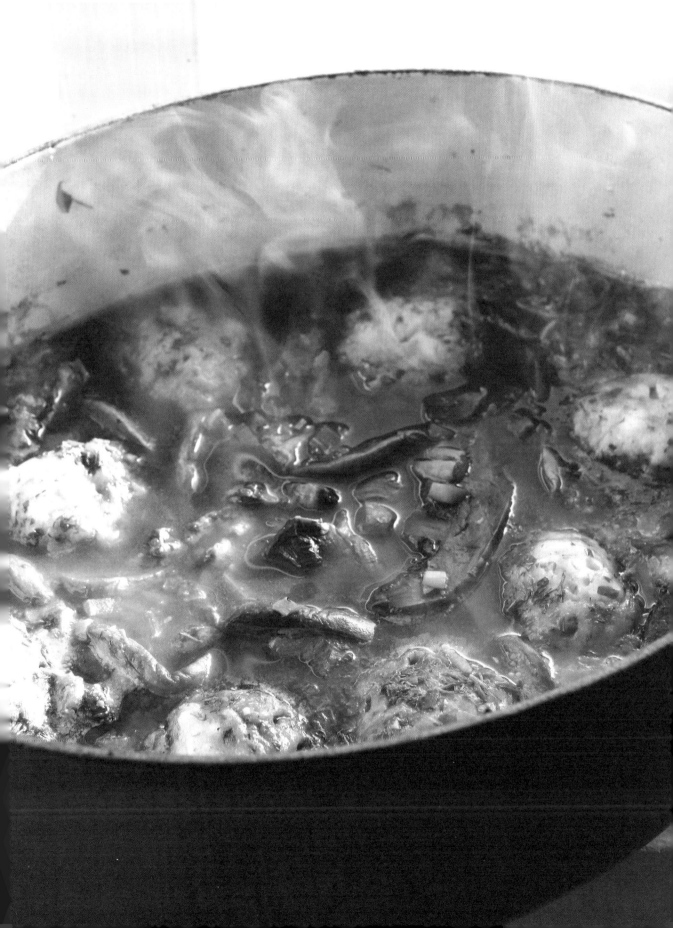

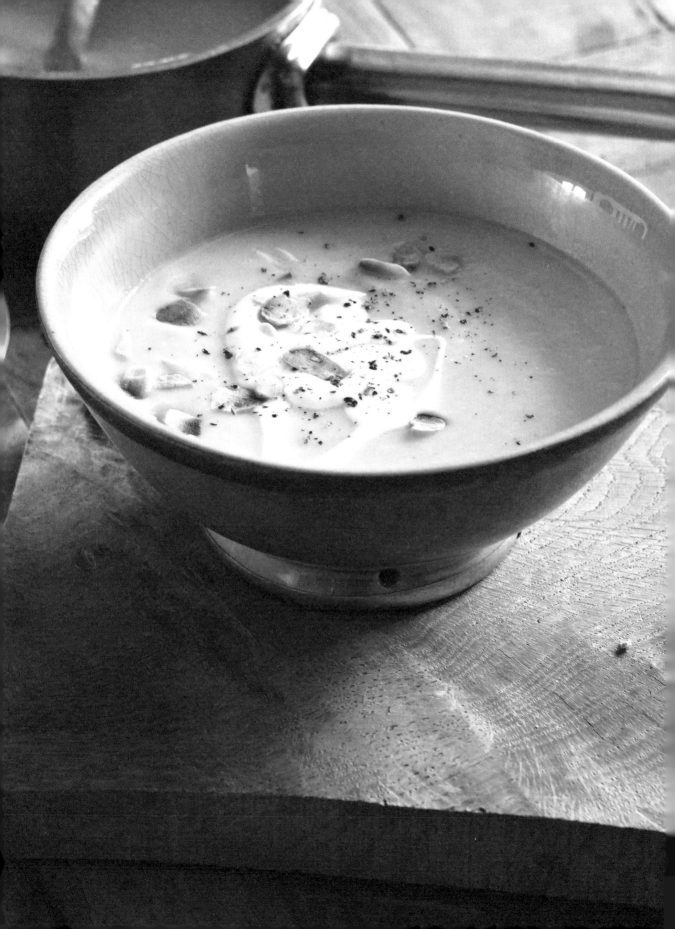

Parsnip and ginger soup

Sweet parsnips and fiery ginger are a winning and warming winter combination.

SERVES 4-6

1 tablespoon olive oil

15g butter

1 large onion, finely chopped

2 garlic cloves, finely chopped

4–5cm piece of ginger, peeled and finely chopped

¼ teaspoon ground cardamom

¼ teaspoon ground cumin

¼ teaspoon cayenne pepper

500g parsnips, peeled and cut into 1cm cubes

800ml vegetable stock (see page 130)

200ml whole milk

Sea salt and freshly ground black pepper

TO FINISH

2–3 tablespoons flaked almonds or pumpkin seeds

1–2 tablespoons double cream or thick, plain (full-fat) yoghurt

Heat the olive oil and butter in a saucepan over a medium-low heat and sauté the onion for about 10 minutes, until soft and translucent. Add the garlic, ginger, cardamom, cumin and cayenne and stir for a couple of minutes. Tip in the parsnips and stir until well coated in the spices. Pour in the stock, season with salt and pepper and simmer until the parsnips are very soft – about 15 minutes.

Allow the soup to cool slightly, then purée in a food processor or blender, or using a stick blender, until smooth. Return the soup to the pan, add the milk and adjust the seasoning. Warm through gently – if the soup is a bit thick, thin it with some hot water from the kettle.

While the soup is warming, toast the almonds or pumpkin seeds in a dry frying pan until just beginning to turn golden.

Serve the soup in warmed bowls with a trickle of cream or yoghurt and the toasted almonds scattered over the top. Finish with a grinding of black pepper.

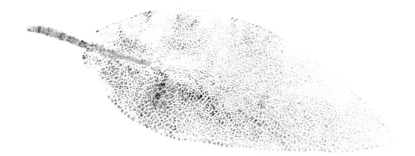

Chestnut and sage soup

This is a rich and elegant soup with a beguilingly velvety texture. A small portion makes a lovely starter, while a larger serving, with some bread and perhaps a crisp green salad, is a satisfying lunch or supper. You can use vac-packed pre-cooked chestnuts for this, or fresh, whole chestnuts, blanched, peeled and simmered until tender.

SERVES 4-6

3 tablespoons olive oil, plus extra to trickle

15g butter

1 medium onion, chopped

6 sage leaves, roughly chopped, plus extra to finish

1 small garlic clove, finely chopped

1 litre vegetable stock (see page 130)

400g cooked, peeled chestnuts

100ml crème fraîche

Sea salt and freshly ground black pepper

Heat 1 tablespoon of the olive oil and the butter in a saucepan over a medium-low heat and sweat the onion for about 10 minutes, until soft and translucent. Add the sage and garlic and sauté for a minute.

Pour in the stock and add most of the chestnuts – reserve a handful for finishing. Season with salt and pepper, increase the heat and simmer for 15 minutes, stirring from time to time.

Remove from the heat and cool slightly, then purée until very smooth in a blender or food processor, or using a stick blender. Return the soup to the pan, add the crème fraîche and adjust the seasoning if necessary. Warm through gently – do not let it boil.

Meanwhile, slice the reserved chestnuts. Heat the rest of the olive oil in a small frying pan over a medium heat and sauté the sage leaves for a few seconds until crisp, then drain on kitchen paper.

Ladle the soup into warmed bowls, scatter on the chestnuts and sage leaves and add a trickle of olive oil. Finish with a generous grinding of black pepper. Serve immediately.

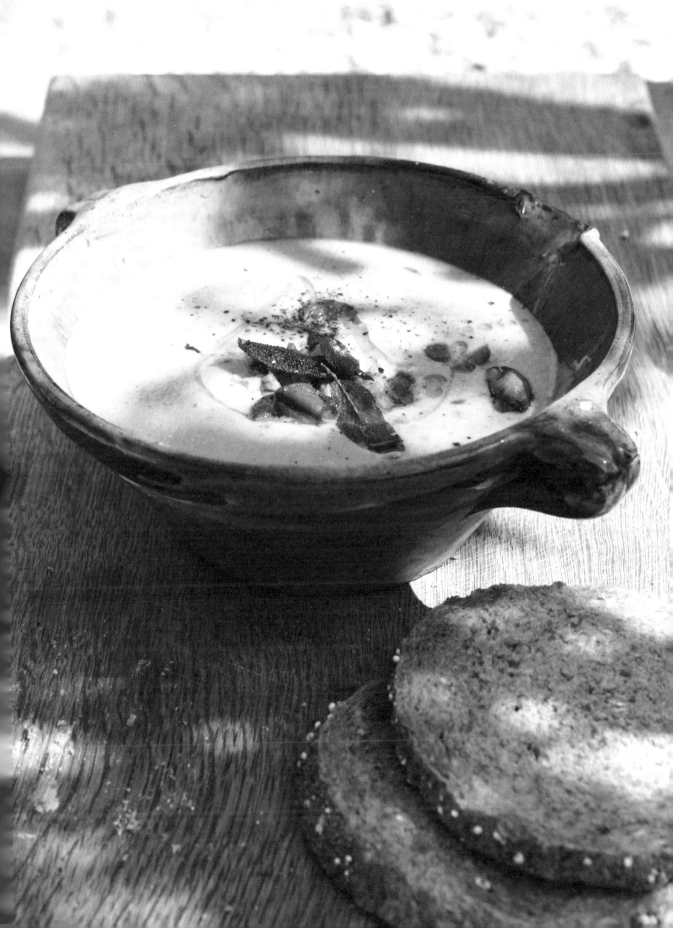

Pearl barley broth

This is a substantial soup – serve it with a salad and some bread and it's a meal in itself. As the barley simmers with the vegetables, it thickens the broth and gives it a creamy texture. You can certainly use pearled spelt in place of pearl barley.

SERVES 4-6

15g butter

2 large onions, finely chopped

1 bay leaf

A few sprigs of thyme, leaves only, chopped

1 small celery stalk, finely chopped

1 small carrot, finely chopped

1 small parsnip, finely chopped

¼ teaspoon ground coriander

A few gratings of nutmeg

A good pinch of cayenne pepper

A pinch of ground mace

100g pearl barley (or pearled spelt), rinsed

1.5 litres vegetable stock (see page 130)

A small handful of parsley, finely chopped

Sea salt and freshly ground black pepper

FOR THE CROÛTONS (OPTIONAL)

4 tablespoons olive oil

About 200g slightly stale white bread

Heat the butter in a large saucepan over a medium-low heat and gently sweat the onions with the bay leaf and thyme for about 15 minutes, until soft and translucent. Add the celery, carrot and parsnip and sauté for a further 5 minutes. Stir in the coriander, nutmeg, cayenne and mace.

Add the barley or spelt, pour in the stock and add some salt and pepper. Simmer gently for 25–30 minutes, or until the grain is very soft. Remove the bay leaf.

You can serve the broth like this or, to make it a little thicker, scoop out a couple of ladlefuls and purée them in a blender or food processor, or with a stick blender, until smooth, then return the puréed soup to the pan and warm through. Stir in the parsley and adjust the seasoning if necessary. Keep over a very low heat if you are making croûtons.

For the croûtons, cut the bread into 2cm cubes. Heat the olive oil over a medium heat in a large frying pan. Add the bread and sizzle gently until golden, turning occasionally, then drain on kitchen paper.

Ladle the soup into warmed bowls and scatter the hot croûtons on top to serve.

ALTERNATIVE FINISHES

• Instead of serving the soup topped with croûtons, sauté some sliced mushrooms in a little butter or olive oil until they give up some of their moisture and start to take on some colour. Scatter the fried mushrooms over the soup just before serving.

• The soup is also very good simply served with a trickle of cream and chopped parsley scattered over the top.

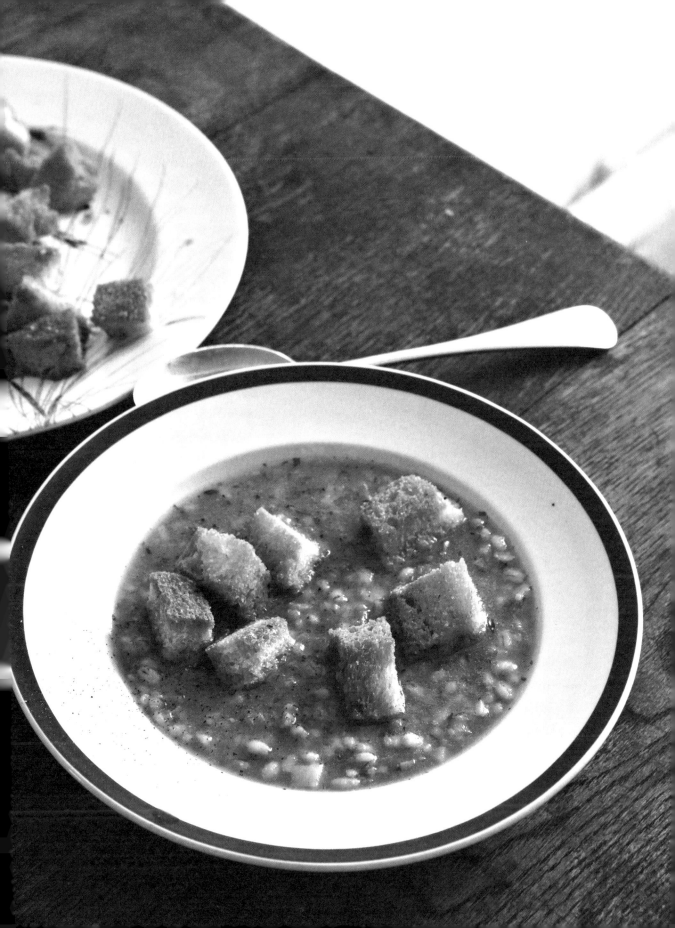

Puy lentil and spinach soup ﮭ

Earthy, nutty Puy lentils and a generous quantity of garlic give this simple soup a hearty and satisfying depth of flavour.

SERVES 4

2 tablespoons olive or rapeseed oil

3 shallots, or 1 onion, finely chopped

1 carrot, finely chopped

A few sprigs of thyme, leaves only, roughly chopped

3 garlic cloves, finely chopped

3 tomatoes, cored, deseeded and diced

150g Puy lentils, rinsed

1.3 litres vegetable stock (see page 130)

A small bunch of parsley, finely chopped

100g baby spinach

Sea salt and freshly ground black pepper

TO SERVE

1–2 tablespoons extra virgin olive or rapeseed oil

Parmesan, hard goat's cheese or other well-flavoured hard cheese (optional)

Heat the oil over a medium-low heat in a large saucepan. Add the shallots or onion, carrot and thyme and sauté gently for 5 minutes. Add the garlic and tomatoes and sauté for a further minute.

Tip in the lentils, stir, then add the stock and a little salt and pepper. Bring the soup to the boil, reduce the heat and simmer for about 25 minutes, or until the lentils are tender. Add the parsley and spinach and simmer for a further 5 minutes.

Check the seasoning, then spoon into warmed bowls, trickle over a little oil and shave over some cheese, if you like.

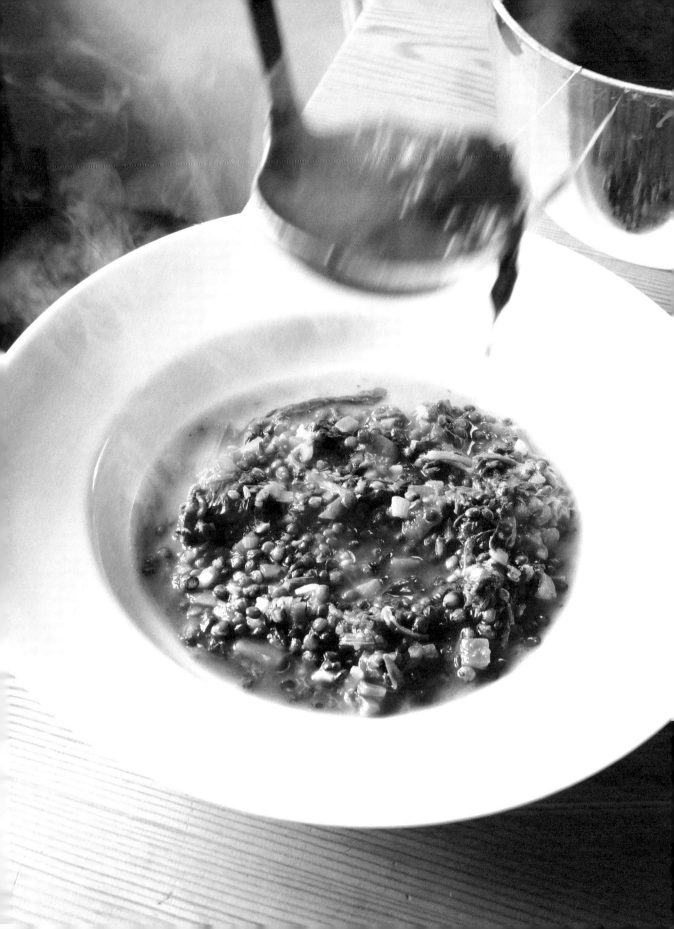

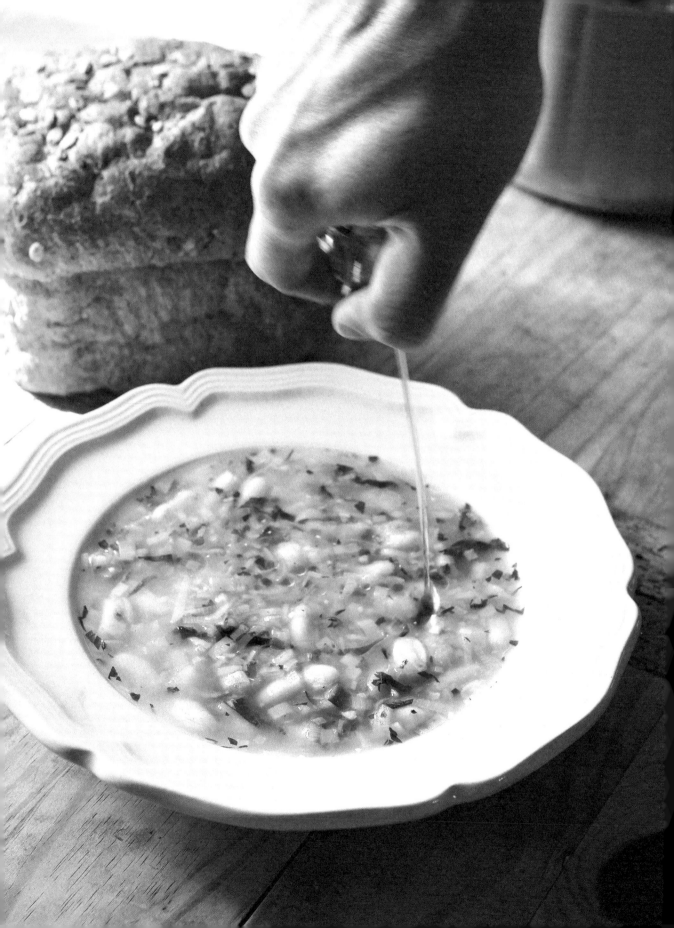

Cannellini bean and leek soup with chilli oil

The chilli oil gives this soup a deliciously piquant finish. Once made, the oil will keep, sealed in an airtight container in the fridge, for a couple of weeks, and you can use it to add a bit of heat to marinades and salad dressings or to trickle over pizzas. However, if you don't have time to make it, you can simply trickle a little extra virgin olive oil over the soup and finish with some shavings of Parmesan, pecorino or hard goat's cheese.

SERVES 4-6

4 medium leeks, trimmed (white and pale green part only)

1 tablespoon olive oil

15g butter

A few sprigs of thyme, leaves only, roughly chopped

1 bay leaf

3 garlic cloves, finely chopped

1.3 litres vegetable stock (see page 130)

2 x 400g tins cannellini beans, drained and rinsed

A handful of oregano, roughly chopped

A bunch of parsley, roughly chopped

Sea salt and freshly ground black pepper

FOR THE CHILLI OIL

4 red chillies, deseeded and sliced

200ml olive oil

A few sprigs of thyme, leaves only

1 garlic clove (unpeeled), bashed

First, make the chilli oil. Put the chillies in a small saucepan with the olive oil, thyme leaves and unpeeled garlic clove. Heat slowly until the oil is simmering very, very gently and cook the chillies until soft, about 20 minutes. Remove from the heat and cool.

For the soup, halve the leeks lengthways, wash well and slice thinly. Heat the olive oil and butter in a saucepan over a medium-low heat. Add the leeks, with the thyme and bay leaf, and sweat gently, stirring from time to time, for about 15 minutes, until very soft. Add the garlic and stir for a minute.

Add the stock and cannellini beans, the oregano and half the parsley. Season with salt and plenty of pepper, increase the heat and bring to a simmer. Cook gently for 20 minutes.

Remove the bay leaf, taste and adjust the seasoning if necessary and stir in the rest of the parsley. Serve in warmed bowls with a trickle of chilli oil over the top.

Curried sweet potato soup ♥

This is a warming soup for a cold evening, the heat of the spices softened by the sweetness of the coconut milk and lime.

SERVES 4-6

2 tablespoons olive or rapeseed oil

2 onions, chopped

4 garlic cloves, finely chopped

4–5cm piece of ginger, peeled and grated

1–2 red chillies, to taste, deseeded and finely chopped

1 tablespoon garam masala

2 teaspoons curry powder

3 sweet potatoes (about 700g), peeled and cut into 2cm dice

1 litre vegetable stock (see page 130)

400ml tin coconut milk

A small handful of coriander, roughly chopped

Juice of 1–2 limes (a good tablespoonful)

Sea salt and freshly ground black pepper

TO FINISH

A few tablespoons plain (full-fat) yoghurt (optional)

A small handful of coriander, roughly torn

Heat the oil in a saucepan over a medium-low heat. Add the onions and sauté for about 10 minutes, until soft and translucent. Add the garlic, ginger, chillies, garam masala and curry powder, and stir for a minute.

Tip in the sweet potatoes and stir until they're well coated in the spices. Add some salt and pepper and pour in the stock. Increase the heat and bring to a simmer. Cook gently until the sweet potatoes are very tender – about 15 minutes.

Remove the soup from the heat, cool slightly and then purée in a blender or food processor, or with a stick blender, until very smooth. Return to the pan, stir in the coconut milk and warm through gently.

Take off the heat and add the coriander and lime juice. Taste and adjust the seasoning if necessary. Serve the soup topped with a good dollop of yoghurt, if you like, and scatter over some torn coriander. Finish with a little black pepper.

VARIATION

Curried red lentil soup ♥

Sweat the onions as above, but add some chopped carrot and celery, and a couple of bay leaves. Add the aromatics and spices, along with 180g red lentils (in place of sweet potatoes). Simmer in about 1.3 litres vegetable stock for 25–30 minutes until the lentils are very soft, then purée until very smooth. Return to the pan, add the juice of ½ lemon, season with salt and pepper and warm through gently. If the soup is a little thick, thin with some hot water from the kettle. Serve, as above, topped with yoghurt, if you like, and coriander. A sprinkle of cumin seeds, lightly toasted in a dry frying pan, is a lovely finishing touch.

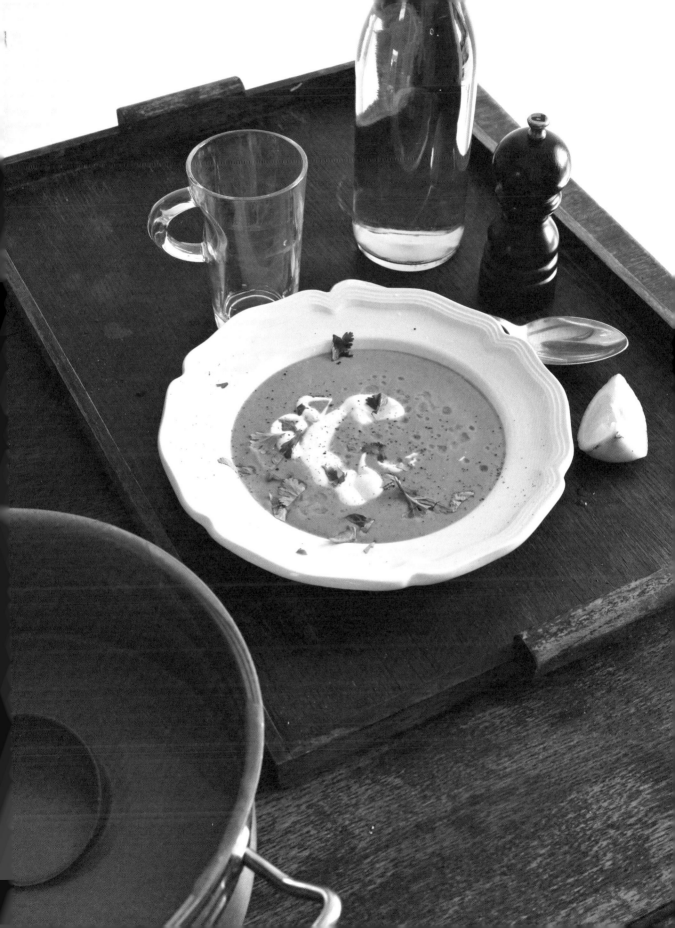

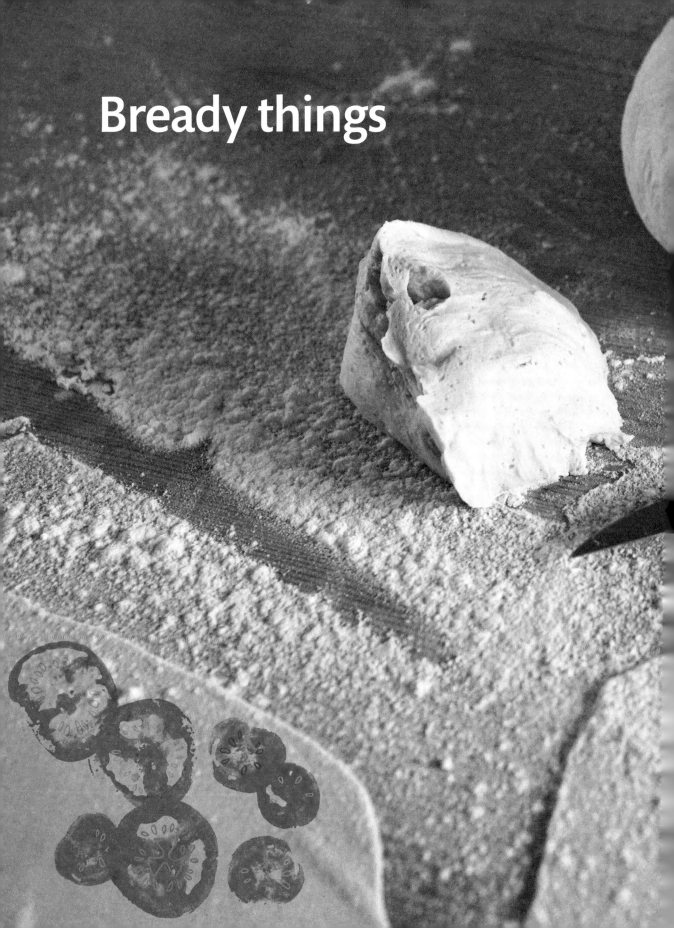

Bready things

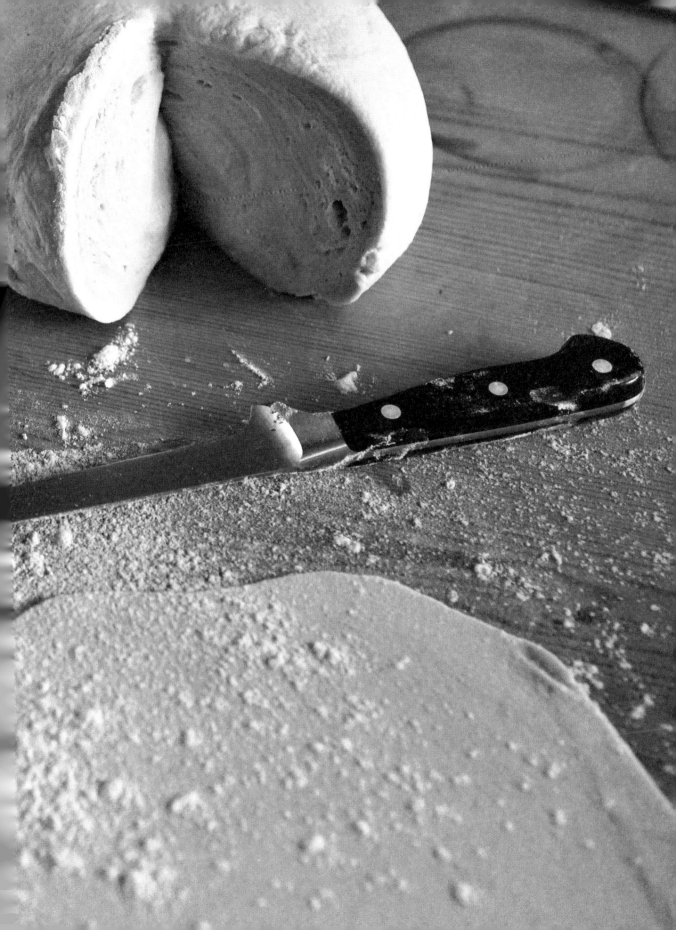

For the versatile cook, bread is not just there to mop up the juice on the plate, although of course it will always be welcome to perform that role; it's a useful and adaptable ingredient in its own right. And when you concentrate more on vegetables in your cooking, and less on meat, the importance of bread is greater still, as is its potential.

Bread has always been a good friend to the vegetable eater. Take a look at cultures that rely primarily on vegetarian food, and you'll often find that they have developed an exciting range of breads to complement it. I'm thinking particularly of the Indian subcontinent, where so many regions are largely meat-free, and where you will find puris, parathas, rotis, naans and chapattis. From here on you too should feel entitled to ask a bit more of your bread – and as long as it's good bread, it won't let you down.

For many of us, bread-based meals were the first we learnt how to make, and are the ones we return to time and again when we need good, comforting food, fast – we know a slice of hot buttered toast or a cheese and pickle sandwich will always fill the gap. We may have a few marginally more complex bready recipes up our sleeves, too – cheese on toast, mushrooms on toast, garlic bread, maybe bruschetta – but these hardly scratch the surface. It's time to find out how bread, so often the sidekick, will happily carry the show if given the chance.

This is an ingredient that generally requires little preparation – beyond removing the loaf from the bread bin, and sawing off a slice. The problem is, when it comes to using bread, we're too bound by convention and habit. As the toast with your pâté, the roll with your soup, even the bit of baguette you nibble at in a restaurant while waiting for the real meal to arrive, bread is part of our culinary vernacular. We take it for granted. We are all guilty of having low expectations of bread: we make do with the mediocre stuff, and we get by without asking too much of it. But, actually, if you change your tactics and challenge your loaf a little more often, it will reward you by bringing many delicious new things to your table.

Think of bread less as a journeyman accompaniment, more as a blank canvas waiting to be turned into something fine, and you will soon discover some simple, delicious new dishes. I would say that half a good loaf on the breadboard puts you as close to a satisfying meat-free meal as a packet of pasta simmering in a pan.

Start with what you know and work upwards and outwards from there. If you like cheese on toast, try adding a few leftover vegetables, or some gently sautéed fresh ones, and before long you'll be rolling out all kinds of toothsome toasties and rarefied rarebits. If you love pizza, put aside your default toppings – the ham or salami, even the tomato sauce – and explore the delightfully creative alternatives the veg garden can provide – new potatoes and blue cheese, anyone? If a filled wrap is a familiar lunch, think how much better you can do with fresh ingredients at home, experimenting with veggie foldovers, maybe even using home-made flatbreads (see page 176). And I'm certainly not sniffy about sarnies: try a couple of my favourites (on page 195); or turn to page 402 for a list of the recipes from the book that can be turned into fantastic fillings.

None of these adventures will be fulfilling, of course, if the quality of the bread itself is not top-notch. It doesn't matter how good your rarebit topping is – if you put it on some pappy white-sliced-from-a-packet, you won't get pleasing results. So take the time to look for bread with character and substance. Sourdough is a real favourite of mine, not just for its flavour but for its robust, open texture: it responds so well to being toasted, then generously topped. But there are other good-quality breads to be had: a proper cottage loaf or cobber from a traditional British bakery, as well as the baguettes, ciabatta, focaccia and fougasses that have come our way from the bread-loving continent. Don't forget flatbreads, naans and pittas either – different sizes, shapes and densities point to different culinary possibilities.

Of course, exploring meat-free meals could even be the spur you need to turn to baking your own bread, if you haven't already. I can't recommend it highly enough. In *River Cottage Every Day*, I explained how my own baking odyssey unfolded as I went from a bread novice, rather wary of the whole mixing, kneading, rising and baking palaver, to someone who now eats homemade bread – usually homemade sourdough – almost every day of the week. I'll concede that sourdough does require a certain amount of commitment, but it's by no means the only sort of bread worth making at home. In fact, if you want one recipe that's very simple, very versatile and almost immediately rewarding (taking you from dry ingredients to hot, oil-trickled flatbreads in little more than an hour), my magic bread dough will do the trick. Which is why it's the first recipe in this chapter.

Magic bread dough ♥

I call this 'magic' because it can grant you so many wishes. It is one of those recipes that can be turned to any manner of different endings – all of them delicious. The tender bread dough, made with half strong flour and half ordinary plain flour, is perfect for the pizza recipes on the following pages. In addition, it makes the most irresistible flatbreads, pitta breads, breadsticks and even, if you have any left, soft bread rolls or a simple white loaf. You can also freeze it, either raw or baked, which is why I suggest never making it in less than the following quantity. It's very easy, and very worthwhile, to simply double these measurements.

**MAKES 3 PIZZAS,
8 FLATBREADS, 12 PITTAS
OR UMPTEEN BREADSTICKS**

250g plain white flour

250g strong white flour

1 ½ level teaspoons fine sea salt

1 teaspoon easy-blend
(instant) dried yeast

1 tablespoon rapeseed or olive
oil, plus a little extra for oiling

Put the two flours into a large bowl with the salt and yeast. Mix well. Add the oil and 325ml warm water and mix to a rough dough. Flour your hands a little. Tip out the dough on to a work surface and knead rhythmically for 5–10 minutes, until smooth. This is quite a loose and sticky dough, which is just as it should be – you get better-textured bread this way – so try not to add too much flour if you can help it. It will become less sticky as you knead.

Trickle a little oil into a clean bowl, add the kneaded dough and turn it in the oil so it is covered with a light film. Cover with a tea towel and leave in a warm place to rise until doubled in size – at least an hour, probably closer to two. You can also prove it in a floured, cloth-lined dough basket, like the one in the picture.

When the dough is well risen and puffy, tip it out and 'knock it back' by poking it with your outstretched fingers until it collapses to its former size. It's now ready to be shaped to your will.

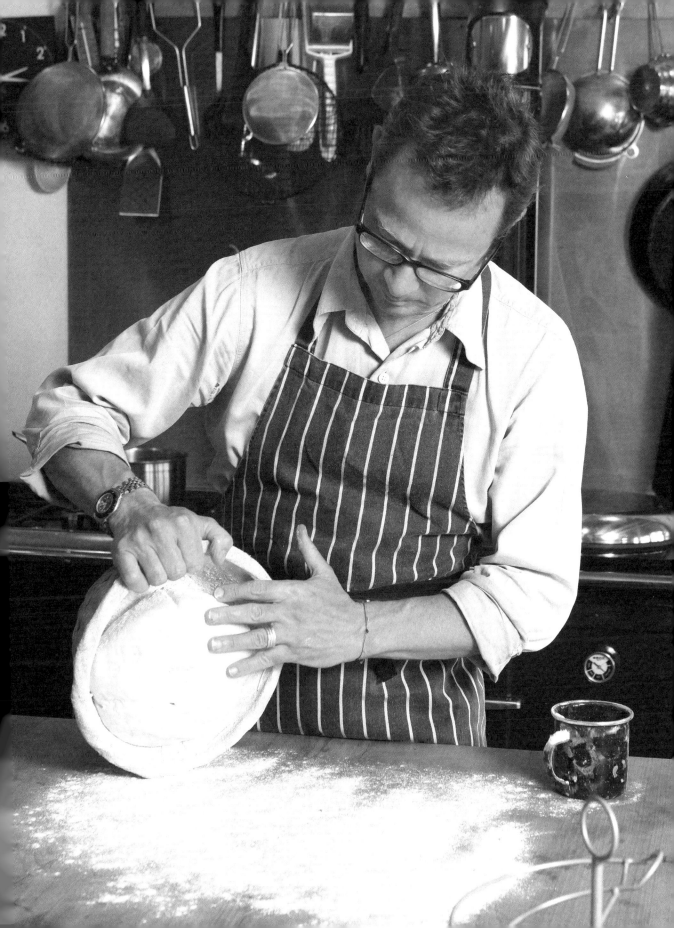

USING THE BREAD DOUGH

Pizzas

This quantity of dough makes 3 pizza bases, each large enough to serve 2–3 people. Follow the instructions in the individual pizza recipes (on pages 180–6).

Flatbreads ♥

This quantity of dough makes about 8 flatbreads. Follow the recipe on page 176, omitting the garlicky oil for plain flatbreads, or if you are using them for wraps or foldovers.

Pitta breads ♥

Take egg-sized balls of knocked-back dough and roll them out on a floured surface into oval shapes, no more than 5mm thick. Transfer to a greased tray and leave for 10–15 minutes, then bake at 220°C/Gas Mark 7 for about 8 minutes, until puffed up and just starting to brown. Take them from the oven and immediately wrap in a clean tea towel. Leave to cool completely before unwrapping (the trapped steam keeps the pittas soft).

Breadsticks ♥

After knocking back, take walnut-sized pieces of dough and roll them out into long, thin rods. Place on a lightly greased baking tray. Leave to rise for 10–15 minutes, then bake at 200°C/Gas Mark 6 for about 10 minutes. Cool on a rack.

Rolls ♥

Take roughly lemon-sized chunks of knocked-back dough (around 125g each) and shape into neat rounds. Place these on a baking sheet and leave until doubled in size – an hour or so. Bake at 220°C/Gas Mark 7 for 15 minutes, until risen and golden.

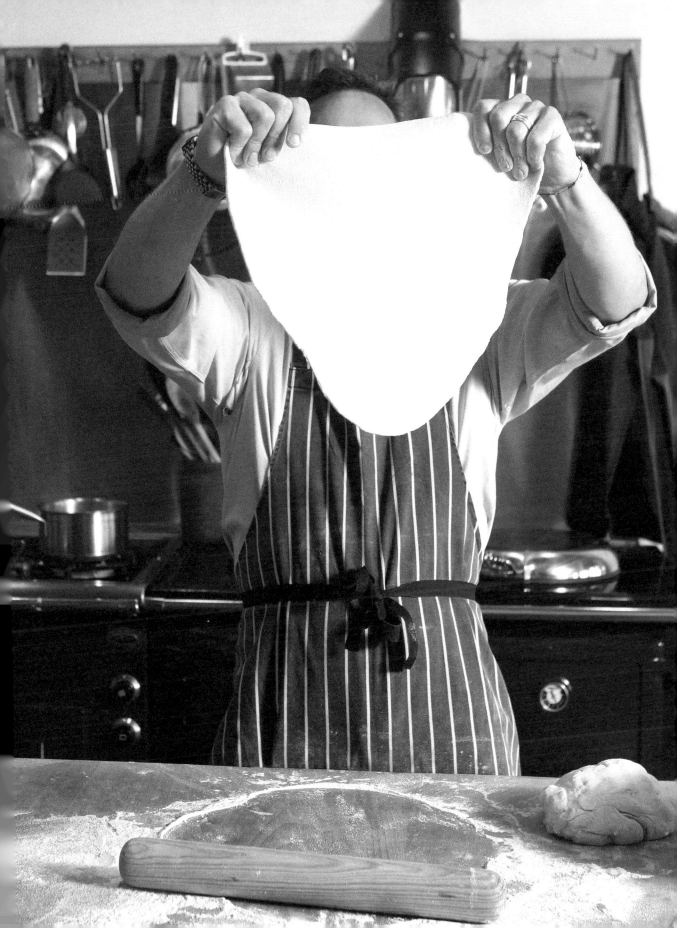

River Cottage garlicky flatbreads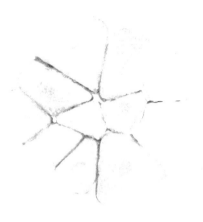

This is perhaps the easiest way to use my magic bread dough. Once you've got the dough risen and knocked back you're just minutes away from these smoky, hot, oily, salty, garlicky wedges. Serve them with any kind of dip or hummus, alongside soup, or with saucy dishes like chachouka (see page 20) or caponata (see page 307), or just on their own before your main course. I bet you won't be able to resist snaffling one or two bits before you've even got them to the table, though...

This is also the recipe to follow for making plain flatbreads - perfect for the foldovers and wraps on pages 188-93, and surprisingly good used as the base of a rarebit or toastie. Just leave out the garlicky oil bit.

MAKES 8 FLATBREADS

1 quantity magic bread dough, risen (see page 172)

A little flaky sea salt

FOR THE GARLIC OIL

About 120ml olive oil

1 fat garlic clove, very finely chopped

First make the garlic oil: combine the olive oil and garlic in a frying pan and place over a medium heat. You're not going to fry it, just warm it through to take the raw edge off the garlic. So as soon as you see the first signs of a sizzle, pour the oil and garlic out of the pan into a small bowl, and leave to cool and infuse for a few minutes.

After punching down the risen dough, take lemon-sized balls (around 125g each) and roll them out into rough circles, 2–3mm thick. Leave to rest for 5 minutes. Meanwhile, heat a heavy-based, non-stick frying pan over a very high heat until smoking hot (I always find it's worth opening the windows or switching on the extractor fan at this point).

Lay one flatbread in the pan and cook for about 2 minutes, until bubbly on top and patched with brown spots (even a touch black) on the base. Flip over and cook for 1–2 minutes more until patchily browned on the other side too. Remove immediately to a warmed plate and trickle with some of the garlicky oil. Scatter with a little sea salt too, if you like. Repeat with all the dough. Cut the oiled flatbreads into wedges to serve.

It's worth using the whole quantity of dough, even if that makes more flatbreads than you need straight away. Extras can be wrapped in a clean tea towel and left until cold. The trapped steam will keep the flatbreads soft and they will make great wraps or bases for various toasted toppings. Either way, eat them within 24 hours, or freeze.

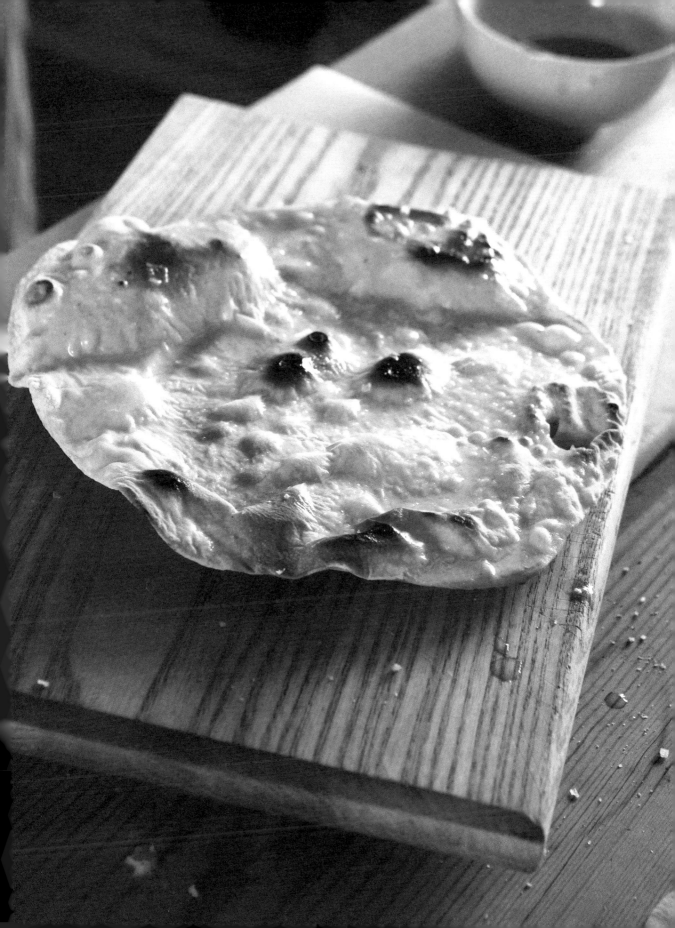

Crostini ♥

Crostini are a fantastic way to use up good bread that's heading towards staleness. I make them most often with sourdough or a good quality baguette, but any decent, fairly open-textured bread will work. Thinly cut and lightly baked, the bread becomes crunchy, crisp and delicious and the perfect vehicle for all manner of toppings. I prefer to stick to fairly finely chopped or puréed toppings – pâtés and dips, pestos or tapenades, or chunky pastes such as the broad bean purée (see below). You could also serve crostini plain, simply for pre-prandial munching, or alongside soup, or break them into rough shards and use as a kind of croûton in salads.

Slightly stale, good quality, robust bread

Olive or rapeseed oil

Sea salt

Preheat the oven to 200°C/Gas Mark 6. Slice the bread very thinly – to a 5mm maximum thickness. Depending on what kind of loaf you are slicing from, you may want to cut larger slices into halves or quarters. If you want small crostini – perhaps to present with various toppings as party food – then cut the slices to the size you want before you bake then. Once baked, they'll be too crisp to cut and will shatter if you try.

Arrange on a baking tray (or two), as close together as possible. Brush or trickle each slice with oil and sprinkle with a little salt. Bake for 5–8 minutes. The slices should be golden and crisp, with a little bit of give still in the centre – they will crisp up further as they cool. Leave to cool, then add your chosen topping. I like to place my toppings over one half of the crostini, leaving the other half uncovered for a final, topping-free, palate-cleansing crunch.

These crostini will keep in an airtight container for a couple of days.

TOPPINGS

Refried beans (page 190) • Garlicky, minty mushy peas (page 387)
Crushed garlicky courgettes (page 200) • Garlicky broad bean purée (page 196)
Lemony guacamole (page 296) • Cannellini bean hummus (page 300)
Baba ganoush (page 303) • Artichoke and white bean dip (page 303)
Cambodian wedding day dip (page 299) • Beetroot and walnut hummus (page 300)
Carrot hummus (page 296) • Herbed goat's cheese (page 316) • Caponata (page 307)
Romesco (page 336) • Pesto (page 256) • Mint pesto (page 266)

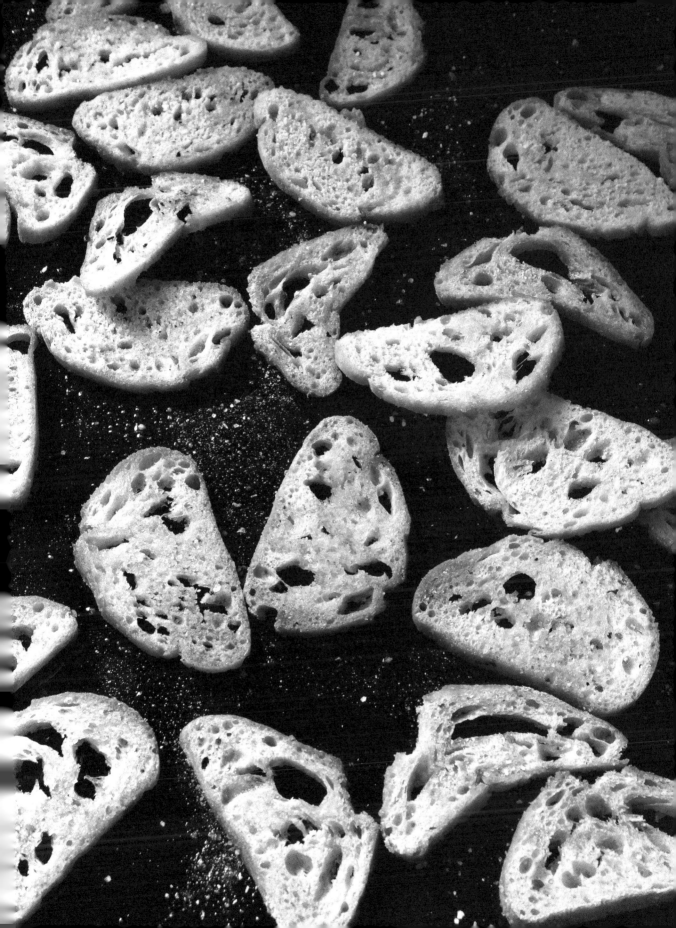

Beetroot pizza with cheddar

I like this smoky-sweet pizza with a slick of tomato sauce on the base. You can use any of the sauces on pages 58, 362 or 366, a good bought tomato sauce or even a tablespoon or two of good quality concentrated tomato purée. Then again, it really wouldn't be the end of the world if you left off the tomato altogether. The beetroot needs to be cooked before you start: use leftovers from either of the roast beetroot recipes on page 92 or 144, or roast it to order. Just scrub a root or two, enfold in a loose foil parcel with some garlic, thyme and a slosh of oil and roast at 200°C/Gas Mark 6 for about an hour.

MAKES 3 PIZZAS, EACH SERVING 2-3

1 quantity magic bread dough (see page 172)

FOR THE TOPPING

3 tablespoons olive oil, plus a little extra to trickle

2 onions, finely sliced

5–6 tablespoons tomato sauce or tomato purée (see above)

About 150g cooked, skinned beetroot (not pickled), thickly sliced

75g medium Cheddar, grated

1 ball of buffalo mozzarella (about 125g)

Sea salt and freshly ground black pepper

Prepare the dough and leave to rise according to the instructions on page 172.

Meanwhile, heat the olive oil in a frying pan over a medium heat and add the onions. Once sizzling, reduce the heat to low and cook gently, stirring from time to time, until they are soft and golden – about 15 minutes. Season with salt and pepper.

Preheat the oven to 250°C/Gas Mark 9, if it goes that high, or at least 220°C/Gas Mark 7. Put a baking sheet in to heat up.

Tip the dough out on to a lightly floured surface and deflate with your fingers. Leave it to rest for a few minutes, then cut it into three. Roll out one piece as thinly as you can.

Scatter a peel (if you have one) or another baking sheet with a little flour and place the dough base on it. Spread one-third of the tomato sauce or purée very thinly over the dough, then spread over a third of the onions. Distribute a third of the beetroot pieces over the onions, then a third of the grated cheese. Scatter over a third of the mozzarella, tearing it into small pieces, then season with salt and pepper.

Slide the pizza on to the hot baking sheet in the oven (for a really crispy crust), or you can simply lay the baking sheet on the hot one in the oven (to avoid the tricky pizza transfer). Trickle with a little olive oil and bake for 10–12 minutes, until the base is crisp and the top bubbling and golden. Repeat with the remaining dough and topping. Serve hot, cut into wedges.

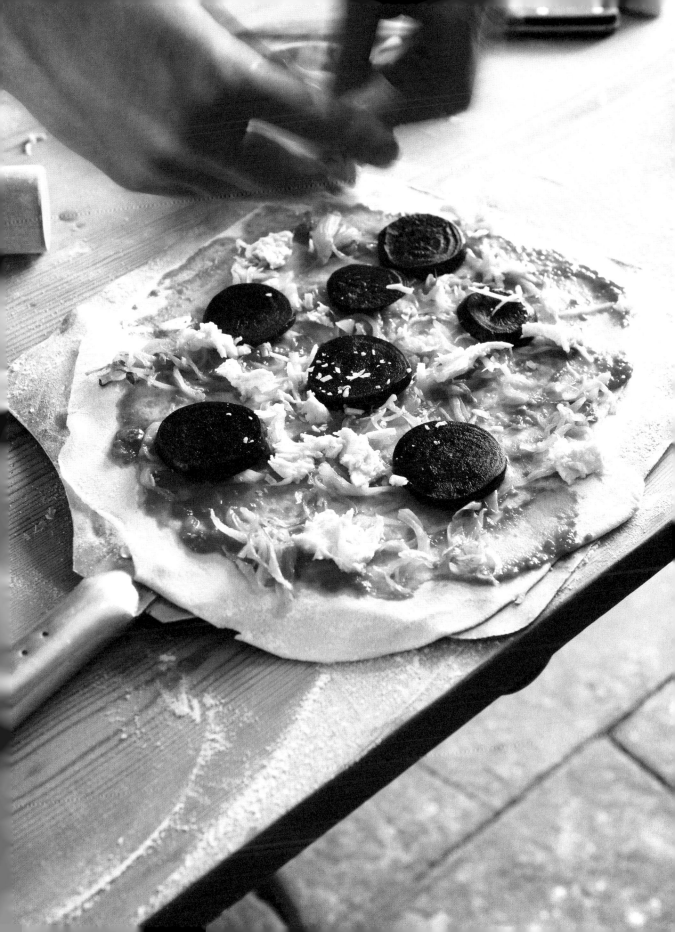

Pizza with new potatoes, rosemary and blue cheese

This pizza really packs a punch and is a lovely way to use up leftover new potatoes. It definitely wants some salad standing by and I love it served with a big, tangled pile of rocket. As ever, for those who are not wild about blue cheese, a crumbly goat's cheese or a combination of ricotta and Parmesan makes a good alternative.

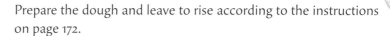

**MAKES 3 PIZZAS,
EACH SERVING 2-3**

1 quantity magic bread dough
(see page 172)

FOR THE TOPPING

3 tablespoons rapeseed or olive oil, plus a little extra to trickle

2 onions, quartered and finely sliced

2 garlic cloves, finely chopped

2 tablespoons finely chopped rosemary

About 200g cold, cooked new potatoes, cut into 2–3mm thick slices

150g blue cheese, such as Dorset Blue Vinny or Harbourne Blue, crumbled or roughly sliced

Sea salt and freshly ground black pepper

Prepare the dough and leave to rise according to the instructions on page 172.

Preheat the oven to 250°C/Gas Mark 9, if it goes that high, or at least 220°C/Gas Mark 7. Put a baking sheet in to heat up.

Meanwhile, heat the oil in a frying pan over a medium heat and add the onions. Once sizzling, lower the heat and cook gently, stirring from time to time, until they are soft and golden, about 15 minutes. Turn off the heat and stir in the garlic, rosemary and salt and pepper.

Tip the dough out on to a lightly floured surface and deflate with your fingers. Leave it to rest for a few minutes, then cut it into three. Roll out one piece as thinly as you can.

Scatter a peel (if you have one) or another baking sheet with a little flour and place the dough base on it. Spread a third of the onion mixture evenly over the dough, then a third of the potato slices, then a third of the cheese. Sprinkle with salt and pepper.

Slide the pizza on to the hot baking sheet in the oven (for a really crispy crust), or you can simply lay the baking sheet on the hot one in the oven (to avoid the tricky pizza transfer). Trickle with a little more oil and bake for 10–12 minutes until the base is crisp and the top bubbling. Repeat with the remaining dough and topping. Serve at once, in generous slices, with lots of rocket or another green salad.

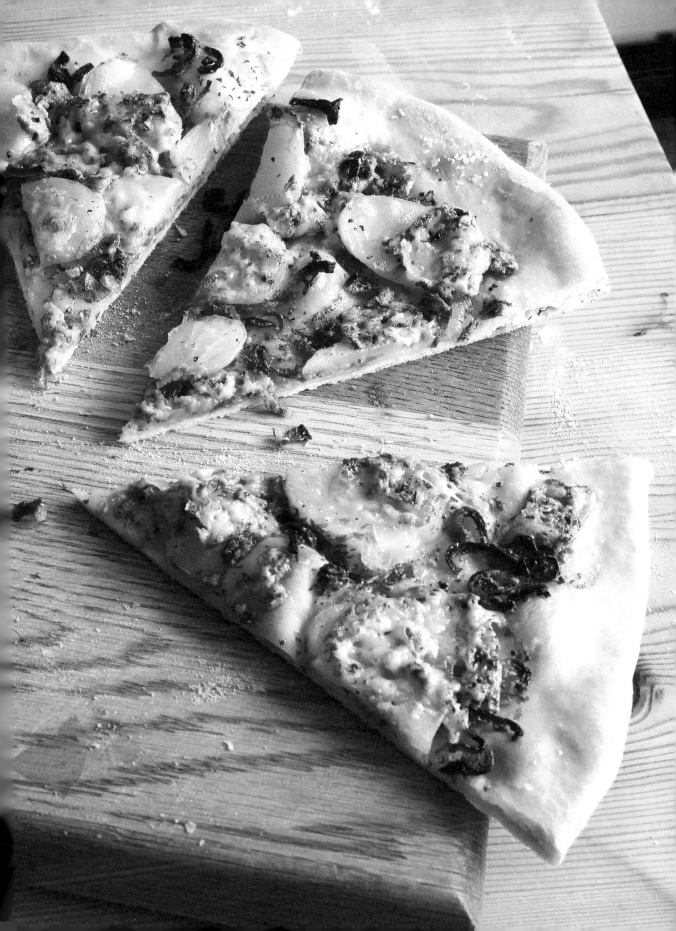

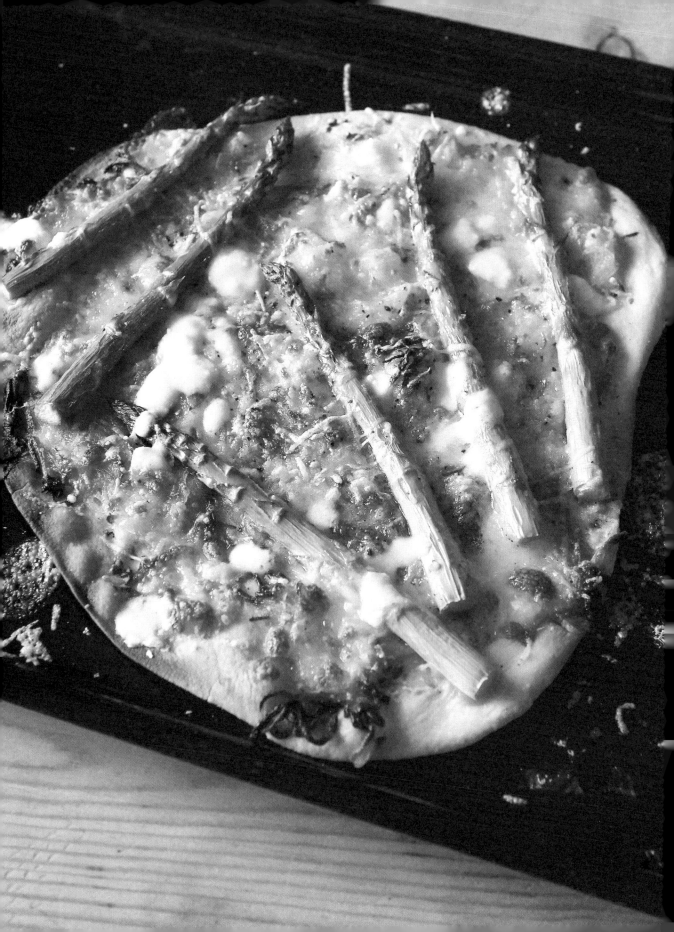

Asparagus pizza

Roasting asparagus on top of a pizza in a super-hot oven makes it deliciously tender and a bit caramelised. Use slender stems that will cook through quickly – or, if you only have thick stems, halve them lengthways.

**MAKES 3 PIZZAS,
EACH SERVING 2–3**

1 quantity magic bread dough (see page 172)

FOR THE TOPPING

3 tablespoons olive oil, plus a little extra to trickle

2 onions, finely sliced

About 350g slender asparagus spears, trimmed

2 balls of buffalo mozzarella (each 125g)

A little grated Parmesan, hard goat's cheese or other well-flavoured hard cheese

Sea salt and freshly ground black pepper

Prepare the dough and leave to rise according to the instructions on page 172.

Preheat the oven to 250°C/Gas Mark 9, if it goes that high, or at least 220°C/Gas Mark 7. Put a baking sheet in to heat up.

Meanwhile, heat the olive oil in a frying pan over a medium heat and add the onions. Once sizzling, reduce the heat to low and cook gently, stirring from time to time, until they are soft and golden – about 15 minutes. Season with salt and pepper.

Tip the dough out on to a lightly floured surface and deflate with your fingers. Leave it to rest for a few minutes, then cut it into three. Roll out one piece as thinly as you can.

Scatter a peel (if you have one) or another baking sheet with a little flour and place the dough base on it. Spread a third of the onions over the dough, then arrange a third of the asparagus over the top. Tear up the mozzarella and distribute a third of it over the asparagus. Scatter over a little grated cheese and some salt and pepper.

Slide the pizza on to the hot baking sheet in the oven (for a really crispy crust), or you can simply lay the baking sheet on the hot one in the oven (to avoid the tricky pizza transfer). Add a generous trickle of oil and bake for 10–12 minutes, until the base is crisp, the edges browned and the asparagus tender. Repeat with the remaining dough and topping. Serve hot, cut into slices or wedges.

Kale and onion pizza

There's no tomato here because I like to emphasise the more unusual flavour of the kale. In the heat of the oven, the kale becomes crisp and dark, and takes on a flavour not dissimilar to that delicious deep-fried 'seaweed' you get in Chinese restaurants. I sometimes add a few sautéed sliced mushrooms to the pizza before it goes into the oven.

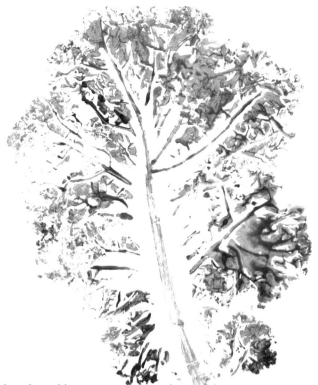

**MAKES 3 PIZZAS,
EACH SERVING 2–3**

1 quantity magic bread dough
(see page 172)

FOR THE TOPPING

3 tablespoons rapeseed or olive oil, plus a little extra to trickle

2 onions, halved and thinly sliced

2 garlic cloves, finely slivered

300g bunch of curly kale or cavolo nero, stalks removed

About 100g mature Cheddar, grated

Sea salt and freshly ground black pepper

Prepare the dough and leave to rise according to the instructions on page 172.

Preheat the oven to 250°C/Gas Mark 9, if it goes that high, or at least 220°C/Gas Mark 7. Put a baking sheet in to heat up.

Meanwhile, heat the oil in a frying pan over a medium heat and add the onions. Once sizzling, reduce the heat to low and cook gently, stirring from time to time, until they are soft and golden, about 10–15 minutes, adding the garlic halfway through.

Shred the kale or cavolo nero leaves into ½–1cm wide ribbons. Stir them into the onions and cook for a further 5 minutes, stirring often, until the leaves have wilted. Season with salt and pepper.

Tip the dough out on to a lightly floured surface and deflate with your fingers. Leave it to rest for a few minutes, then cut it into three. Roll out one piece as thinly as you can.

Scatter a peel (if you have one) or another baking sheet with a little flour and place the dough base on it. Spread a third of the kale and onions on the pizza base, then top with a third of the grated Cheddar.

Slide the pizza on to the hot baking sheet in the oven (for a really crispy crust), or you can simply lay the baking sheet on the hot one in the oven (to avoid the tricky pizza transfer). Trickle with a little more oil and bake for 10–12 minutes. Repeat with the remaining topping and cheese and serve, cut into wedges.

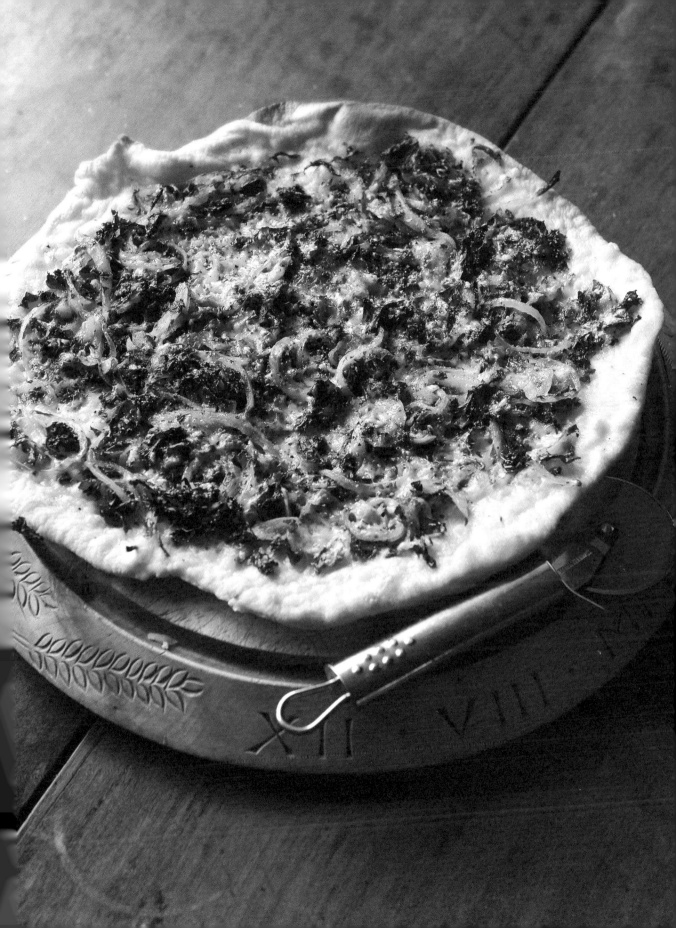

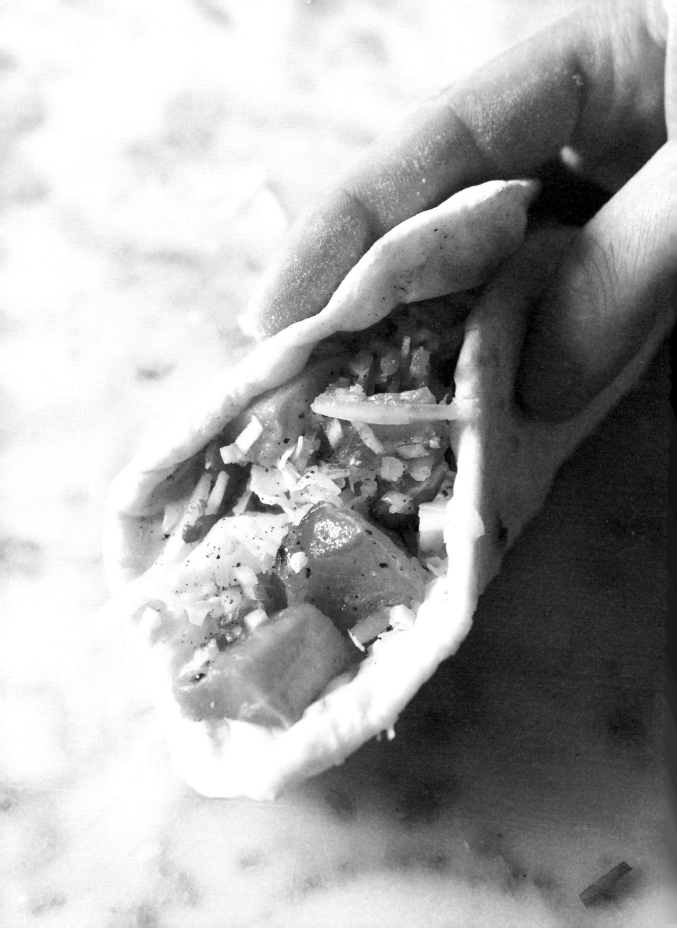

Hot squash fold over

Foldovers are a great way to use freshly made flatbreads (though you can stuff the same filling – or any of those on the following pages – into a warm pitta bread with very pleasing results).

Roasting a small tray of squash or pumpkin is so easy and can be done while the bread dough is rising so, although I couldn't honestly call this a quick meal, it's certainly a very straightforward one. The onion, salad leaves, chilli and cheese allow you to 'dress' this as though it were a kebab – feel free to customise it further, to your taste. Dukka, the spicy seed mix on page 294, is a great addition.

SERVES 4

500g squash or pumpkin, peeled, deseeded and cut into bite-sized chunks

3 garlic cloves (unpeeled), bashed

1 sprig of thyme, leaves only

2 tablespoons rapeseed or olive oil

4 freshly cooked, soft flatbreads (see page 176) or pitta breads

A handful of rocket or other salad leaves

1 small red onion, finely chopped (optional)

1 red chilli, deseeded and finely chopped, or a dash of chilli sauce

50g hard goat's cheese or Cheddar, grated

Extra virgin olive oil, to trickle

Sea salt and freshly ground black pepper

Preheat the oven to 190°C/Gas Mark 5. Put the squash in a roasting tray with the garlic, thyme leaves, oil and plenty of salt and pepper. Toss together well and roast for 50–60 minutes, stirring once, until soft and caramelised.

Lay one flatbread on a board. Place a few leaves in the centre, then spoon on one quarter of the hot squash (or use to fill the pocket of a warmed pitta). Sprinkle over a quarter each of the onion, if using, chilli and cheese, season with salt and pepper and finish with a trickle of extra virgin olive oil. Fold or roll the flatbread tightly, enclosing the filling. Repeat with all the flatbreads.

Leave the foldovers for a minute or two before eating, so the cheese starts to melt.

VARIATIONS

You can do the same thing with all sorts of other roasted veg, including roast potatoes or aubergines – or potatoes *and* aubergines (see page 351). A hot roasted beetroot foldover, with some soured cream or plain yoghurt instead of the cheese, is also quite delicious.

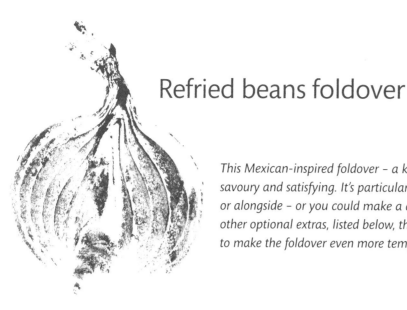

Refried beans foldover

This Mexican-inspired foldover – a kind of burrito, really – is deliciously savoury and satisfying. It's particularly good with some avocado inside or alongside – or you could make a quick guacamole. There are various other optional extras, listed below, that you can stuff in with the beans to make the foldover even more tempting.

SERVES 3

2 tablespoons rapeseed or olive oil

1 small onion, finely chopped

1 garlic clove, chopped

½ red chilli, deseeded and chopped

A pinch of dried oregano (optional)

1 large or 2 medium tomatoes

400g tin cannellini or borlotti beans, drained and rinsed

Cayenne pepper or hot smoked paprika (optional)

3 freshly cooked, soft flatbreads (see page 176) or pitta breads

2–3 tablespoons soured cream

Sea salt and freshly ground black pepper

OPTIONAL EXTRAS

Grated Cheddar or hard goat's cheese

Finely sliced red onion or chopped chives

Sliced, pickled chilli

Sliced or diced avocado, or lemony guacamole (see page 296)

Cayenne pepper or hot smoked paprika

Heat the oil in a small frying pan over a medium heat. Add the onion and fry for about 10 minutes, until soft, adding the garlic and chilli a few minutes before the end, along with the oregano, if using.

Halve the tomato(es) and grate the flesh directly into the pan (discard the skin), then let the mixture bubble and reduce for a few minutes. Add the beans and cook gently, crushing them down with a fork to make a coarse purée. Season well with salt and pepper and add a pinch of cayenne or smoked paprika if you like things spicy.

Put a spoonful of the mixture in the centre of a flatbread (or the pocket of a warmed pitta). Top with a dollop or two of soured cream and any optional extras that you fancy. Fold and eat.

VARIATION

Nachos with refried beans

Instead of serving with the flatbread, by all means open a bag of tortilla chips, and use them to scoop the beans. The soured cream and optional extras all still apply.

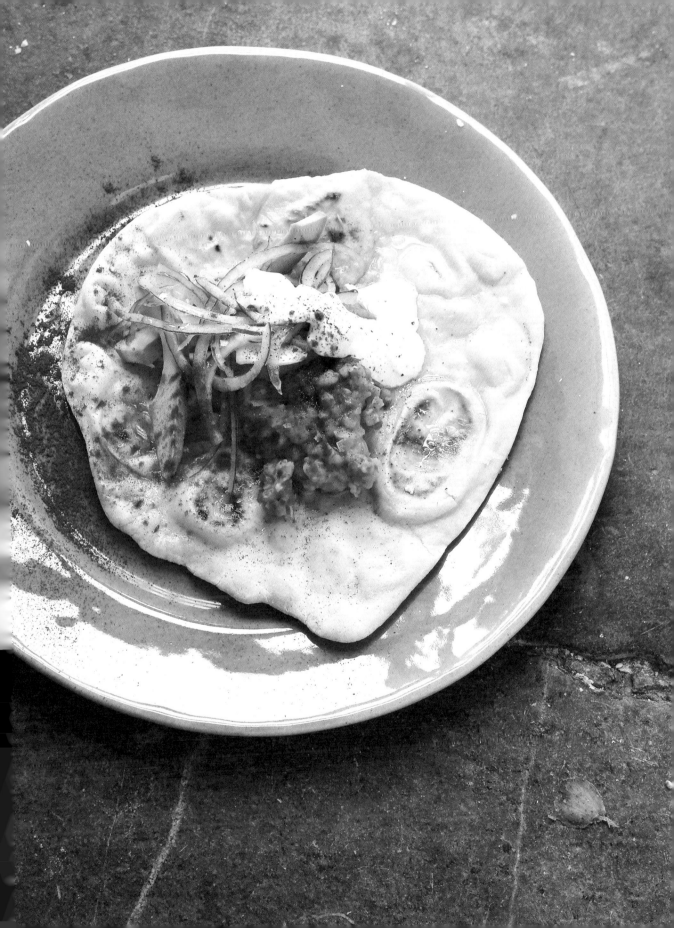

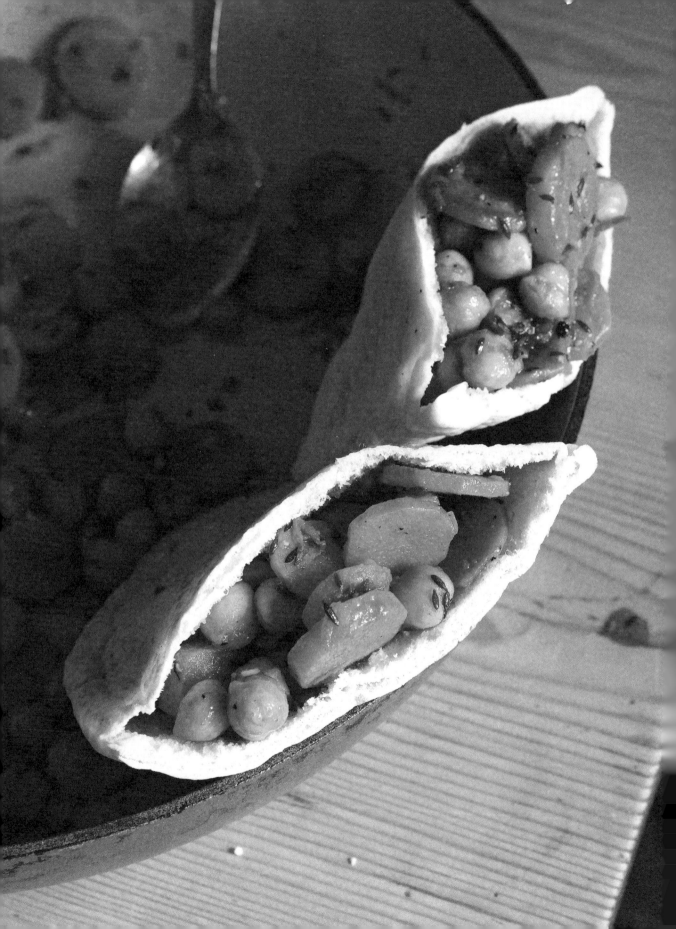

Spicy carrot and chickpea pitta pocket

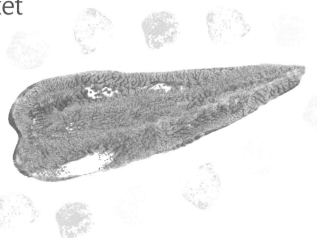

This is one of those recipes that transforms everyday fridge and cupboard staples into something special. The chickpeas don't dominate: they provide a nutty, creamy counterpoint, but the spiced, buttery carrots are the stars of the show. You can also serve it on bruschetta – or indeed bread-free, as part of a vegetable mezze-style feast.

SERVES 4

50g butter

1 tablespoon rapeseed or olive oil

1 heaped teaspoon cumin seeds

4 large carrots (about 500g), peeled and cut into 2–3mm thick slices

1 large garlic clove, finely sliced

Finely grated zest of 1 orange, plus a good squeeze of juice

1 teaspoon hot smoked paprika

400g tin chickpeas, drained and rinsed

4 pitta breads or freshly cooked, soft flatbreads (see page 176)

4 heaped tablespoons plain (full-fat) yoghurt or soured cream

Sea salt and freshly ground black pepper

Heat the butter and oil in a frying pan over a medium heat. Add the cumin seeds and let them fry for a minute or two. Add the carrots and fry for about 8–10 minutes, stirring often, until tender and starting to brown, but still with some bite.

Add the garlic, orange zest, paprika and chickpeas and cook until the chickpeas are hot. Remove from the heat, season with salt and pepper and add a good squeeze of orange juice. Taste and add more salt, pepper and/or orange juice as needed.

Spoon some of the chickpea mixture into the pocket of a warmed pitta (or into the middle of each flatbread) and top with a spoonful of yoghurt or cream. Fold flatbreads, if using. Serve straight away.

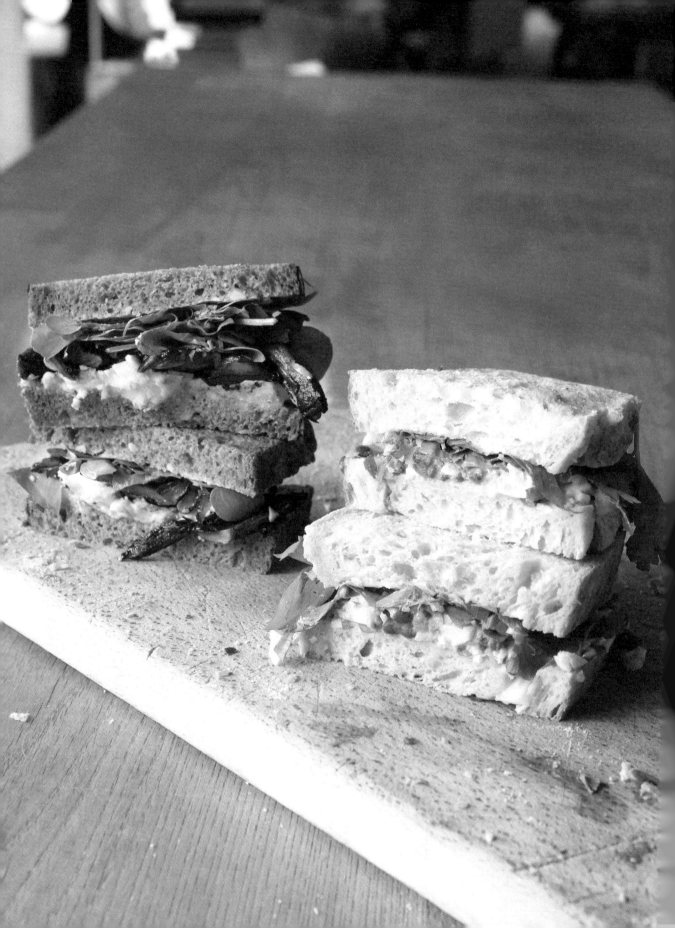

Two veggie sarnies

Do I really need to tell you how to make a sandwich? Of course I don't – but I can certainly give you a few ideas for some great veg-based fillings. On page 402, you'll find a list of the many recipes in this book which can be put to good use in a sandwich. But here are two of my other favourite bespoke veg fillings.

Mushroom, watercress and blue cheese

Hot, garlicky fried mushrooms make a substantial sandwich filling, especially when coupled with a tangy, creamy blue cheese, such as Roquefort or Harbourne Blue.

PER PERSON

2 big flat mushrooms, trimmed

A little soft butter

A dash of olive or rapeseed oil

½ garlic clove, chopped

About 50g blue cheese

A little yoghurt or crème fraîche

A good handful of watercress

2 slices of brown bread

Sea salt and freshly ground black pepper

Thickly slice the mushrooms. Heat a small knob of the butter with the oil in a frying pan over a medium heat. Add the mushrooms, garlic and some salt and pepper, and fry until tender and nicely browned.

Meanwhile, crumble the blue cheese and bind with a little yoghurt or crème fraîche. Remove any tough stems from the watercress. Butter both slices of bread.

Put the cheese mixture on one piece of bread, top with the hot mushrooms and finish with the watercress. Add the second slice of bread, cut in half and serve.

Curried egg, lentils and flat-leaf parsley

Lentils in a sandwich? Why not? The curried mayonnaise and egg hold them nicely, giving you a lovely textured mouthful. Include the raisins for a little fruity sweetness.

PER PERSON

1 hard-boiled large egg

½–1 tablespoon mayonnaise

½–1 teaspoon curry powder

1–2 tablespoons cooked, cold Puy lentils

A few raisins (optional)

2 slices of bread

A little soft butter

A handful of flat-leaf parsley, or lettuce or baby spinach leaves

Sea salt and freshly ground black pepper

Roughly chop the hard-boiled egg and mix with the mayonnaise and curry powder, then stir in the lentils, and raisins if using. Season with salt and pepper to taste – and mix in a little more mayo if you want to loosen it a bit.

Lightly butter the bread. Spread the eggy mixture on one slice, then top with the parsley leaves, lettuce or spinach. Add the second slice of bread and close the sandwich. Slice in half and serve.

Bruschetta with broad beans and asparagus

This is a fantastic celebration of the crossover between the last of the asparagus and the first baby broad beans. Later in the summer, you can use a few French beans, just blanched and still crunchy, instead of the asparagus.

SERVES 4

12–15 asparagus spears, trimmed

200g baby broad beans (podded weight)

A bunch of spring onions

2 tablespoons olive oil

4 large slices of sourdough or other robust bread

1 garlic clove, halved (optional)

Extra virgin olive oil, to trickle

About 50g mild, crumbly goat's cheese

Sea salt and freshly ground black pepper

Bring a pan of salted water to the boil, add the asparagus spears and blanch for 2 minutes. Scoop them out and drain. Let the water come back to the boil. Now add the baby broad beans and blanch for just 30–60 seconds until tender, then drain.

Trim the spring onions, leaving just a little of the green end attached. Slice on the diagonal into 1–2cm pieces. Heat the olive oil in a frying pan over a medium heat, add the spring onions and fry fairly gently for 2–3 minutes, until just starting to soften.

Cut the asparagus spears into 2–3cm pieces and add, along with the broad beans, to the spring onions in the pan. Add salt and pepper and toss the whole lot together over the heat, for just a minute, then take off the heat.

Meanwhile, toast the bread. Rub very lightly with the cut garlic clove, if you like. Trickle the toast with a little olive oil. Crumble the goat's cheese over the veg in the pan and stir very lightly again. Pile this veg mixture on to the toast, trickle with a touch more olive oil, and serve.

VARIATION

Bruschetta with garlicky broad bean purée, ricotta and mint
This works with larger, more floury broad beans or bought frozen ones. Cook 600g podded broad beans in boiling water until tender. Drain and, as soon as they are cool enough to handle, pop the beans out of their skins. Melt 30g butter with 2 tablespoons rapeseed or olive oil over a very low heat, add 2 finely chopped garlic cloves and warm gently for a minute or two. Add the beans to the garlicky butter and then blitz to a coarse purée, or mash. Add a little more butter if needed. Pile the warm purée on to hot bruschetta, prepared as above, then scatter over 50g crumbled ricotta, a trickle of extra virgin oil and some chopped mint.

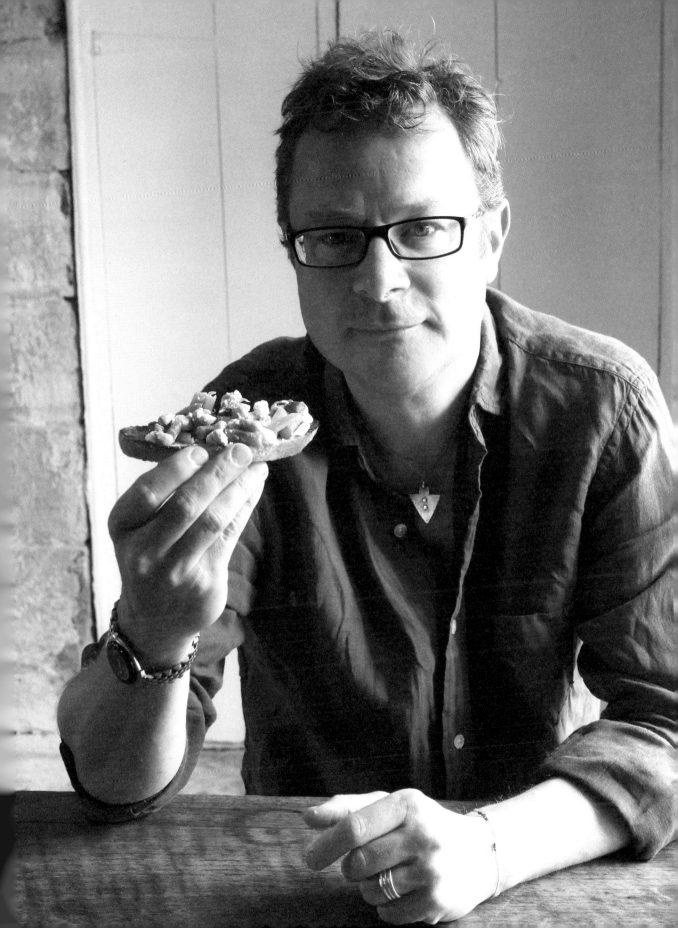

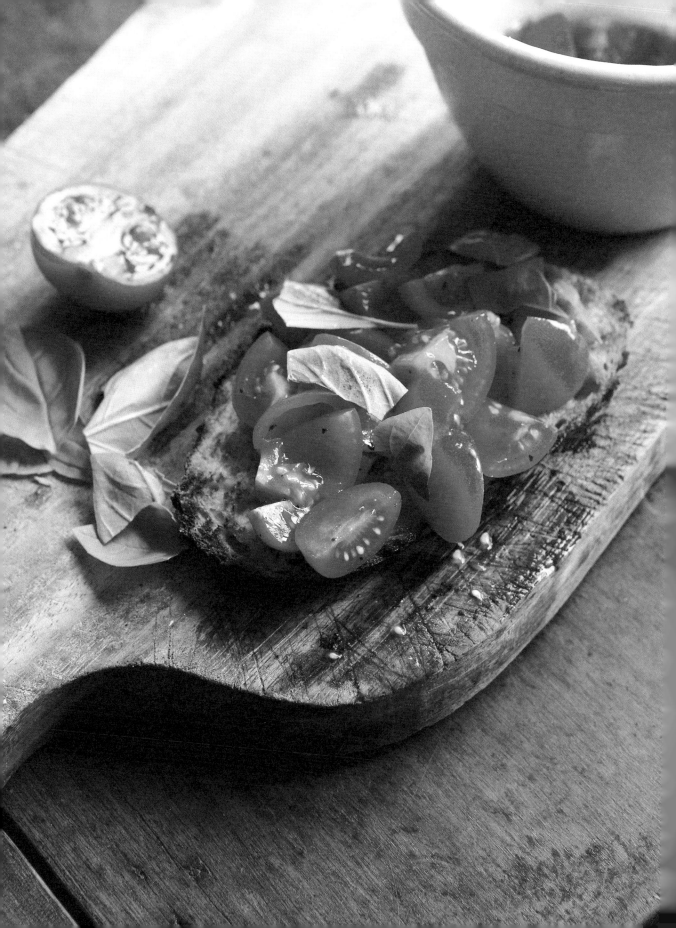

Tomato bruschetta ♥

This is one of the best ways to enjoy really ripe, flavoursome tomatoes – any kind
from tiny cherries to big, beefy slicers. You can add cheese if you want to – shaved
hard goat's cheese, perhaps, or torn buffalo mozzarella, but it's very good just as it is.

SERVES 2

250g ripe, sweet tomatoes

2 tablespoons extra virgin olive
oil, plus extra to trickle

A pinch of sugar

2 large slices of sourdough
or other robust bread

1 garlic clove, halved

A handful of basil, roughly torn,
or chives, chopped

Sea salt and freshly ground
black pepper

Cut the tomatoes into small chunks. For cherry tomatoes, this
generally means quarters – or eighths if they are on the larger side.
Big tomatoes should be cut into similarly small pieces – slice them
thickly, then cut the thick slices into 6–8 pieces. Put them in a bowl
with the olive oil, a pinch of sugar and plenty of salt and pepper.
Toss together well.

Toast the bread and, while still hot, lightly rub the halved garlic clove
over it. Trickle the toast with a little oil. Pile the tomatoes on to the
toast, scatter over the basil or chives, give it another little trickle of oil,
then serve straight away.

Celery and blue cheese bruschetta

Much as I love celery in a supporting role, I like to see it as the star ingredient from
time to time. Avoid using the outer stems, which may be a bit coarse and fibrous
– save those for stocks. If you don't fancy blue cheese, use goat's cheese or Parmesan.

SERVES 2

3–4 medium celery stalks

2 slices of sourdough or other
robust bread

1 garlic clove, halved

Rapeseed or extra virgin olive
oil, to trickle

About 75g blue cheese,
crumbled

1–2 teaspoons clear honey

Sea salt and freshly ground
black pepper

Check out the celery by snapping a stem in half. If it's a bit too fibrous,
use a potato peeler to strip the tougher fibres from the outside of the
stem. Slice the celery finely, on the diagonal.

Toast the bread. While still hot, rub lightly with the cut surface of the
garlic clove. Trickle over a little oil, then pile the celery on to the toast.
Scatter on the crumbled cheese, then some salt and pepper, and finish
with a fine trickle of honey. Serve straight away.

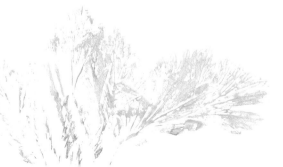

Bruschetta with cavolo nero

Cabbage on toast? Try it: this is a simple way to appreciate the earthy taste of lovely, dark cavolo nero. If you can't get that particular leaf, any good kale will work – or spring greens, Brussels tops or the greener outer leaves of a Savoy cabbage.

SERVES 2

About 150g cavolo nero or greens (see above)

1 large garlic clove

2 slices of sourdough or other robust bread

1–2 tablespoons extra virgin rapeseed or olive oil

Parmesan, hard goat's cheese or other well-flavoured hard cheese shavings

Sea salt and freshly ground black pepper

Strip the cavolo nero leaves from their stems and put into a saucepan. Cut off a third of the garlic clove and set aside; roughly chop the rest and add to the pan. Cover with water, add salt and bring to the boil. Lower the heat and simmer for 4–5 minutes – a little longer if need be – until the cavolo nero is tender. Drain well in a colander.

Tip the cavolo nero and garlic on to a board and chop together roughly. Return to the hot pan, season well with salt and pepper and toss in a tablespoon or so of oil.

Toast the bread and rub lightly with the reserved bit of garlic clove. Trickle with a little more oil. Pile the cavolo nero and cheese shavings on to the bread and serve.

Courgette bruschetta

This old favourite appears in the original River Cottage Cookbook *– garlicky, slightly bashed-up courgettes remain one of my all-time favourite toppings for bruschetta.*

SERVES 2

2 tablespoons olive or rapeseed oil

250g small courgettes, sliced

1 small garlic clove, crushed, plus another, halved, for the bread

A squeeze of lemon juice

2 thick slices of robust bread, such as sourdough

Extra virgin rapeseed or olive oil, to trickle

1–2 sprigs of thyme, leaves only

40–50g mild, crumbly goat's cheese

Sea salt and freshly ground black pepper

Heat the oil in a large frying pan over a medium heat, then add the courgettes, crushed garlic and a pinch of salt. Once sizzling, turn the heat down a little and cook, stirring often, for at least 15 minutes until the courgettes are very soft. You want to drive off their moisture without letting them brown. As they start to soften, you can bash them up a bit with a spatula or spoon. When you have a concentrated, tender, courgettey mess, take them off the heat.

Season with a little more salt if necessary, plus some black pepper and a squeeze of lemon juice. Leave the courgettes to cool slightly while you prepare the bread.

Toast the bread and, while still hot, rub lightly with the halved garlic clove. Trickle with some extra virgin oil, then pile the courgettes on top. Sprinkle over the thyme leaves and crumble over the goat's cheese. Add a final trickle of oil and serve.

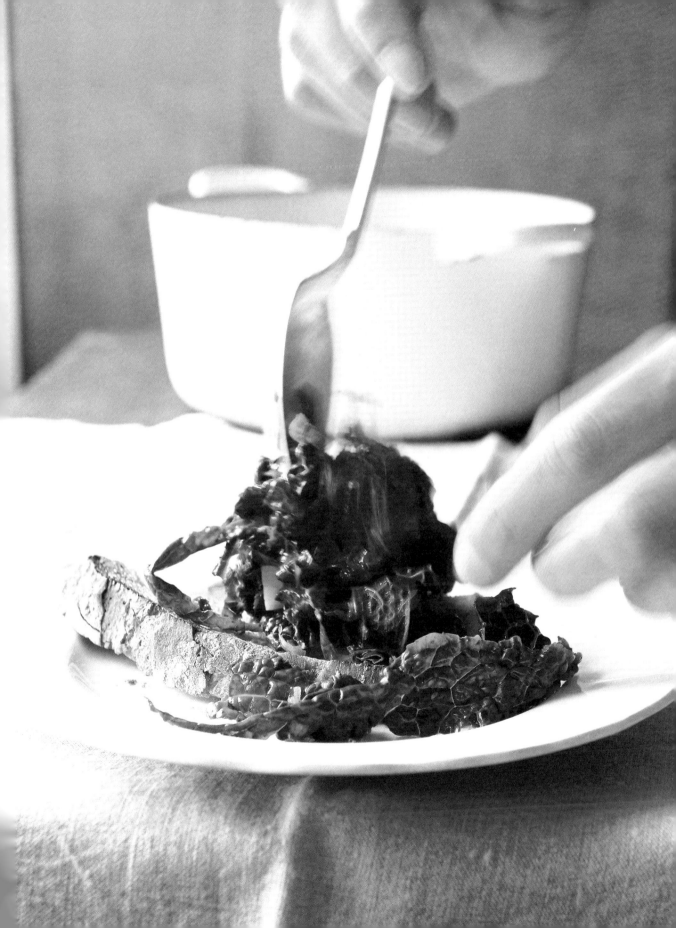

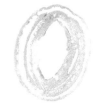

Leek and cheese toastie

Over the years, I've experimented and improvised all kinds of leek-based, cheesy toast toppings. Most of them have been a delight, even if I say so myself, but this is perhaps the simplest and most midweek-friendly.

SERVES 2

15g butter

2 medium leeks, trimmed (white and pale green part only), washed and sliced

A couple of sprigs of thyme, leaves only, roughly chopped (optional)

3 tablespoons double cream

50g strong Cheddar, grated

2 thick slices of sourdough or other robust bread

Sea salt and freshly ground black pepper

Melt the butter in a small frying pan over a medium heat and add the leeks. As soon as they are sizzling, turn the heat down quite low and sweat gently, stirring often, for about 10 minutes until tender. Stir in the thyme, if using, and cream and cook for a minute or two longer until the cream is bubbling. Take off the heat and stir in two-thirds of the cheese. Add salt and pepper to taste.

Preheat the grill. Toast the bread lightly. Spread the leek mixture thickly over the bread and top with the remaining grated cheese. Grill until bubbling and golden, and serve straight away.

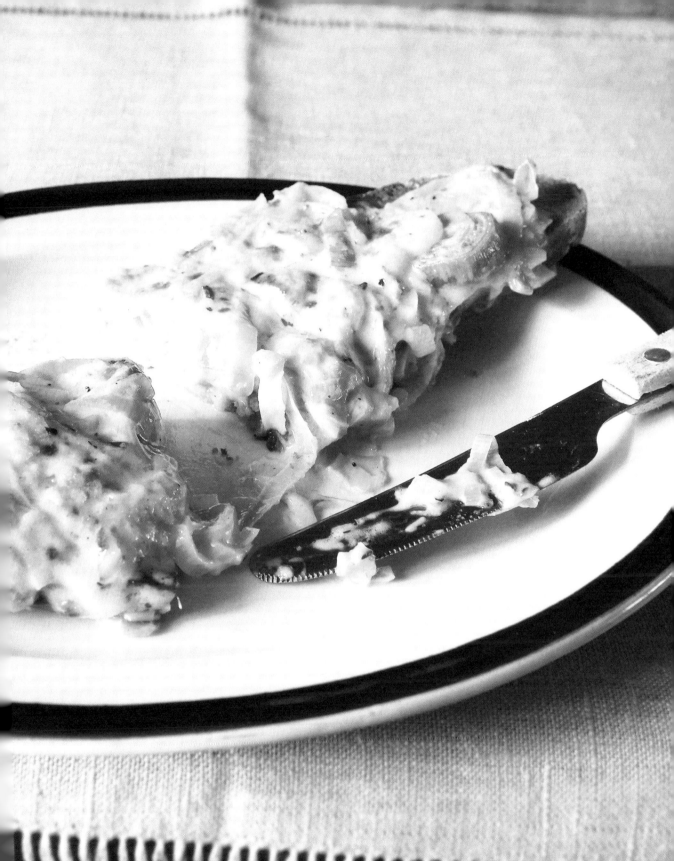

Squash and walnut toastie

If you're roasting squash or pumpkin, do a little extra and have this quick lunch the day after. You could use other leftover roasted veg too, such as celeriac, beetroot or carrots, and different nuts, such as hazelnuts, cashews or pine nuts. No nuts is fine too...

SERVES 2

A handful of walnuts

1 tablespoon rapeseed or olive oil

A knob of butter

200–250g leftover roasted squash or pumpkin

A couple of sprigs of thyme, leaves only (optional)

50g blue cheese (or Cheddar or goat's cheese), crumbled

2 thick slices of sourdough or other robust bread

A trickle of clear honey

Sea salt and freshly ground black pepper

Heat a non-stick frying pan over a medium heat. Add the walnuts and toast gently, tossing the pan, for a few minutes until they start to smell toasty and take on a little colour. Tip out of the pan; set aside.

Return the pan to the heat and add the oil and butter. When foaming, add the squash and cook for 3–4 minutes, crushing it down a bit, until heated through. Stir in the thyme, if using, then take off the heat. Add the nuts and the crumbled cheese, and stir roughly into the squash. Taste and add a little salt and some pepper if you think it needs it.

Preheat the grill to medium and lightly toast the bread. Pile the squash mixture on to the bread, packing it down a little and making sure some chunks of cheese are on top. Trickle over a little honey and grill until golden brown and bubbling. Serve straight away, with some salad leaves if you like.

Apple and blue vinny toastie

This simple blend of tart apple and salty, savoury cheese is immensely satisfying, and makes a great quick lunch. A spoonful of mayonnaise helps to bind the mix but isn't essential. And if blue cheese isn't your thing, try a good tangy Cheddar.

SERVES 2

2 small, tart eating apples, such as Cox's, OR 1 medium cooking apple, such as a Bramley

100g Dorset Blue Vinny or other crumbly blue cheese

1 tablespoon mayonnaise (optional)

2 slices of sourdough or other robust bread

1 garlic clove, halved

Sea salt and freshly ground black pepper

Grate the apples, skin and all, into a bowl. Grate or finely crumble the cheese and add this too, along with some black pepper and a little salt (the blue cheese will already be quite salty). Add the mayonnaise if you like, and mix well.

Preheat the grill to medium. Lightly toast the bread. Rub the cut garlic clove lightly over the toasted bread, for just a hint of garlic. Spread the apple and cheese mixture in a thick, even layer on the toast. Put under the grill, not too close to the heat, and let the mixture heat up gently so the apple gets a chance to soften. After 5 minutes or so, when the apple is softening and the cheese is melted, bring the toasties closer to the heat and grill until golden brown and bubbling. Serve at once.

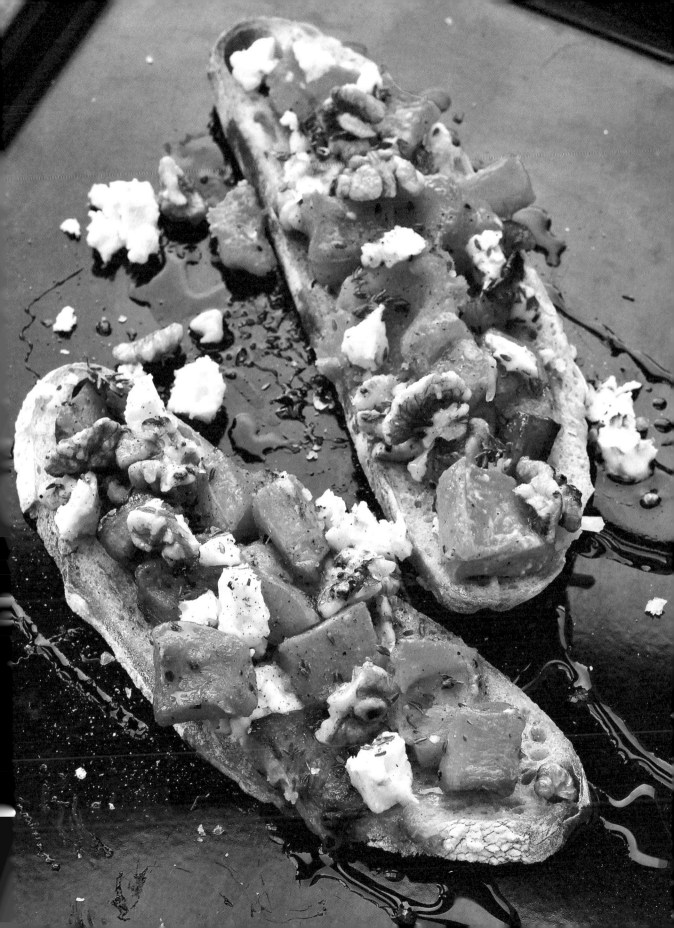

The vegiflette toastie

My very easy tartiflette toastie, which appears in River Cottage Every Day, *was inspired by the classic, rich and greedy Swiss mountain dish of cheese, ham, cream and spuds. This is an equally irresistible, meat-free version. The classic cheese for a tartiflette is Reblochon, but Camembert, Stinking Bishop and other well-flavoured 'washed rind' cheeses all work well. And, frankly, so do most goat's cheeses and even Cheddar.*

Indulgent, creamy, cheesy combinations like this are well-complemented by a few bitter salad leaves, and here I've actually made them an integral part of the toastie topping.

SERVES 2

2 tablespoons rapeseed or olive oil

2 smallish, cold, cooked potatoes, thickly sliced

8–10 leaves of chicory, radicchio or other bitter salad leaf, roughly sliced

2–3 tablespoons double cream or crème fraîche

2 thick slices of sourdough or other robust bread

About 50g (3–4 slices) cheese (see above)

Sea salt and freshly ground black pepper

Heat the oil in a non-stick frying pan over a medium heat. Add the potatoes and cook for a few minutes, turning every now and then, until starting to turn golden. Add the sliced chicory or other salad leaves and cook for a minute or so, until they are starting to wilt. Add the cream and let it bubble and reduce for a minute or two, then season with salt and pepper to taste.

Preheat the grill and toast the bread lightly. Heap the mixture from the pan on to the toast. Lay the cheese slices on top and grill until bubbling. Serve straight away.

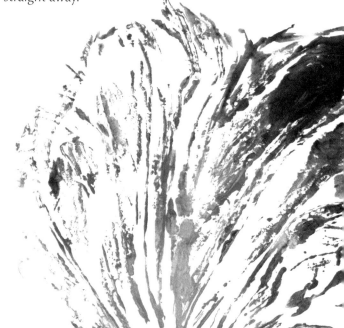

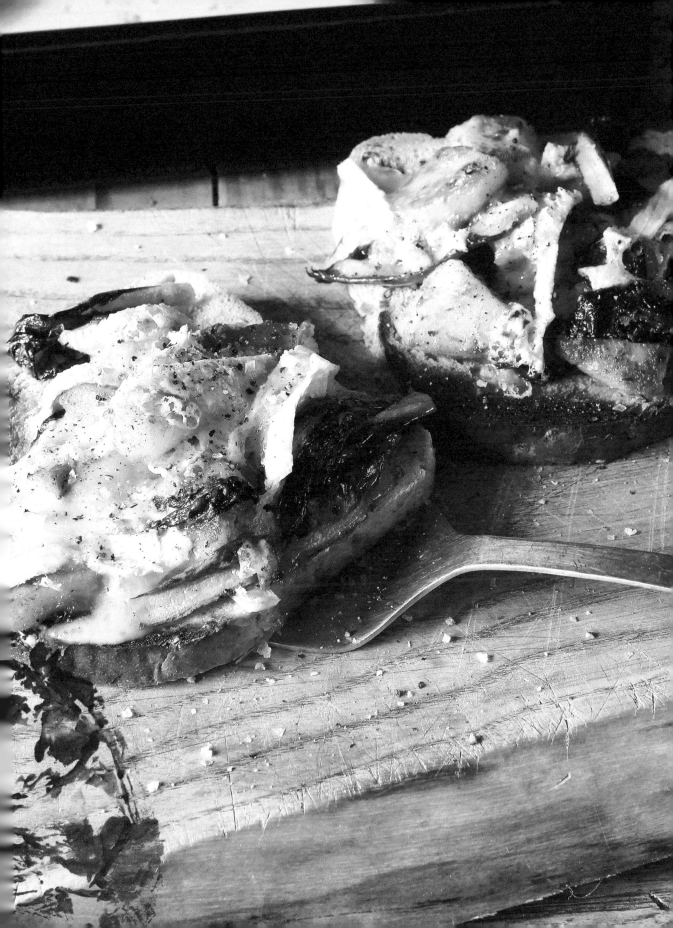

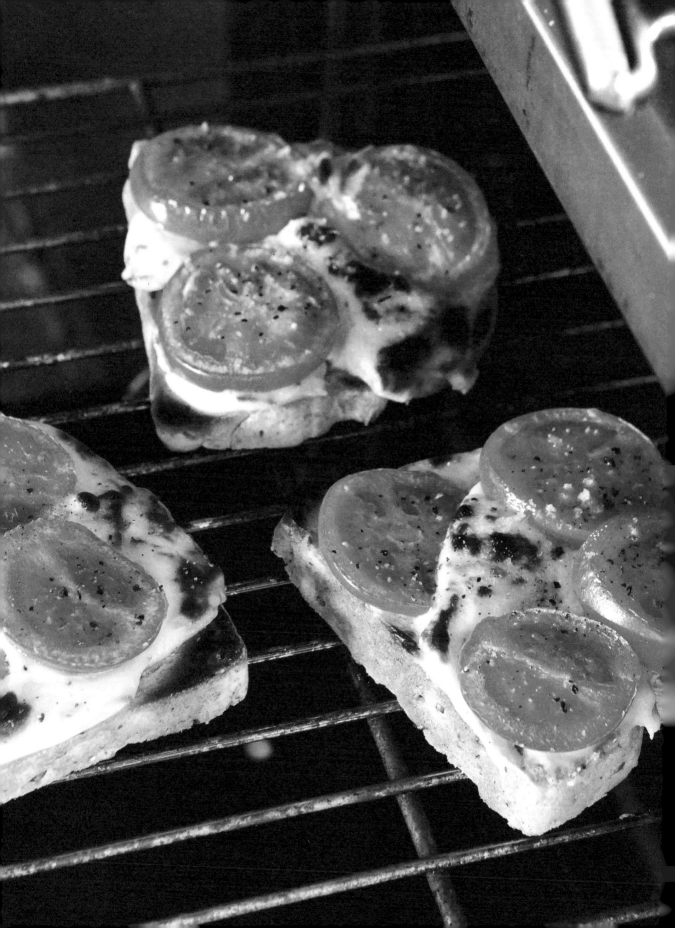

Various rarebits

Welsh rarebit is so much more than cheese on toast. My version is based on a simple béchamel sauce with cheese added. Other recipes include beer, and you might like to replace some or all of the milk with warmed good bitter or ale. Rarebit can be customised with various veg too (see below). It's also worth trying it on a homemade flatbread instead of toast. The result – somewhere between cheese on toast and an indulgent pizza – is fantastic.

SERVES 4

300ml whole milk

1 bay leaf (optional)

½ onion (optional)

50g unsalted butter

50g plain flour

150g fairly strong Cheddar, grated

½ teaspoon English mustard, or to taste

A dash of Worcestershire sauce (optional)

4 slices of good bread or 4 small flatbreads (see page 176)

Sea salt and freshly ground black pepper

Put the milk in a saucepan, with the bay leaf and onion if you have them to hand, along with a grinding of black pepper. Bring the milk to just below a simmer, then turn off the heat.

Melt the butter in another pan over a medium-low heat. Stir in the flour to make a smooth roux and let it bubble and seethe for a couple of minutes. Remove from the heat. If you've infused the milk with the bay and onion, strain them out. Add the milk to the roux in three or four lots, beating well after each addition to create a smooth sauce.

Return the thick sauce to a low heat and cook for another 2 minutes. Turn off the heat and stir in the cheese until melted, then add the mustard and season with salt and pepper to taste, adding a dash of Worcestershire sauce if you like (not for vegetarians).

Preheat the grill to medium-high. Toast the bread. If you're serving your rarebit just as it comes, then spread the cheese sauce thickly on the toast. Alternatively, add your veggie extras (see below) before spreading on the toast. Either way, grill the rarebit reasonably slowly, not too close to the heat, so the thick sauce is bubbling hot all the way through before the top gets too brown. Serve straight away.

ALTERNATIVE TOPPINGS

Tomato rarebit (shown left)
Top the cheese sauce with a few thick slices of tomato before placing under the grill.

Celery rarebit
Finely slice 4 celery stalks and sauté them in a knob of butter for 5 minutes, until tender but still a bit crunchy. Season and stir into the rarebit mixture before spreading on toast and grilling.

PSB rarebit
Lay some stems of lightly cooked purple-sprouting broccoli across your toast and smother with the sauce.

Poached egg on toast

You may have your own preferred method for poaching an egg – in which case, stick to it. This is mine. I concede that there are no actual vegetables involved in this recipe: I'm including it not just because it makes such a very fine, quick meal in its own right, but because a perfectly poached egg is an excellent finishing touch or accompaniment to a great many of the dishes in this book. Frankly, there's barely a recipe in this chapter that I would want to discourage you from serving with a poached egg on top. Indeed, if on reading any of the recipes in this book, you find yourself thinking, 'I wonder what that would be like with a poached egg?'... well, there's only one way to find out.

The absolute most important thing is to make sure the egg you use is fresh. Old eggs almost invariably produce raggedy poached whites.

SERVES 1

1 large egg, at room temperature

1 slice of bread

Butter

Sea salt and freshly ground black pepper

Pour a 4–5cm depth of water into a saucepan and bring to the boil. Meanwhile, break the egg carefully into a mug or small jug, taking care not to damage the yolk.

When the water is at a rolling boil, stir it fast in one direction with a wooden spoon to create a vortex or whirlpool in the centre. When you have a distinct vortex, remove the spoon and immediately tip the egg straight into the centre. Turn off the heat, put a lid on the pan and leave it for exactly 2½ minutes. Meanwhile, lightly toast your bread and butter it.

Remove the lid. Use a slotted spoon to carefully scoop up the egg. Check that the white is set, with no jellyish clear bits left – if there are, return it to the water for 30 seconds. Give the egg half a minute in the spoon for the water to drip and steam away. You can dab carefully with a piece of kitchen paper to help get rid of the water.

Slide the egg carefully on to the hot toast, sprinkle with a little salt and pepper, and serve.

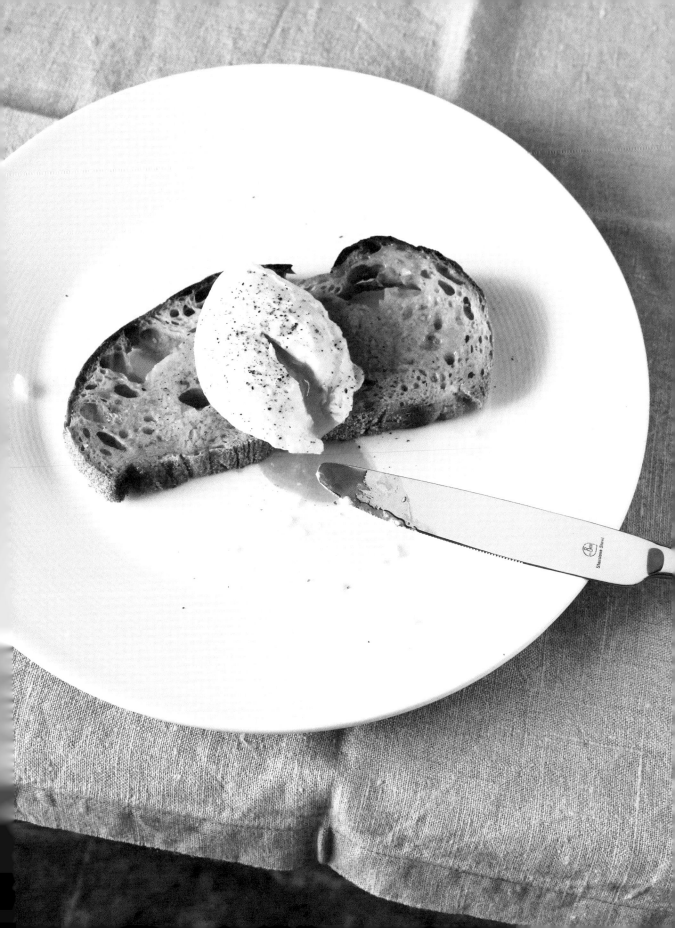

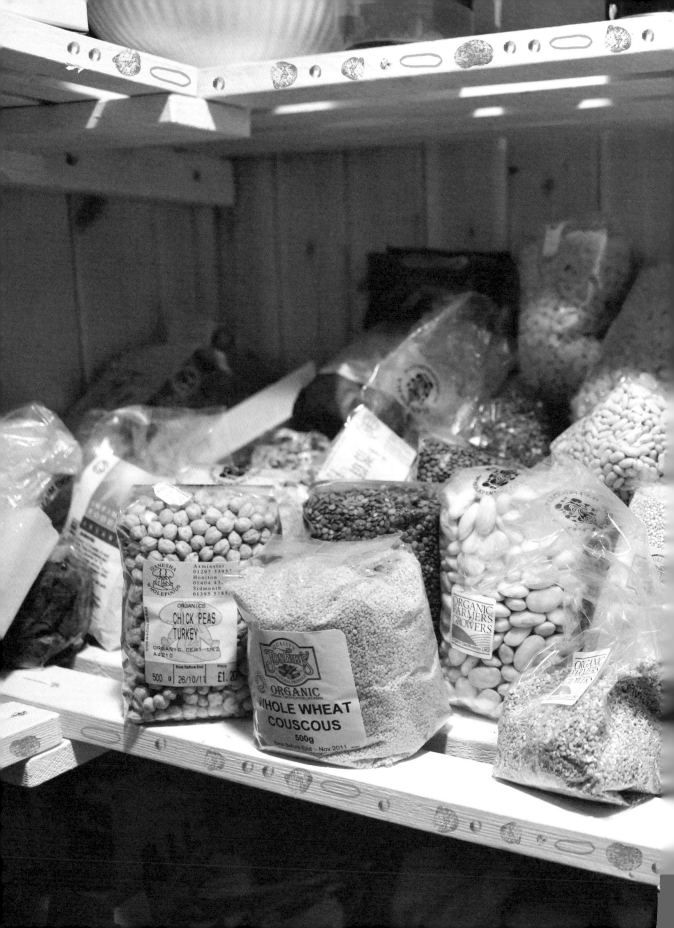

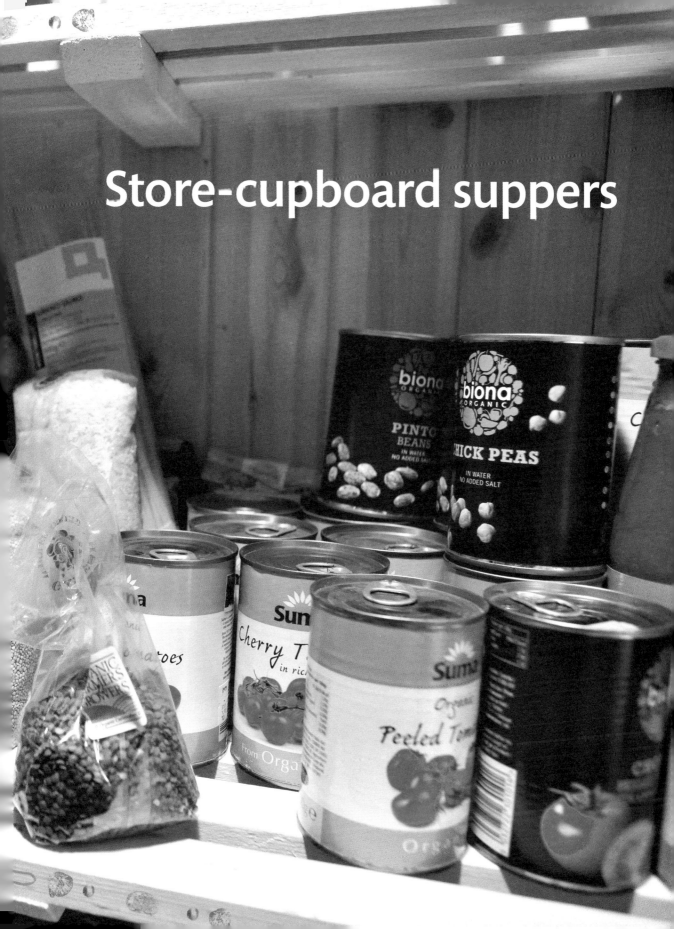

Store-cupboard suppers

There will always be occasions when you're really pushed for time, or tired and hungry, and you crave something filling and satisfying but simple and quick. When you are in that frame of mind, the temptation can be strong to reach for the sausages or bacon. But really, you don't have to default to meat just because you're in a hurry.

With a well-stocked store cupboard, and the fridge in a supporting role, you can pretty much throw together meat-free meals from things readily to hand, even when there are no actual fresh vegetables in the house. You'll find a list of some key store-cupboard ingredients that I always like to have waiting in the wings on pages 400–1. But I think it's worth going into a bit of detail here about the ones that are particularly steadfast friends to the weary and the time-poor.

First of all, my shelves always harbour a few tins of beans, chickpeas and/or lentils. You'll find pulses popping up in various recipes throughout the book, but in this chapter they are the focus of some very fast and tasty meals. They are such great standbys – instantly ready, and offering a substantial dose of both protein and starch. It's just a matter of building a dish around them with a few well-chosen, contrasting flavours and textures.

My second crucial ingredient is eggs. I try to make sure there are always half a dozen in the house. If the tally falls below this, I become panicky, and I'll threaten the hens with early retirement into the stockpot, even as I head down to the village shop. It goes (almost) without saying that an egg offers a nutritious little package; one that boiled, poached or fried, can top off not just a plate of toast soldiers, but also a hearty salad or even a tray of roasted veg, so that where you might have had a snack or a side dish, you find you've got yourself a meal. And when it comes to mid-week quickies, eggs can be more than the last-minute meal-maker. They can be the central 'planned' ingredient too, as the upcoming frittata recipes testify.

Then there's quick-cook noodles. These can be the base of meals so effortless that you don't even need to get a saucepan out. I've discovered that it's amazingly easy to create a fast, hot meal based around noodles and your kettle. Okay, it wasn't my discovery. But I have had fun re-working the concept of the instant noodle meal to exclude nasties such as MSG, and embrace some genuinely virtuous ingredients. These are particularly great one-dish, one-person meals – the sort you might find yourself eating in the kitchen, standing up, perhaps before you've even got your coat off. And they can be taken to work, as a just-add-boiling-water instant lunchbox.

Puff pastry, tucked away in the freezer, is an ingredient I turn to more and more these days. It's now possible to buy very good all-butter, and even organic, puffs that are a world away from the bog-standard margarine-based ones, which so often have a rather stale flavour. What's more, puff pastry is often sold in ready-rolled sheets. They defrost in minutes and then offer you a blank canvas – ready and waiting for the tastes and textures of a few well-chosen veg, a pinch of herbs and perhaps a scattering of cheese and a trickle of good extra virgin olive or rapeseed oil. A little bit indulgent but, once in a while, why not?

The good old potato is, of course, a slightly more ordinary starchy standby. Spuds are a mid-week mainstay for many of us, and I hope to do them justice in this chapter. They can be cooked from scratch, which may not be exactly quick, but is certainly straightforward – you'll find my current favourite twists on chips and jacket potatoes on pages 225 and 226. But in my house, more often than not, potatoes appear mid-week as leftovers.

I rarely cook spuds without deliberately adding a few more than are needed immediately, so they can go into the fridge and stand by for supper duty. Re-hashed (quite literally sometimes) in the frying pan, they never fail to please. Although cooked potatoes may be the most versatile of leftover veg, they are by no means the only ones. Almost any leftover roots, along with leftover greens, beans and peas, can be improvised into a frittata, or bubble and squeak, or some variation of the theme.

There are other incredibly useful things – onions, frozen peas, well-flavoured cheese (you can't beat a good Cheddar), dried lentils, couscous, pasta and rice of course – which extend my arsenal of ever-ready ingredients. The list may sound mundane, but the uses to which they are put are anything but. Your store cupboard should be a rich source of delicious goodies that, even in the absence of lovely fresh veg, can feed you warmly, generously, and without recourse to meat. So keep it well stocked but – and this bit is vital – make sure there's as much coming out of it as there is going in. The larder is not an emergency bomb shelter; don't be afraid to use it, even in peacetime.

Tomato, thyme and goat's cheese tart

*This is a very simple tart to make, using good-quality ready-made puff pastry.
I've suggested various cheese and herb options below, but the basic principle
is the same: crisp pastry, soft caramelised tomato, tangy cheese.*

SERVES 4-6

A little sunflower oil

½ teaspoon fine cornmeal
or polenta (optional)

375g all-butter, ready-made
puff pastry

Beaten egg, for brushing

About 350g tomatoes

1 garlic clove, finely chopped

A little extra virgin olive or
rapeseed oil

100g rinded goat's cheese

A handful of thyme sprigs,
leaves only

Sea salt and freshly ground
black pepper

Preheat the oven to 190°C/Gas Mark 5. Lightly oil a baking sheet and
scatter over a little fine cornmeal or polenta, if you have some – this
helps to keep the pastry really crisp.

Roll out the pastry fairly thinly and trim to a rectangle about 30 x 25cm.
Put it on the baking sheet. Cut a 1cm strip from each edge. Brush
these strips with a little beaten egg, then stick on to the edges of the
rectangle, to form a slightly raised border. Brush the edges with a little
more egg.

Thinly slice the tomatoes across into 2–3mm slices; discard the stalky
top and skinny bottom slices. Scatter the garlic over the pastry, then
arrange the sliced tomatoes on top, overlapping them only slightly.
Season with salt and pepper and trickle with a little oil. Bake for about
15 minutes, until the tomatoes are tender and lightly browned.

Take the tart out of the oven, scatter over the cheese and thyme, add
another twist of pepper and a trickle of oil, and return to the oven. Bake
for another 10 minutes or so, until the cheese is melty and bubbly and
the pastry golden brown. You can serve this hot, but I think it's better
half an hour or so after it comes out of the oven, with a green salad.

VARIATIONS

Basil and mozzarella tart
Replace the goat's cheese with 1 ball of buffalo mozzarella (about 125g),
torn into small pieces. Replace the thyme with a couple of tablespoons
of shredded basil – but add this after the tart is cooked, not before.

Rosemary and pecorino tart
Replace the goat's cheese with a generous grating of pecorino or
Parmesan, and the thyme leaves with 1 tablespoon chopped rosemary.

Blue cheese and chives tart
Replace the goat's cheese with crumbled blue cheese. Omit the thyme.
Scatter a chopped handful of chives over the tart once it is cooked.

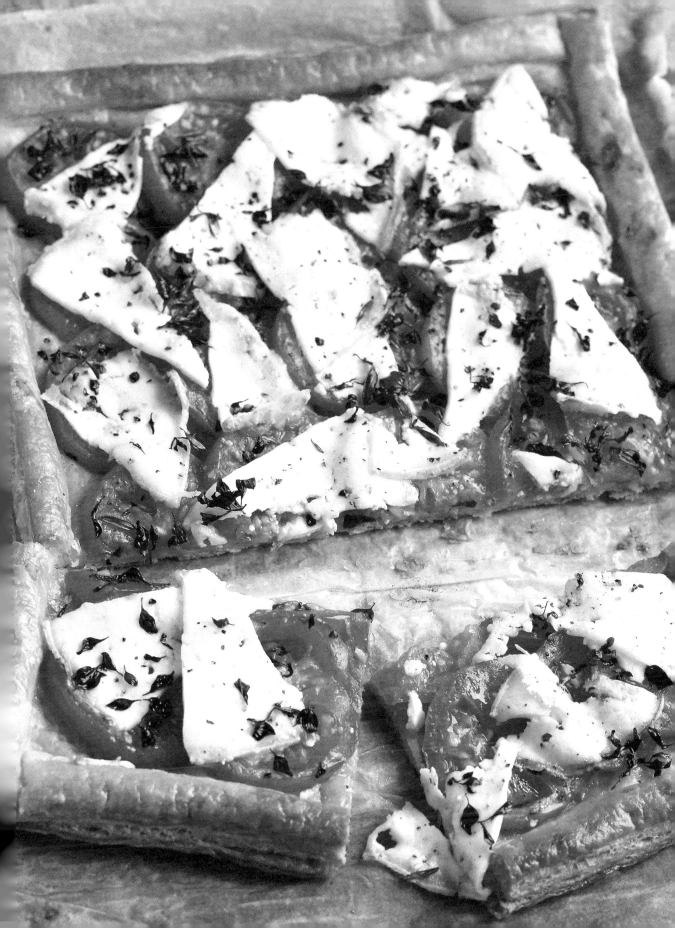

Upside-down onion tart

This is now a favourite 'cupboard's-bare' recipe, shown to me by my friend Sarah Raven. With just two ingredients – onions and puff pastry – you can produce, in a short space of time, something rather smart and very tasty. It's another tarte tatin variation, of course.

SERVES 4

About 200g all-butter, ready-made puff pastry

3–4 medium onions (about 350g)

A small knob of butter

1 tablespoon rapeseed or olive oil

1 tablespoon balsamic vinegar

Sea salt and freshly ground black pepper

Preheat the oven to 190°C/Gas Mark 5. Roll out the pastry to a 3–4mm thickness and cut out a 20cm circle. Wrap the pastry disc and place it in the fridge.

Peel the onions and slice each one into 6 or 8 wedges, keeping them attached at the root end. Heat the butter and oil in a 20cm tarte tatin pan or ovenproof frying pan over a medium heat. Add the onions, arranging them roughly in a concentric pattern. Sprinkle with salt and pepper and cook for about 15–20 minutes, turning once or twice, until they are fairly tender, and starting to caramelise around the edges.

Trickle the balsamic vinegar over the onions and cook for a couple of minutes more, so the vinegar reduces a little. Remove from the heat and make sure the onions are fairly evenly spread around the pan.

Lay the pastry disc over the onions and put the pan into the oven. Bake for 20 minutes, until the pastry is fully puffed up and golden.

Invert the tart on to a plate, so the sticky caramelised onions are facing up, on top of the crispy pastry. Serve straight away, ideally with a green leafy salad. You could also crumble or grate over a favourite cheese.

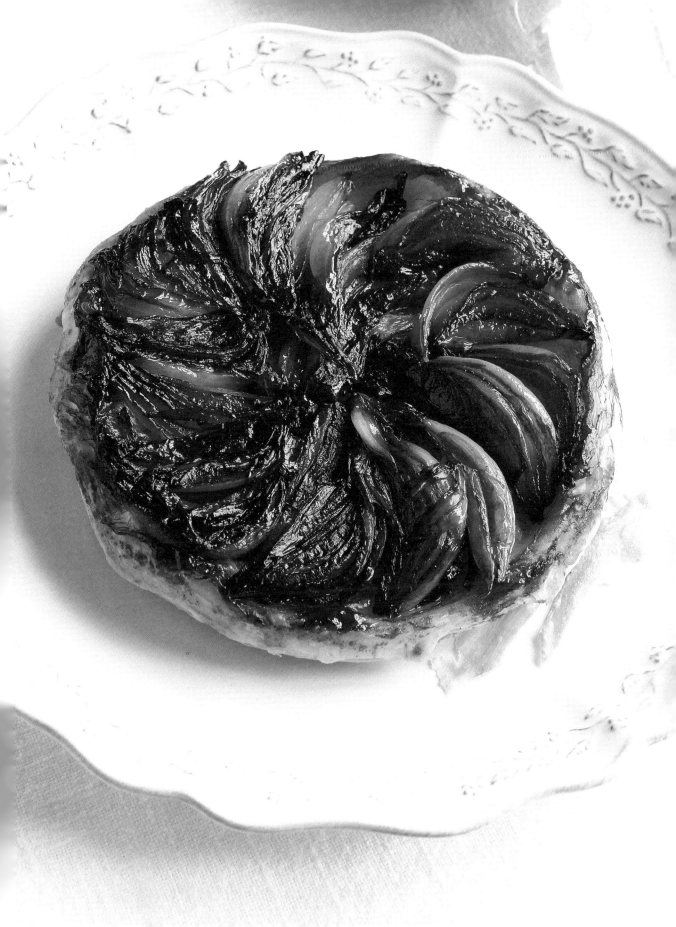

Spring onion galette

This is a really tasty, quick supper. The spring onions should be just charred in places and slightly chewy on the outside, yet steamed-tender in the middle.

SERVES 4

375g all-butter, ready-made puff pastry, ready rolled if you like

About 500g spring onions (3 large bunches)

3 tablespoons olive oil, plus a little extra for oiling

50g Parmesan, mature Cheddar or hard goat's cheese, grated

Sea salt and freshly ground black pepper

Preheat the oven to 200°C/Gas Mark 6. Roll out the puff pastry, if it isn't ready-rolled, to a rectangle, 4–5mm thick. Lay the pastry on a lightly oiled baking sheet.

Trim off the root ends of the onions and the green ends, leaving 2–3cm of the tender green part attached. Strip off the outer layer too if it looks a bit tired. Rinse briefly and pat dry. If the onions are slender, use them whole; halve thicker ones lengthways. Put the onions in a bowl, add the olive oil, cheese and some salt and pepper and toss together thoroughly.

Lay the spring onions on the pastry in a single layer, leaving a 2–3cm clear margin around the edges. Dot any remaining cheese and oil over the onions and bake for 25 minutes. Serve hot or warm.

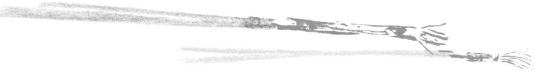

Cheesy peasy puff turnover

Another quick corner-shop special and an ideal way to use pastry left over from another recipe. Choose a well-flavoured (not too strong) cheese and don't be afraid to use up odds and ends – a little Parmesan never goes amiss.

SERVES 2–3

A little sunflower oil (optional)

About 200g all-butter, ready-made puff pastry

About 75g frozen peas or petits pois

About 75g mature Cheddar, hard goat's cheese or other well-flavoured hard cheese, grated

1 large egg, beaten

Sea salt and freshly ground black pepper

Preheat the oven to 200°C/Gas Mark 6. Lightly oil a baking sheet or line with a non-stick liner.

If your puff pastry isn't ready-rolled, roll it out and trim to a square, roughly 20cm. Place it on the baking sheet. Carefully place the frozen peas in the centre and scatter over a little salt and pepper. Scatter the grated cheese evenly over the peas.

Brush the edges of the pastry with beaten egg. Trickle most of the rest of the egg over the cheese and peas, leaving a teaspoonful or so. Fold the pastry over to form a large triangle and pinch the edges together firmly to seal. Brush the pastry with the remaining egg and bake for 20 minutes, or until golden brown. Serve hot.

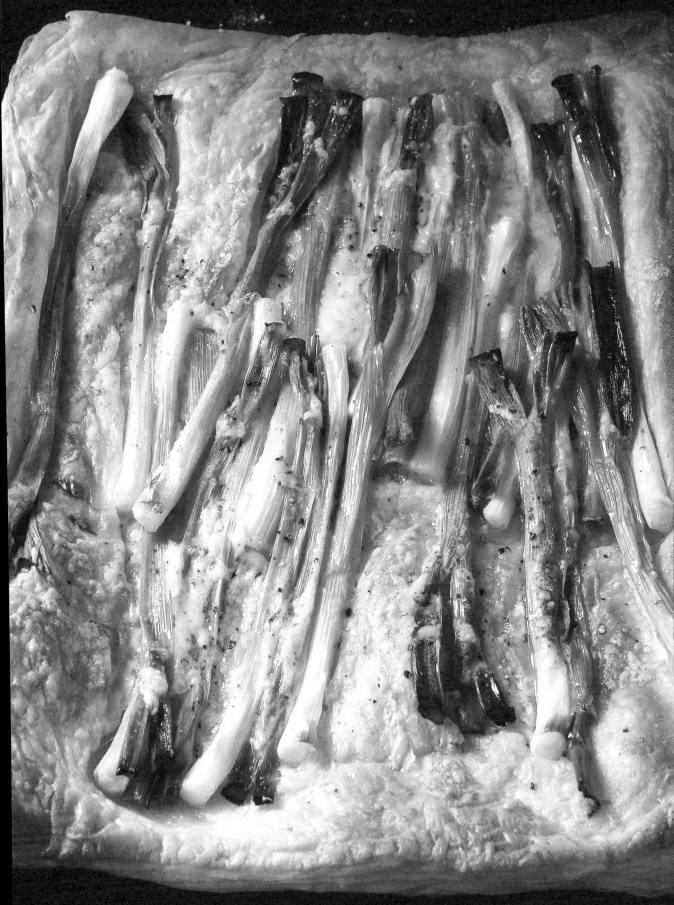

Green beans, new potatoes and olives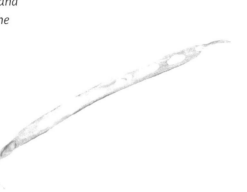

Straightforward it may be, but this is one of my favourite recipes in this chapter. It's such a simple combination: just two vegetables mixed with a few aromatic ingredients, which form a sort of deconstructed tapenade. It's very easy to throw together, looks glossy and gorgeous, and always seems to hit the spot: a perfect summer supper.

SERVES 2-3

500g small new potatoes

200g French or other green beans, trimmed and cut into 3–4cm lengths

2 tablespoons olive oil

2 garlic cloves, thinly slivered

50g stoned black olives, very roughly chopped

A good handful of basil, shredded

A generous squeeze of lemon juice

Sea salt and freshly ground black pepper

Cut the potatoes into 2 or 3 pieces each. Put them in a saucepan, cover with water, add salt and bring to the boil, then lower the heat. Simmer for about 8 minutes, until tender, adding the beans for the last 2 or 3 minutes. Drain well and return to the hot pan.

Meanwhile, heat the olive oil in a small pan over a low heat. Add the garlic and cook very gently for a couple of minutes, without letting it colour. Add the chopped olives and cook for a minute more. Remove from the heat.

Tip the oil, garlic and olives into the pan with the potatoes and beans. Add the basil, a generous squeeze or two of lemon juice, and some salt and pepper. Toss together and serve warm.

VARIATION
Potatoes and 'deconstructed pesto'
Omit the beans. Heat the garlic in the oil, as above, then toss with the drained potatoes and loads of shredded basil (a good bunch), some lemon juice and plenty of slivered or finely grated Parmesan, hard goat's cheese or other well-flavoured hard cheese.

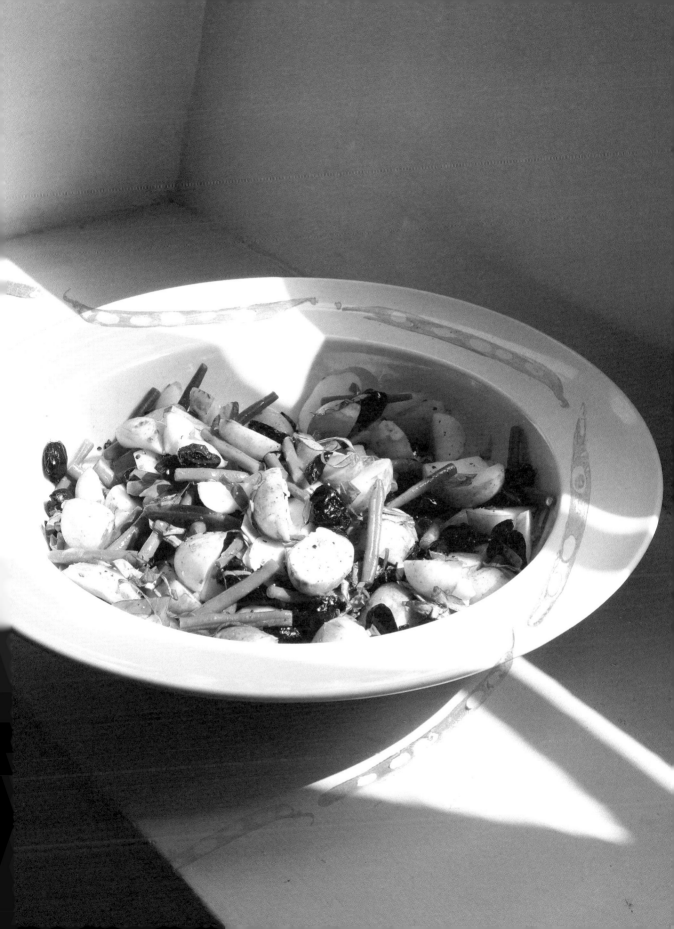

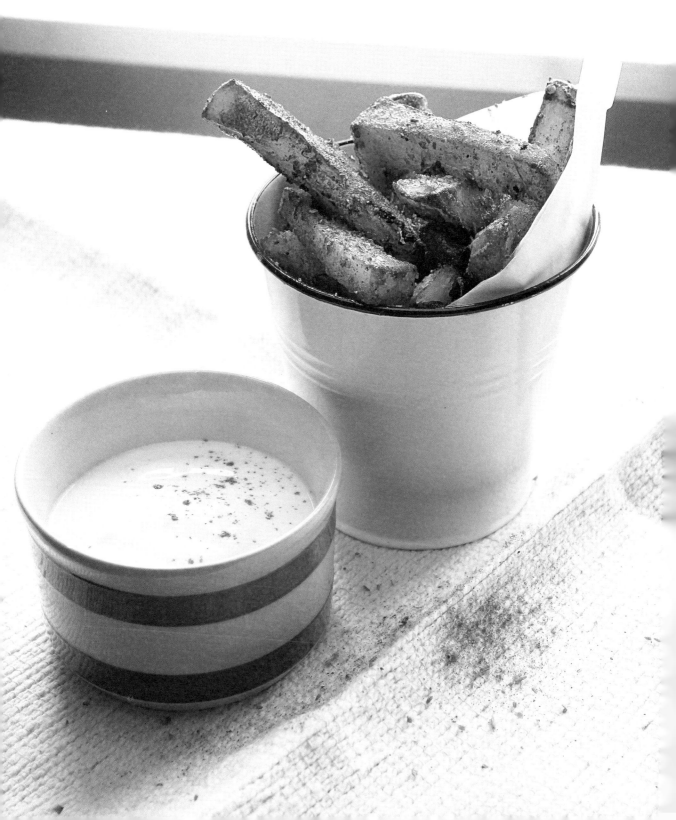

Spicy merguez oven chips with yoghurt dip

It's impossible to resist these spicy chips. You can use floury or waxy potatoes – either will be good – but floury ones such as Maris Piper or King Edward will give you more crumbly, crispy bits.

SERVES 4

About 1kg potatoes

5 tablespoons rapeseed or olive oil

FOR THE MERGUEZ SPICE MIX

1 teaspoon cumin seeds

1 teaspoon fennel seeds

1 teaspoon coriander seeds

1 teaspoon caraway seeds (optional)

10–12 black peppercorns

1 teaspoon sweet smoked paprika

A pinch of cayenne pepper

¼ teaspoon fine sea salt

FOR THE DIP

6 heaped tablespoons plain (full-fat) yoghurt

A scrap of garlic (about ¼ clove), crushed with a little salt

A pinch of cayenne, to sprinkle

Preheat the oven to 200°C/Gas Mark 6. Give the potatoes a good scrub (you don't need to peel them), then cut into thick chips. Put them into a saucepan and cover with cold water. Bring to a rolling boil and boil for 1 minute, then immediately drain well.

Meanwhile, for the spice mix, crush the cumin, fennel, coriander and caraway seeds, if using, with the black peppercorns to a powder, using a pestle and mortar. Combine with the paprika, cayenne and salt.

Pour the oil in a large, shallow roasting dish and put into the oven for 5 minutes to heat up.

Set aside about 1 heaped teaspoon of the spice mix. Add the rest to the drained potatoes and toss together. Take the hot roasting dish from the oven, add the spiced potatoes and turn to coat in the oil. Roast for 35–45 minutes, giving a stir halfway through, until golden and crisp.

Meanwhile, for the dip, stir the remaining spice mix into the yoghurt with the crushed garlic. Transfer to a serving bowl and sprinkle with a pinch of cayenne.

Test one of the spicy chips to see if they need sprinkling with a little more salt, then serve them hot, with the cool yoghurt dip.

VARIATION

Roasted new potatoes with harissa

Cut 750g new potatoes into even-sized chunks and spread out in a large roasting dish. Add 3 tablespoons rapeseed or olive oil and some salt and pepper and toss the potatoes to coat well. Roast at 190°C/Gas Mark 5 for 30–40 minutes until the potatoes are starting to turn golden brown and crisp. Take out, give them a good stir, then add 1 tablespoon harissa and toss to coat. Return to the oven for about 10 minutes until the harissa just starts to caramelise. Serve hot, scattered with chopped parsley. You can just eat these as they are or add some crumbled ricotta, Puy lentils (see page 237) or a poached egg (see page 210).

Twice baked potatoes

The jacket potato remains one of the best stand-by options when you find yourself tired, hungry and lacking the will to try something new. This way of preparing them is still simple but turns them from a predictable to a rich and indulgent supper. There are lots of different ways to jazz them up, as you'll see from my suggestions below.

SERVES 4

4 large baking potatoes

40g butter

180ml soured cream or crème fraîche

120g mature Cheddar, grated

2–3 spring onions, trimmed and thinly sliced

Sea salt and freshly ground black pepper

Preheat the oven to 200°C/Gas Mark 6. Place the potatoes on a baking sheet and cook for about an hour, until tender when pierced with a knife. Remove from the oven but leave the oven on.

When the potatoes are just cool enough to handle, carefully halve them lengthways – you might want to wrap them in a tea towel when you do this – and scoop out most of the insides into a bowl, leaving a shell about 5mm thick. Return these shells to the oven to crisp up while you make the filling (don't let them cook for more than 10 minutes).

Mash the scooped-out potato with the butter, then stir in the soured cream or crème fraîche, Cheddar and spring onions. Season generously with salt and pepper. Spoon the mixture back into the shells and bake until heated through, about 10–15 minutes. Cool slightly before serving.

VARIATIONS

• Instead of Cheddar, mash a little crumbled blue cheese, such as Stilton or Blue Vinny, and the leaves from a few thyme sprigs, into the potato.

• Cook, drain, squeeze and chop some spinach. Add to the potato with a handful of grated Gruyère and a grating or two of nutmeg.

• Sauté some chopped onion until soft and turning golden, add 1 or 2 crushed garlic cloves, 1 teaspoon curry powder and a handful of peas. Mix into the mash, adding, if you like, some cubes of paneer, cottage cheese or cream cheese, before spooning back into the potato shells and baking.

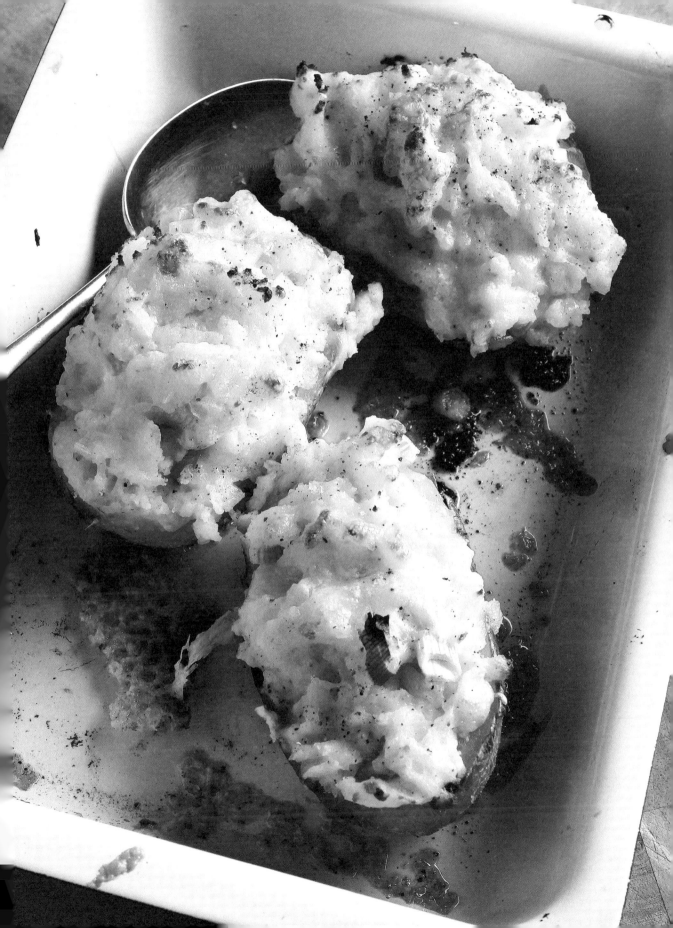

Curried bubble and squeak^v

Bubble and squeak is surely one of the finest leftovers dishes known to man. This is just a mildly spicy riff on the theme – but a great one, nonetheless. Some recipes bind everything together, perhaps with an egg, to form a fryable cake but I prefer a more rough and tumble approach, like a hash. This is good as it is, but absolutely excellent with a poached egg.

SERVES 3–4

2–4 tablespoons rapeseed or sunflower oil

1 onion, quartered and finely sliced

1 garlic clove, crushed

1 heaped teaspoon curry powder or paste

About 400g cold, cooked potatoes (boiled, baked, roast or mashed), in rough chunks

About 200g cold, cooked cabbage, greens, kale or Brussels sprouts, roughly shredded or chopped

Sea salt and freshly ground black pepper

Heat 2 tablespoons oil in a large, non-stick frying pan over a medium heat. Add the onion and fry for 6–7 minutes, until soft and just starting to colour. Add the garlic and curry powder or paste and cook for another 2 minutes.

Add the potato chunks and cook for a few minutes, stirring often, until they start to colour. You may want to add a little more oil at this stage and you'll probably need to use the edge of a spatula to scrape up some of the lovely crusty bits from the bottom of the pan. Add the cabbage or greens and cook, stirring, for a further 2–3 minutes.

Season with salt and pepper and serve straight away, topping each portion with a poached egg (see page 210) if you like.

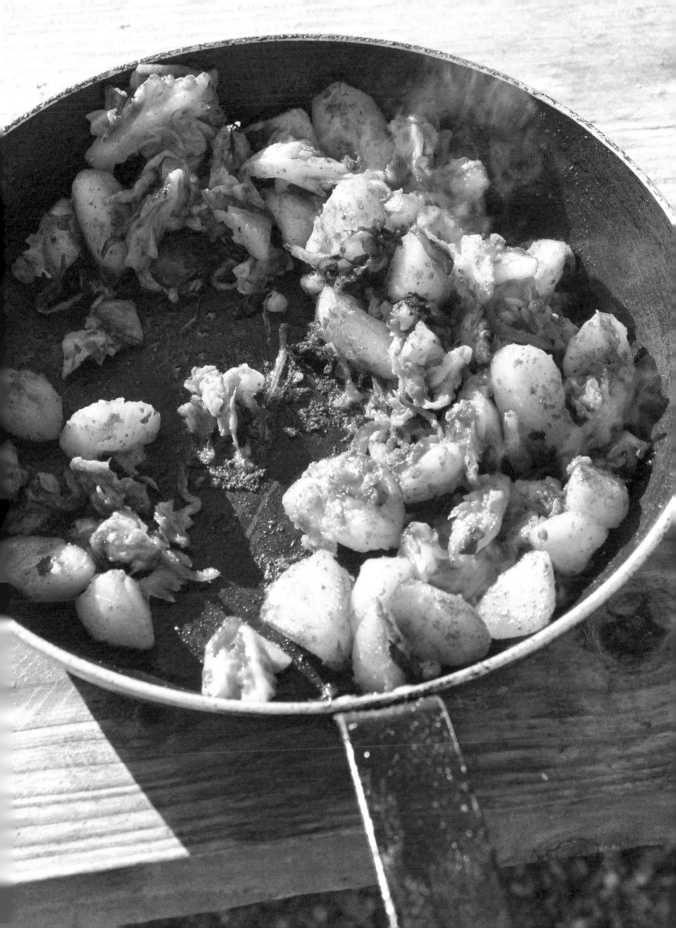

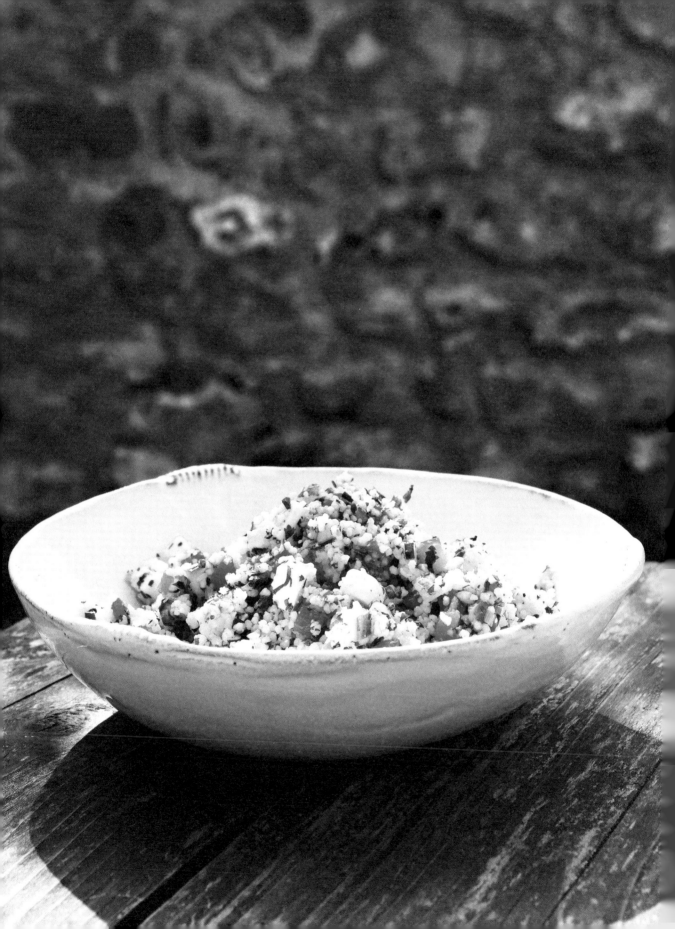

Quick couscous salad with peppers and feta

Although you can cook the couscous especially, this is the sort of thing I often throw together with what's left over from the day before. In fact, I nearly always cook more couscous than I need to be sure that I have leftovers for a dish like this. Do vary the flavourings: try basil, coriander or mint with – or in place of – parsley, and spice it up with a pinch or two of dried chilli flakes if you like. It pays to be generous with the herbs: some Middle-Eastern couscous dishes are almost green with the amount of herbs used, and that's the way I like them.

SERVES 4

250g couscous

2 tablespoons olive oil

Juice of ½ lemon

280g jar chargrilled red peppers in olive oil, drained and cut into 1cm dice

1 small cucumber, cut into 1cm dice

1 small red onion, finely chopped

200g feta cheese, cut into 1cm cubes

A large handful of flat-leaf parsley, finely chopped

Sea salt and freshly ground black pepper

Cook the couscous according to the instructions on the packet. As soon as it's cooked, trickle over the olive oil and lemon juice, season with salt and pepper, and fork the couscous gently to separate the grains. Leave to cool a little, and fork again.

While the dressed couscous is still just warm, or cool (but not hot), add the red peppers, cucumber, onion, feta and parsley and toss gently until thoroughly combined. Taste and add more salt and pepper if it needs it, and trickle over a little more olive oil if it tastes at all dry. Serve still slightly warm, or at room temperature.

VARIATIONS

Tomato and olive couscous ♥

Prepare the couscous as above, forking it with the olive oil, lemon juice, salt and pepper. While still warm, toss with 300g cored, deseeded and diced tomatoes or halved cherry tomatoes, 125g roughly chopped stoned black olives, 6 finely chopped trimmed spring onions, 100g toasted pine nuts and a finely chopped small handful each of parsley and basil. Check the seasoning and add a little more olive oil if needed.

Moroccan spiced couscous ♥

Prepare the couscous as above, adding ½ teaspoon each ground cumin and coriander and ¼ teaspoon ground cinnamon to the cooking water. Fork with the olive oil, lemon juice, salt and pepper. While still warm, toss with a drained, rinsed 400g tin of chickpeas, 40g chopped dried apricots, 40g sultanas, 40g toasted chopped almonds or pistachios and a finely chopped handful each of parsley and coriander. You can also add leftover roast veg, such as carrots or squash, cut into cubes. Taste and add more salt and pepper and a little more olive oil if needed.

Frittata with summer veg and goat's cheese

A traditional frittata is a lovely way to celebrate the arrival of early summer veg. If you have some cooked new potatoes to hand, or indeed any other leftover veg, you can use them here – but cooking them from scratch doesn't take long. I like to use two or three different green veg.

SERVES 4-6

400g new potatoes

About 300g mixed summer veg, such as asparagus, French beans, shelled young broad beans, shelled or frozen peas (defrosted), broccoli

2 tablespoons rapeseed or olive oil

2 bunches of spring onions, trimmed and roughly chopped

A good handful of chives and/ or flat-leaf parsley, chopped

7 large or 8 medium eggs

About 75g medium-strong goat's cheese (hard or soft, it doesn't matter)

Sea salt and freshly ground black pepper

Cut the new potatoes into 5mm slices. Put them into a large pan, cover with plenty of water, add salt and bring to the boil. Meanwhile, if using, cut French beans and asparagus into 3–4cm lengths; cut broccoli into small florets.

When the potatoes come to the boil, add the green vegetables. Once the water has returned to the boil, reduce the heat and simmer for 3–4 minutes, by which time all the veg should be just tender. Drain well.

Preheat the oven to 180°C/Gas Mark 4, or preheat the grill to medium. Heat the oil in a large non-stick frying pan (about 28cm) over a medium heat. Add the spring onions and sweat for about 5 minutes, until soft. Add the drained vegetables and herbs and toss with the onions. Turn the heat to medium-low.

Beat the eggs together with plenty of salt and pepper and pour over the veg in the pan. Cook gently, without stirring, until the egg is about two-thirds set, with a layer of wet egg still on top. Crumble or roughly chop the cheese and scatter over the surface of the frittata, then transfer the pan to the oven or grill for a further 4–5 minutes, until the egg is all set and the top is starting to colour.

Leave to cool slightly, then slide the frittata out on to a plate or board. Serve warm or cold, cut into slices.

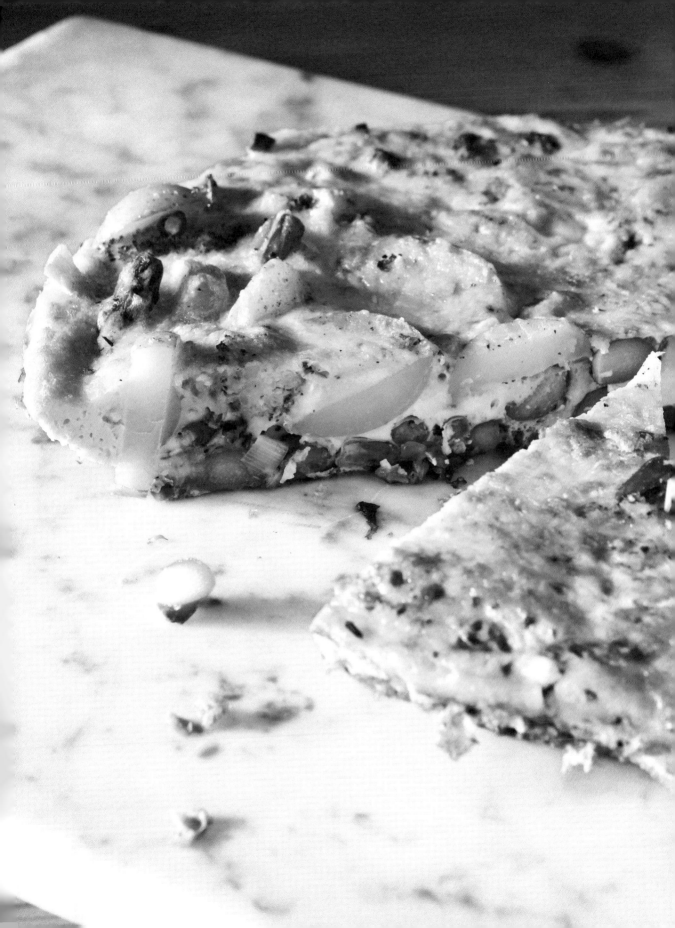

Oven-roasted roots frittata

This is a great way to use up odds and ends of fresh veg, and leftovers too. You can use more or less whatever you fancy from the list, though I do think some kind of onion is essential. As the egg is poured straight into the roasting dish full of hot veg, you don't need to fry this frittata at all, but it helps to have a heavy ceramic or cast-iron dish, which retains the heat well. And the eggs should be at room temperature, not cold from the fridge.

SERVES 4–6

About 600g mixed winter veg, such as shallots or onions, carrots, squash or pumpkin, parsnip, celeriac, beetroot, potatoes

1 large garlic clove, finely chopped

3 tablespoons rapeseed or olive oil

7 large or 8 medium eggs

A handful of mixed herbs, such as curly parsley, chives and thyme, finely chopped

About 20g Parmesan, hard goat's cheese or other well-flavoured hard cheese, grated

Sea salt and freshly ground black pepper

Preheat the oven to 190°C/Gas Mark 5. Meanwhile, prepare your chosen veg: peel shallots or onions and quarter or thickly slice; peel carrots and cut into 5mm slices; peel squash or pumpkin, deseed and cut into 2–3cm cubes; peel parsnip, celeriac and beetroot and cut into 1–2cm cubes; cut potatoes into 1–2cm cubes.

Put all the veg into an ovenproof dish, about 23cm square. Add the garlic, oil and plenty of salt and pepper and toss well. Roast for about 40 minutes, stirring halfway through, until the veg are all tender and starting to caramelise in places.

Beat the eggs together with the chopped herbs and some more salt and pepper. Take the dish from the oven, pour the egg evenly over the veg and scatter over the grated cheese. Return to the oven for 10–15 minutes until the egg is all set and the top is starting to colour. If your oven has a grill, you can use that to accelerate the browning of the top.

Leave to cool slightly, then slide the frittata out on to a plate or board. Serve warm or cold. Perfect lunchbox fare…

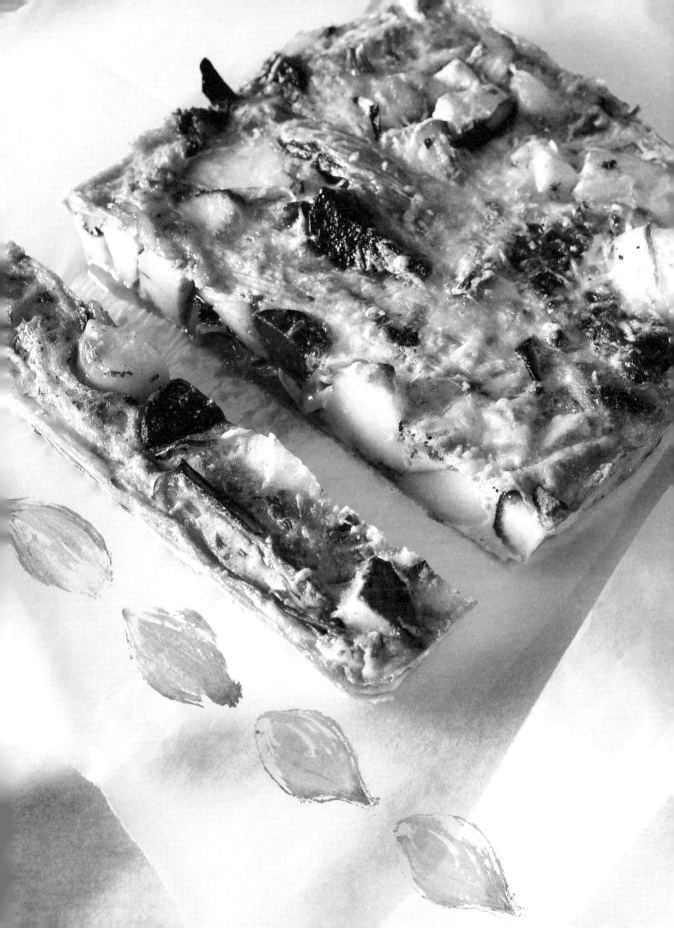

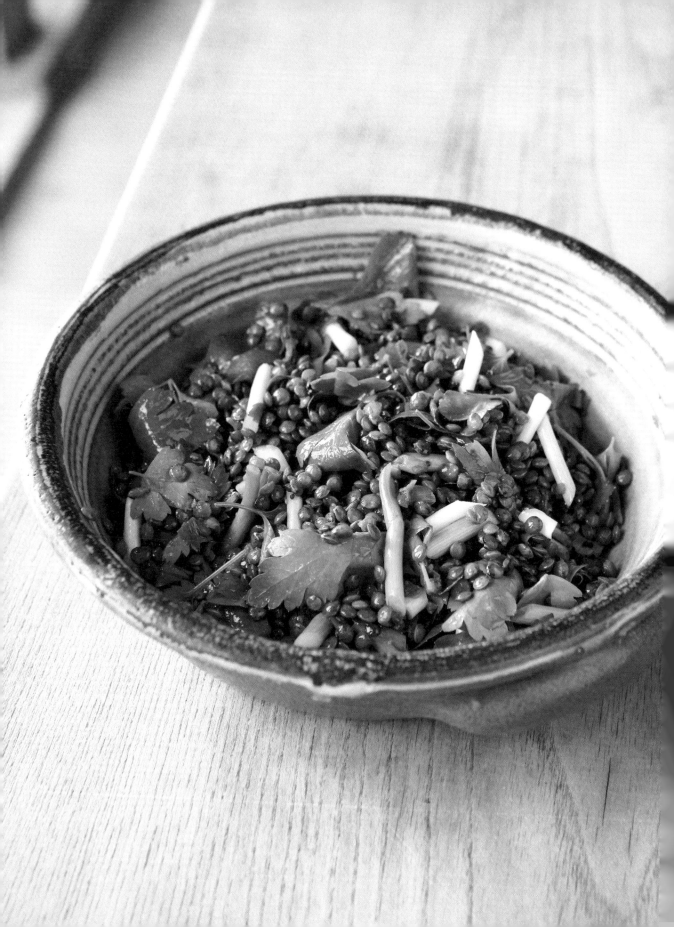

Dressed puy lentils ♥

These lovely, speckled green lentils are an absolute mainstay of my cooking. They get their distinctive earthy flavour from the volcanic soils around Puy in the Auvergne region of France. Their firm, nutty texture makes them great for adding to salads, or jumbling up with all manner of tasty companions.

SERVES 4–6

250g Puy lentils

Light vegetable stock (see page 130) or water

1 bay leaf

2 garlic cloves, bashed

A few parsley stalks (optional)

2 tablespoons olive oil

A squeeze of lemon juice

Salt and freshly ground black pepper

Put the lentils in a saucepan and add plenty of water. Bring to the boil and simmer for a minute only, then drain. Return the lentils to the pan and pour on just enough stock or water to cover them. Add the bay leaf, garlic and parsley stalks, if using. Bring back to a very gentle simmer, and cook slowly for about half an hour, until tender but not mushy.

Drain the lentils and discard the herbs and garlic. Dress with the olive oil and lemon juice, and season with salt and pepper to taste. Serve warm or cold.

FOUR WAYS WITH LENTILS

Lentil and parsley salad ♥ (shown left)
For the dressing, make a mustardy vinaigrette: shake 3 tablespoons olive oil, 1 tablespoon cider vinegar, 1 teaspoon mustard, a pinch each of salt and sugar and a few twists of black pepper together in a screw-topped jar. Toss the warm or cold lentils with the leaves from a good bunch of flat-leaf parsley, 3 trimmed spring onions, cut into short lengths, and the vinaigrette.

Summer garden lentils niçoise
Toss the warm lentils in a mustardy vinaigrette (see above) and mix in some crisp, cooked French beans, finely diced shallot or red onion, chopped black olives and quartered cherry tomatoes. Serve warm with poached eggs on top, or cold with quartered hard-boiled eggs.

Lentil and tomato salad
Toss the warm or cold lentils with honey roasted cherry tomatoes (see page 343) and a handful of rocket. You could finish with some shavings of Parmesan or hard goat's cheese too, if you like.

Lentils with beetroot and feta
Dress the warm lentils with olive oil and some balsamic vinegar and toss with wedges of roasted beetroot and cubes of feta or goat's cheese.

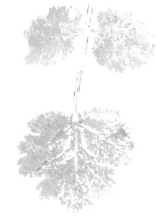

Dhal 🌱

A simple, red lentil dhal is such a great complement to so many vegetable dishes – not just curries or biryanis, pakoras or bhajis, but even simple fare such as shredded, stir-fried greens and a scoop of rice. It's a delicious way to add protein to a veg-based meal too. This easy but authentic example is based on a recipe from the wonderful Indian chef Udit Sarkhel.

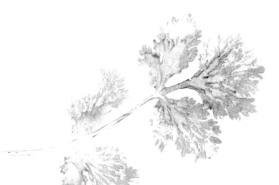

SERVES 4

250g red lentils

1 teaspoon ground turmeric

¾ teaspoon fine sea salt

2 tablespoons sunflower oil

1 teaspoon cumin seeds

1 onion, halved and thinly sliced

TO FINISH (OPTIONAL)

A small bunch of parsley or coriander, or a couple of sprigs of mint, roughly chopped

Put the lentils in a pan with 800ml cold water and bring to the boil. Skim off any scum, then stir in the turmeric and salt. Lower the heat and simmer, uncovered, for about 15 minutes, stirring or whisking vigorously every now and then, until the lentils have broken down completely and you have a purée – the consistency of a thick soup or thin porridge. You can whisk in a little hot water from a just-boiled kettle if you need to thin it a bit. Keep warm in the pan.

When the dhal is just about done, heat the sunflower oil in a frying pan over a medium heat. Add the cumin seeds and fry for a couple of minutes until browned and fragrant. Add the onion and fry fairly briskly for 5–10 minutes until golden brown, even just a smidge burnt.

Tip the mixture on to the hot lentils in the pan, cover and leave for 5 minutes, then stir in the onions and cumin. Taste and adjust the seasoning. This is very good with coriander, parsley or mint sprinkled on top – but that's not essential.

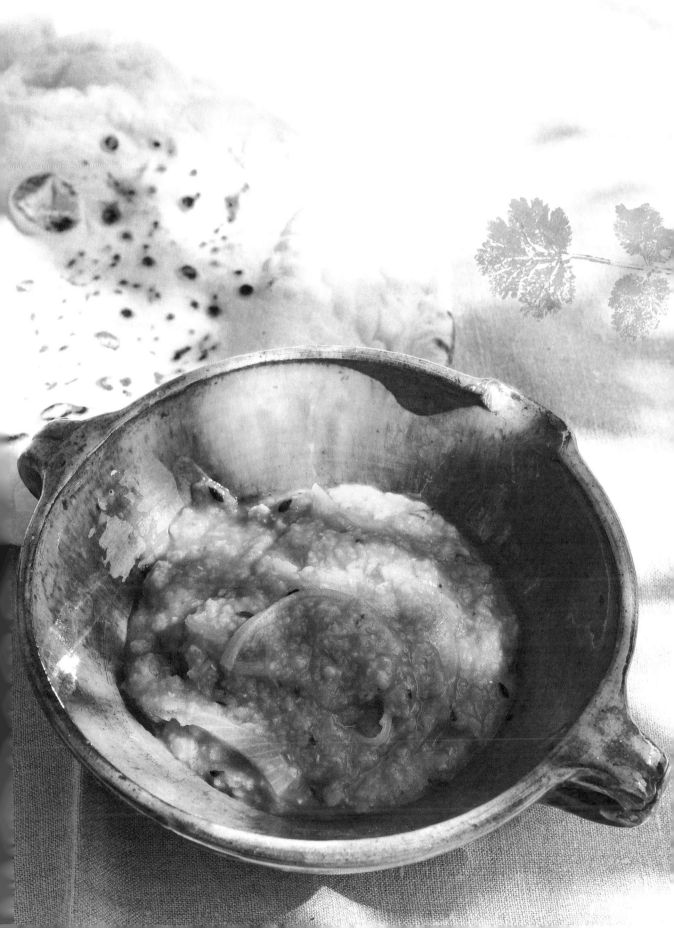

White beans with artichokes ♥

Decent, oil-preserved, char-grilled or roasted artichoke hearts, available from delis and some supermarkets, are a great store-cupboard standby. They're full of flavour and their oil is useful too.

SERVES 2

150g grilled/roasted artichoke hearts in oil, cut into wedges, plus 1 tablespoon of the oil

1 garlic clove, slivered

400g tin cannellini or other white beans, drained and rinsed

Juice of ½ lemon

A good handful of salad leaves

Sea salt and freshly ground black pepper

A little crumbled or shaved goat's cheese or Parmesan, to finish (optional)

Heat 1 tablespoon oil from the artichokes in a small frying pan over a medium-low heat. Add the garlic and fry gently for a minute or two. Add the artichokes and heat for a minute or so, then stir in the beans. Heat, stirring, for 2–3 minutes, until everything is hot. Remove from the heat, add the lemon juice and season with salt and pepper to taste (the artichokes may already have contributed some salt).

Arrange the salad leaves on two plates and top with the hot beans and artichokes. Finish with the goat's cheese or Parmesan, if you like, and serve warm.

VARIATION

White bean salad with tomatoes and red onion ♥
Here's another very quick but really quite substantial beany supper. To make a creamy dressing, whisk 3 tablespoons rapeseed or olive oil, 1 tablespoon lemon juice, ½ teaspoon English mustard, a pinch of sugar and some salt and pepper together in a large bowl. Finely slice ½ small red onion and add to the dressing with a drained and rinsed 400g tin of white beans. Add about 150g ripe, sweet tomatoes (any kind, but cherry tomatoes are good), cut into smallish pieces (or halved, if cherry type). Serve with parsley sprinkled on top, or salad leaves underneath – or both – and some bread on the side.

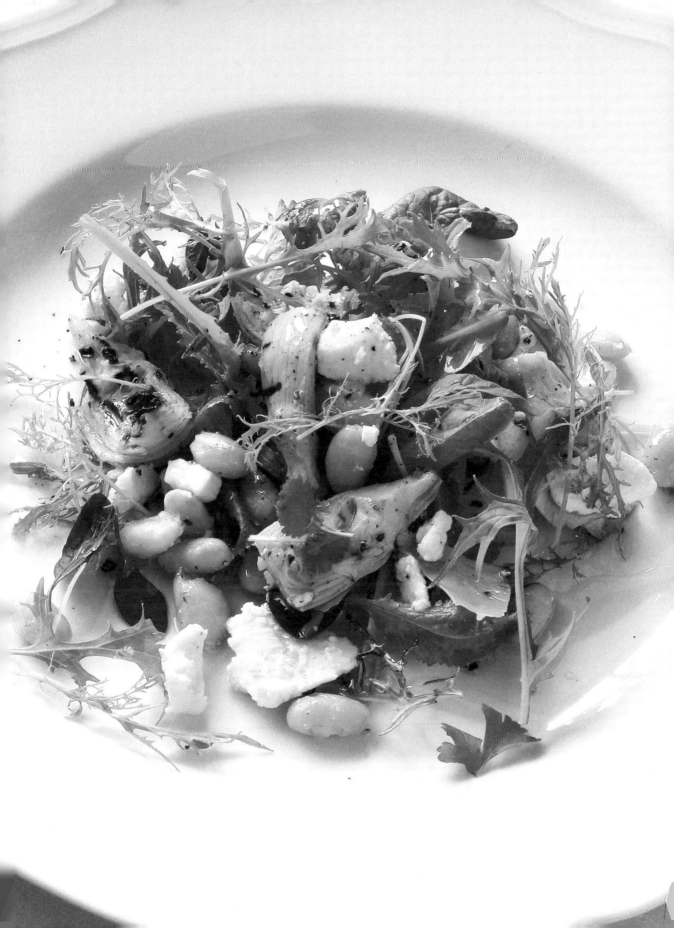

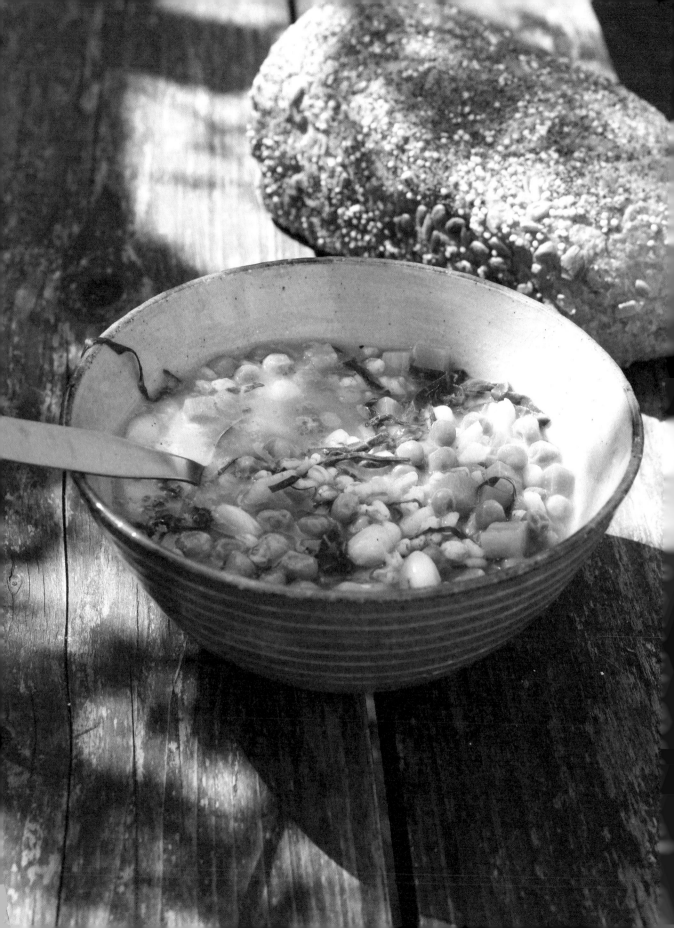

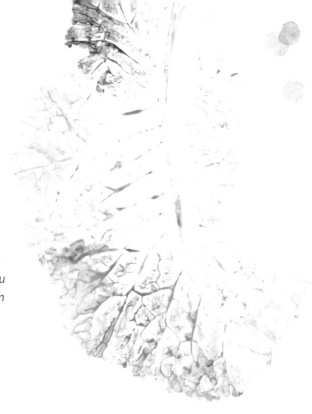

Raid-the-larder bean and spelt broth

This is a quick but sustaining broth. The stock, spelt and beans form the heart of it and the fresh veg you then add pretty much depends on you – or what's in the fridge/freezer/garden.

SERVES 2

750ml vegetable stock (from a cube or bouillon powder is fine)

50g pearled spelt (or pearl barley)

A few leaves of cabbage, kale or greens or a couple of handfuls of spinach, washed

1 medium carrot, peeled and diced

100g frozen peas or petits pois

400g tin cannellini or other white beans, drained and rinsed

Sea salt and freshly ground black pepper

Extra virgin olive oil, to finish

Bring the stock to the boil in a saucepan. Add the spelt (or barley), reduce the heat and simmer until almost tender, about 15 minutes (or a bit longer for barley).

Meanwhile, remove any tough stalks or ribs from the greens or spinach and shred the leaves roughly.

Add the carrot, peas and tinned beans to the broth. Once it returns to a simmer, add the greens or spinach and cook for a further 2–3 minutes, until just tender. Season with salt and pepper to taste, then ladle into bowls. Finish with a generous trickle of olive oil and serve.

VARIATIONS

Try diced parsnip instead of carrot, or sliced green beans instead of peas. Almost any shredded greens will work, even Brussels sprouts or lettuce.

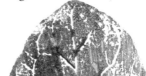

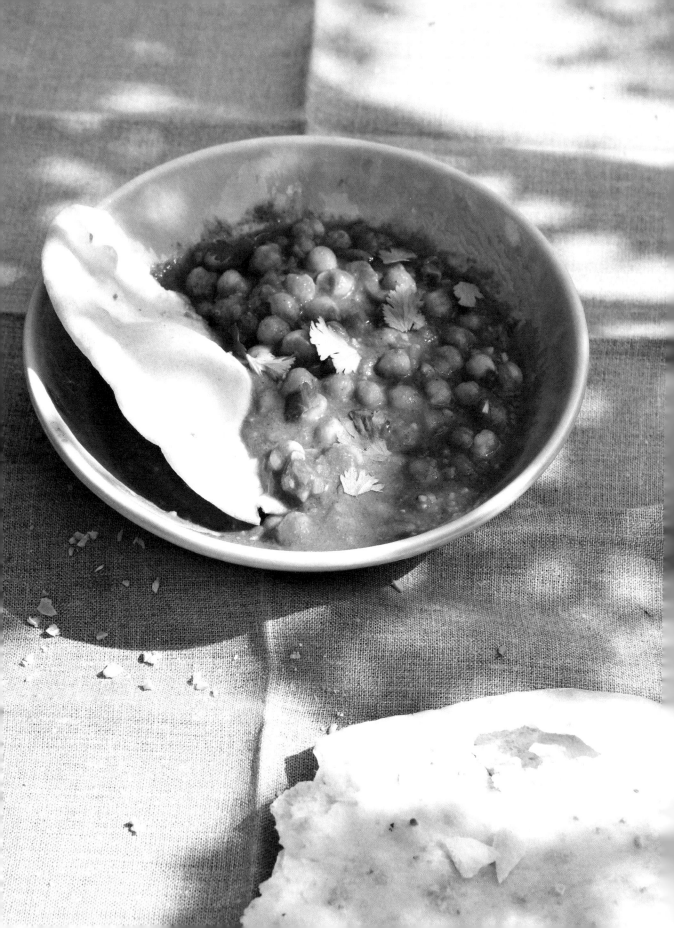

Chickpea ketchup curry ᵛ

*I have no problem with using
'cheaty' ingredients when a quick
meal is called for – as long as
they are good quality cheats.
I cadged the idea of basing a
curry on a decent tomato ketchup
from a Martha Stewart recipe.
The sauce lends bags of spice and
a delicate, mango-chutney-like
sweetness to the dish. The logical
variation – a ketchup bean chilli
– is also a winner.*

SERVES 2

2 tablespoons sunflower oil

1 small onion, thinly sliced

2cm piece of ginger,
finely grated

A pinch of dried chilli flakes

1 garlic clove, crushed

2 teaspoons curry powder
or paste

400g tin chickpeas, drained
and rinsed

5 tablespoons tomato ketchup

Juice of ½ lemon

Sea salt and freshly ground
black pepper

A handful of coriander,
to finish

Heat the oil in a frying pan over a medium-low heat. Add the onion
and sweat for around 8 minutes, until soft and golden, then stir in the
ginger, chilli flakes, garlic and curry powder or paste. Fry, stirring, for
1–2 minutes more.

Add the chickpeas, tomato ketchup and enough water to just loosen to
a thick sauce consistency. Simmer gently for about 5 minutes, then stir
in the lemon juice. Taste and add salt and pepper if needed.

Serve in warmed bowls scattered with coriander leaves. Plain rice,
quick-cook noodles, naan or flatbreads are all good accompaniments.

VARIATION

Ketchup chilli
This spiced-up bean chilli is unbelievably simple and really good.
Use a 400g tin of kidney (or other) beans instead of the chickpeas, and
2 teaspoons sweet paprika (or 1 teaspoon each of sweet and hot) instead
of the curry powder. This is great served on rice, baked potatoes or
toast, or with tortillas or tostadas, and with toppings such as soured
cream, grated cheese, guacamole ...

Quick chickpea pasta

Wholesome, hearty and quick, this is a lovely store-cupboard supper just as it is. Or, you could jazz it up a little if you like, perhaps adding some frozen petits pois along with the chickpeas, or some chopped fresh herbs at the end.

SERVES 2

125g small pasta shapes, such as orecchiette or conchigliette

400g tin chickpeas, drained and rinsed

3 tablespoons olive oil

1 garlic clove, slivered

1 red chilli, deseeded and finely chopped

A good squeeze of lemon juice

Sea salt and freshly ground black pepper

Parmesan, hard goat's cheese or other well-flavoured hard cheese, grated, to serve

Bring a pan of water to the boil, salt it well, then add the pasta and cook according to the packet instructions. About 2 minutes before the end, add the chickpeas to the pan, to heat through with the pasta.

Meanwhile, heat the olive oil in a small pan over a very gentle heat. Add the garlic and chilli and cook very gently for 2–3 minutes, without letting the garlic colour. Remove from the heat.

Drain the pasta and chickpeas well. Stir in the garlic, chilli and oil. Add salt and pepper and a good squeeze of lemon juice, to taste. Serve topped with plenty of grated cheese.

Chickpeas with cumin and spinach ^v

This delicately spiced quickie is very good with some warm pitta or flatbreads.

SERVES 2

2 tablespoons sunflower or rapeseed oil

1 small onion, sliced

1 garlic clove, chopped

½ red chilli, deseeded and finely chopped, or a pinch of dried chilli flakes

1 teaspoon ground cumin

Grated zest of 1 lemon

4–6 large fresh plum tomatoes or a 400g tin plum tomatoes

About 150g spinach, washed

400g tin chickpeas, drained and rinsed

Sea salt and freshly ground black pepper

Heat the oil in a saucepan over a medium-low heat. Add the onion and sweat gently for about 8 minutes, stirring occasionally, till tender and golden. Add the garlic, chilli, cumin and lemon zest and cook for another 1–2 minutes.

Halve the fresh tomatoes and grate their flesh directly into the pan, discarding the skins. Alternatively, finely chop tinned tomatoes, discarding any skin and stalky ends, then add to the pan. Stir well and bring the mixture to a simmer, then simmer gently for a few minutes, until saucy.

Meanwhile, remove any tough stalks from the spinach and roughly shred larger leaves. Add to the pan and stir over the heat until wilted, then add the chickpeas and some salt and pepper. Cook for a few minutes, just to heat the chickpeas through, then taste and adjust the seasoning if needed. Serve with warm flatbreads or pitta.

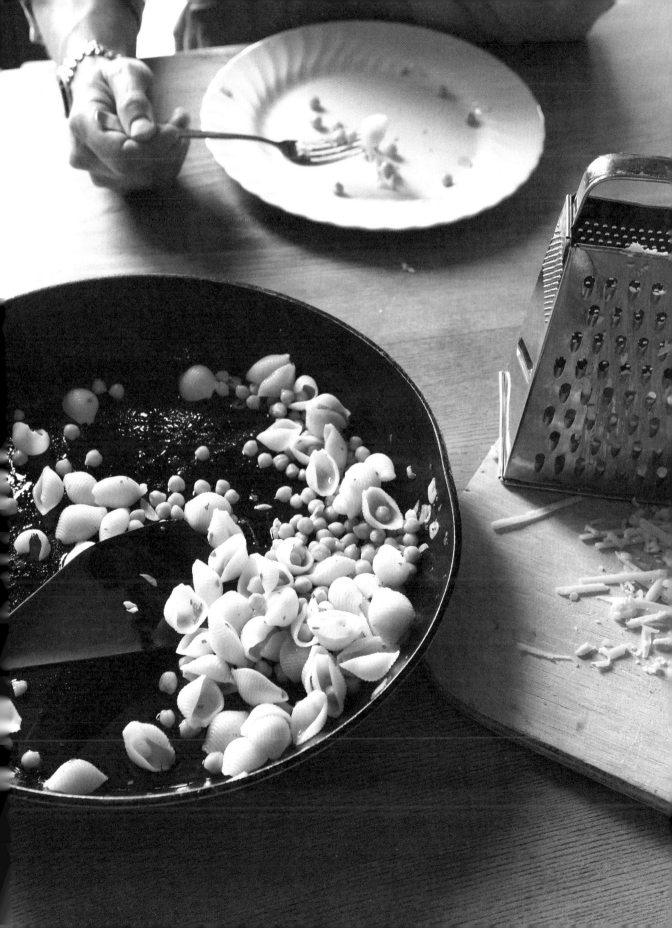

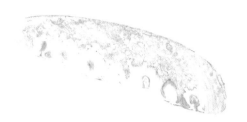

DIY 'pot' noodles

I first experimented with these when I was looking at ways to improve workday lunches. However, the concept works equally well as a fast and very satisfying supper. It's important to find the right kind of noodle – one that will soften nicely in boiling water from the kettle without the need for pan-cooking. I find flat, thin, quick-cook egg noodles fit the bill very well. The 'pot' should be covered once the water is added… with this in mind, a sealable heatproof jar, such as a kilner, is ideal.

SERVES 1

1 nest of thin, quick-cook egg noodles

1 teaspoon vegetable bouillon powder, or ¼ veg stock cube

A good pinch of soft brown sugar

1 small carrot, peeled and very thinly sliced or cut into fine julienne

3–4 spring onions, trimmed and finely sliced

6 sugar snap peas, shredded, or a few frozen petits pois

1 leaf of spring greens or green cabbage or a couple of leaves of pak choi, stalk removed, finely shredded

½ teaspoon freshly grated ginger

½ garlic clove, grated

¼ red or green chilli, deseeded and finely chopped

2 teaspoons soy sauce

Juice of ½ lime

Put all the ingredients, except the soy sauce and lime, in a 'pot'. Pour over boiling water to just cover everything, pressing the ingredients down. Cover and leave for 8–10 minutes, stirring once or twice, then add soy sauce and lime juice to taste, and eat.

VARIATION

Curried mushroom pot

This works 'instantly' with raw mushrooms and defrosted frozen peas; you can of course add other finely sliced or shredded cooked veg too. Mix ½ teaspoon cornflour with 1 teaspoon curry powder and put into a 'pot' with a nest of thin, quick-cook egg noodles, 3–4 finely sliced mushrooms, 1 tablespoon defrosted frozen peas, 1 finely grated small garlic clove and a finely grated 1–2cm piece of ginger, along with about 25g paneer (Indian cheese) if you can get hold of some. Season with salt and pepper. Pour over boiling water to just cover everything, pressing the ingredients down. Cover and leave for 8–10 minutes, stirring once or twice, then eat.

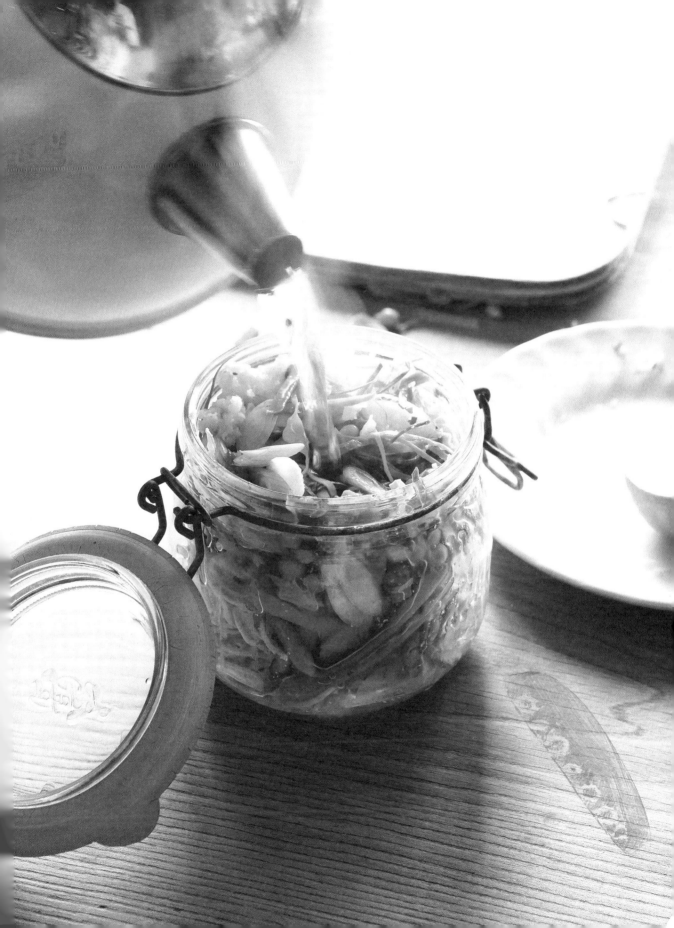

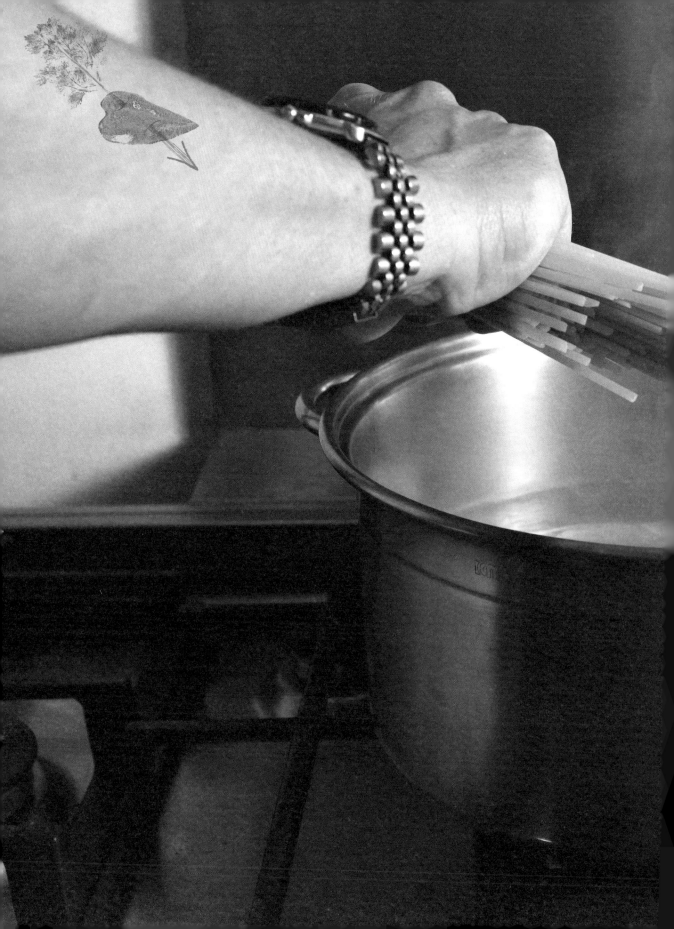

Pasta & rice

When tummies are rumbling and time is tight, pasta, rice and what I think of as their sister ingredients – grains such as spelt, barley and quinoa – are ideal. You don't really need to cook them – you can just ask a helpful pan of simmering water to do it for you. Even a risotto, which requires a bit of hands-on cooking, needn't be more than half an hour in the making. So, while not all the recipes here are as quick as those in the store-cupboard suppers chapter, they're certainly pretty undemanding.

Pasta is an easy fallback – too easy, maybe – in danger of losing its charm, and selling itself short. Personally, if forced to choose, I would rather eat rice than pasta every day. That's because I accept rice as a kind of neutral ballast and flavour carrier, whereas pasta is, or should be, a little more than that. Served up with the right sauce, something that fits its shape and coats its curves, it's a proper treat. In the interests of eating it a little less but enjoying it a lot more, it's worth thinking about how to get the very best out of pasta.

In most of the recipes, I've suggested a particular pasta shape that I think would go well with the other ingredients. I do believe the form of the pasta makes a difference to the eating experience – but I would never want to become a pasta pedant. For myself, I'm perfectly happy to replace linguine with spaghetti, or macaroni with penne, or conchiglie with farfalle. I certainly wouldn't avoid a pasta recipe simply because I didn't have the right shape in the cupboard.

When it comes to cooking pasta, be generous with the salt you add to the water. Most of that salt will remain in the water, of course, but the pasta will absorb and be seasoned by some of it in a way that cannot be replicated by adding salt later. Some Italian cooks swear by the 1000:100:10 ratio, which means 1000g of water (ie 1 litre) per 100g of pasta, and 10g of salt. I think that's a bit too much, but I'd certainly put 20–25g (ie a good tablespoon) of salt in roughly 4–5 litres of boiling water, in which I'll usually cook 350g or so of pasta to feed four or five of us.

Cooking time is the other crucial variable. Perfect pasta should be, as I'm sure you know, *al dente* – or 'to the tooth'. I recommend that you start testing it a good minute or two before the cooking time suggested on the packet is up. You aren't looking for any kind of chalky uncooked-ness in the pasta, just a little bit of resistance. Pasta cooked to this degree really is much nicer to eat than when it is softened to the point of collapse – and it holds sauces and dressings better as well.

I want to say a bit more about rice, too. It's a grain I'm turning to more frequently. I find it, paradoxically, a light way to fill up – satisfying but somehow never heavy. An increasing number of people have problems digesting wheat and opt for rice instead – you can even buy rice pasta, though it's not as good as wheat pasta. Whether or not you have specific issues with wheat, I think it's a good idea to vary the starches you eat. Making sure rice appears on your table as often as bread or pasta is one way to do that.

Rice cooking for many seems to be freighted with anxieties, but it needn't be. You might consider investing in a proper rice-cooker. They are surprisingly inexpensive and I've been impressed with the results from these machines – the grains emerge tender and well separated. (I'm sceptical of the word 'fluffy' being applied to rice. Surely that's for kittens?) When cooking rice in a saucepan I still rely on the simple tea-towel-under-the-lid absorption method used in the vegeree on page 276. I don't claim to understand why that tea towel makes a difference but it works for me. However you cook 'plain' rice, such as long-grain or basmati, thoroughly rinsing the rice *before* cooking, to remove all excess starch, is important – as is simmering the rice gently, rather than boiling.

Risotto rice is a different proposition, of course, because here you want to keep all the starch that clings to the grains, to thicken it into a lovely soupy texture. Cooking risotto is not difficult, but you do need to get a bit of a feel for it, to catch the rice at the right point of done-ness. That's a matter of personal taste, of course, but I like just the faintest hint of chalkiness in the middle of the grain. It's something that simply comes with practice – I hope the comforting risotto recipes in this chapter will keep you keen.

The other grains you'll find here include quinoa – a fantastically proteinaceous little Latin American seed, which I heartily recommend. It might take you two or three goes to be won over – it did me – but I bet you'll end up a fan. Then there's spelt – the whole, pearled grains of which have almost completely sidelined pearl barley in my cooking (though of course you can use that instead). I use a locally produced, organic spelt grain that cooks very easily to a nutty, nubbly finish. It also soaks up a flavourful stock to great effect: the 'speltotto' is now a pillar of my kitchen and I urge you to give it a go.

I have found that forgoing meat more often, and excluding it deliberately from dishes that are built around pasta, rice and other grains, has heightened my enjoyment of these brilliant ingredients. I hope it'll do the same for you.

Pasta with raw tomato ᵛ

This wonderfully simple raw tomato sauce can be tweaked and flavoured to your taste: sometimes I use mint instead of basil, or add a little finely chopped raw red onion or fennel, or replace the capers with sliced olives. Feel free to have fun with it and use several different varieties of tomato if you like.

SERVES 4

750g large, ripe tomatoes

1 garlic clove, finely chopped

1 tablespoon baby capers, rinsed

½ small red chilli, deseeded and finely chopped, or a pinch of dried chilli flakes

About 10 large basil leaves, shredded

100ml extra virgin rapeseed or olive oil

350g pasta shapes, such as small penne, conchigliette or orecchiette

Sea salt and freshly ground black pepper

Parmesan or hard goat's cheese, to serve (optional)

Put the tomatoes into a bowl, cover with boiling water and leave for just 1 minute, then remove and peel off their skins. Quarter and deseed the tomatoes, putting all the seeds and clinging juicy bits into a sieve over a bowl.

Roughly chop the deseeded tomato flesh and put into another bowl. Press the juice from the seeds in the sieve, adding it to the chopped tomatoes. Add the garlic, capers and chilli, half the shredded basil and the oil and toss to mix. Add a little salt and pepper (the capers may be quite salty). Set aside somewhere fairly cool, but not the fridge, for about an hour to allow the flavours to mingle.

Put a large pan of well-salted water on to boil. Add the pasta to the boiling water and cook until *al dente*, then drain well. Combine the pasta with the raw tomato sauce, then taste and adjust the seasoning.

Serve scattered with the remaining shredded basil and add a grinding of black pepper. You can add a few shavings of Parmesan or hard goat's cheese, but I prefer it without.

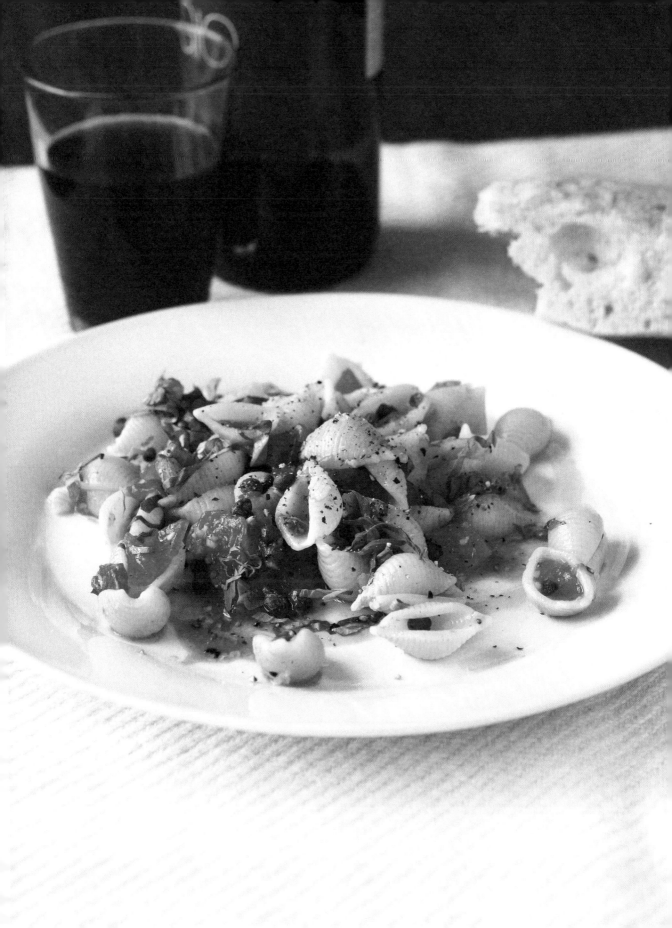

Pasta with new potatoes, green beans and pesto

This is a traditional Ligurian pasta dish: substantial but not as heavy as you might think. The green olives are authentic, but you can easily leave them out; I often do. A decent, ready-made pesto would work here, but the dish is taken to a whole new level if you make your own. I've used a combination of basil and parsley for the pesto but you can use all basil or all parsley if you prefer.

SERVES 4

300g new potatoes

300g pasta, such as trofie, orecchiette or penne

200g French or other green beans

50g stoned green olives, roughly sliced or chopped (optional)

FOR THE PESTO

50g pine nuts or walnuts, lightly toasted

A large bunch of basil (about 30g), leaves only

A large bunch of parsley (about 30g), leaves only

A few mint leaves (optional)

1 garlic clove, chopped

50g Parmesan, hard goat's cheese or other well-flavoured hard cheese, finely grated

Finely grated zest of ½ lemon

100–150ml extra virgin olive oil

A good squeeze of lemon juice

Sea salt and freshly ground black pepper

TO SERVE

Extra virgin olive oil, to trickle (optional)

Extra cheese (as above)

First make the pesto: put the toasted nuts into a food processor along with the herbs, garlic, grated cheese and lemon zest. Blitz to a paste, then, with the motor running, slowly pour in the olive oil until you have a thick, sloppy purée. Scrape the pesto into a bowl and season with salt, pepper and a good squeeze of lemon juice. This will keep in the fridge for a few days.

Put a very large pan of well-salted water on to boil. Meanwhile, cut the potatoes into thick matchsticks (the size of thin chips). Add the potatoes and pasta to the pan and cook until the pasta is *al dente* – probably 10–12 minutes, which should be the right amount of time for the potatoes too. If the pasta is a type that cooks very quickly, put the potatoes in a few minutes before. (If using very freshly dug new spuds, they'll cook quicker, 6–7 minutes, so add halfway through the pasta cooking). In the meantime, cut the beans into lengths that roughly match the size of the pasta. Add them to the pan about 4 minutes before the end of cooking.

Drain the pasta and vegetables, and let them steam off for a minute or two, then add the pesto and mix thoroughly but gently. Check the seasoning (it will probably benefit from a generous grinding of black pepper).

Divide between warmed serving bowls and scatter over the green olives, if using. Grate over some cheese and trickle over a little extra virgin olive oil if you like. Have extra cheese for grating on the table.

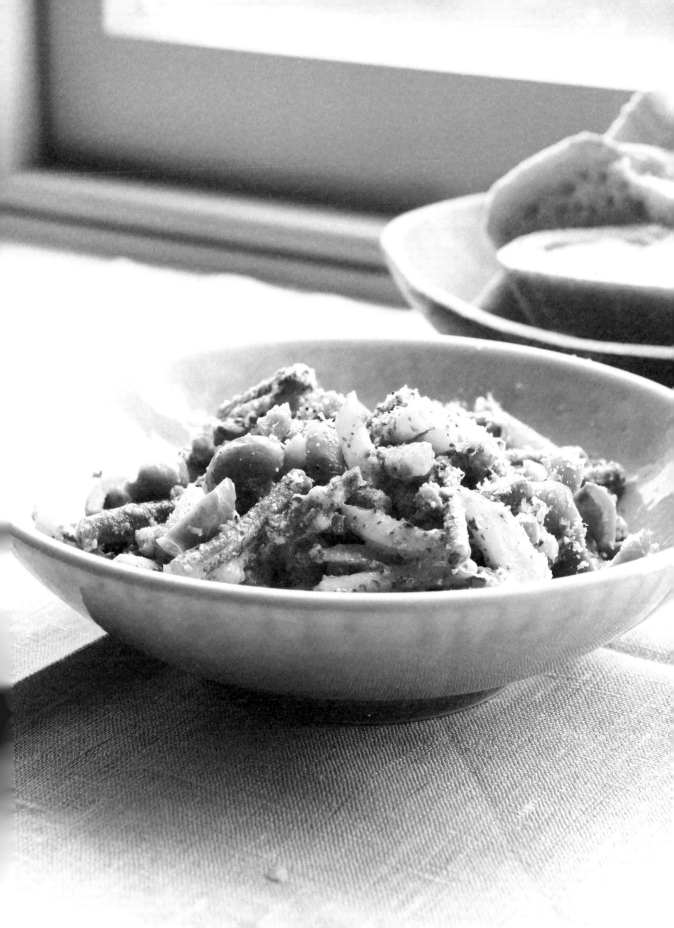

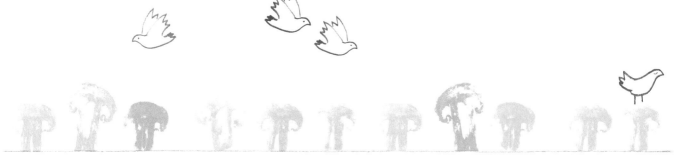

Mushroom risoniotto

Risoni (or orzo) is a tiny rice-shaped pasta with a unique charm. There's something deeply satisfying about its texture, and it's quicker and easier to cook than rice. Here, it's combined with a rich mushroom ragout for a warming autumn or winter dish. Use a dark and flavoursome variety of mushroom, such as chestnut, open-cap or field mushrooms, and include a few wild mushrooms if you have some to hand.

SERVES 2

2 tablespoons rapeseed or olive oil

A knob of butter

500g mushrooms (see above), cleaned, trimmed and thickly sliced

150g risoni or orzo pasta

2 garlic cloves, chopped

A few sprigs of thyme, leaves only

1 teaspoon balsamic vinegar

About 75ml dry white wine

About 50ml double cream or crème fraîche

Sea salt and freshly ground black pepper

A good handful of flat-leaf parsley, chopped, to serve

Put a large pan of well-salted water on to boil, so that you're ready to cook the pasta while the sauce is coming together.

Heat 1 tablespoon of the oil and half the butter in a large frying pan over a medium-high heat. Add half the mushrooms and cook briskly, stirring often, until all the liquid released has evaporated and the mushrooms are starting to caramelise. Transfer to a dish and repeat with the rest of the oil, butter and mushrooms. (Cooking in two batches like this avoids overcrowding the pan and ensures the mushrooms do not stew.)

When the second batch of mushrooms are nearly cooked, add the pasta to the pan of boiling water and cook until *al dente*.

Return the first lot of mushrooms to the frying pan. Add the garlic, thyme and balsamic vinegar and cook, stirring, for a minute or two. Add the wine and cook until there is almost no liquid left. Add the cream or crème fraîche, reduce the heat a little and stir until it is just about simmering. Season with salt and pepper to taste.

Drain the pasta as soon as it is cooked, add to the mushroom mixture and toss well. Serve scattered with lots of chopped parsley.

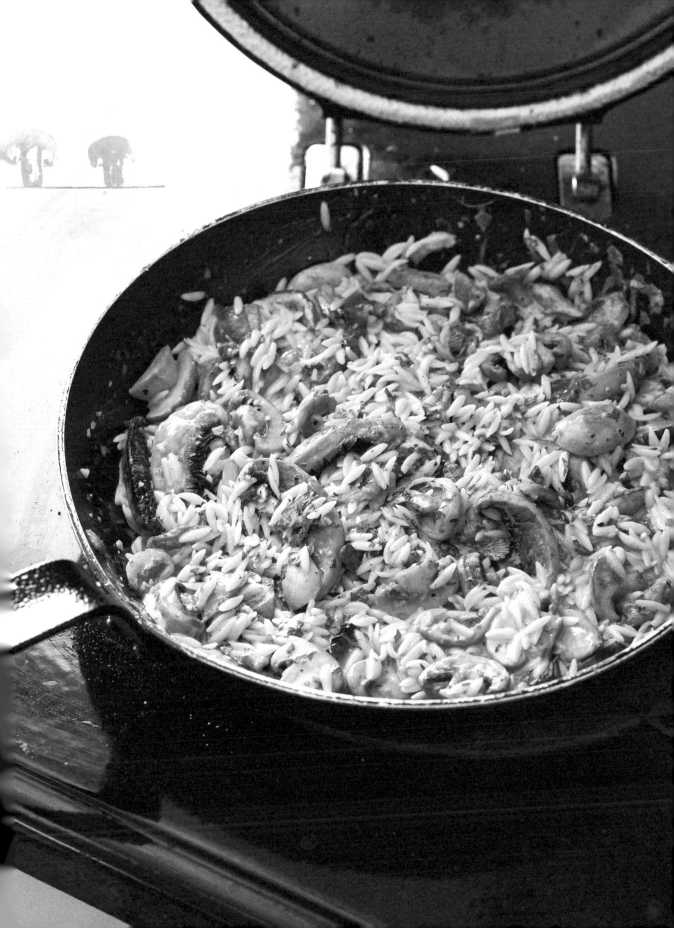

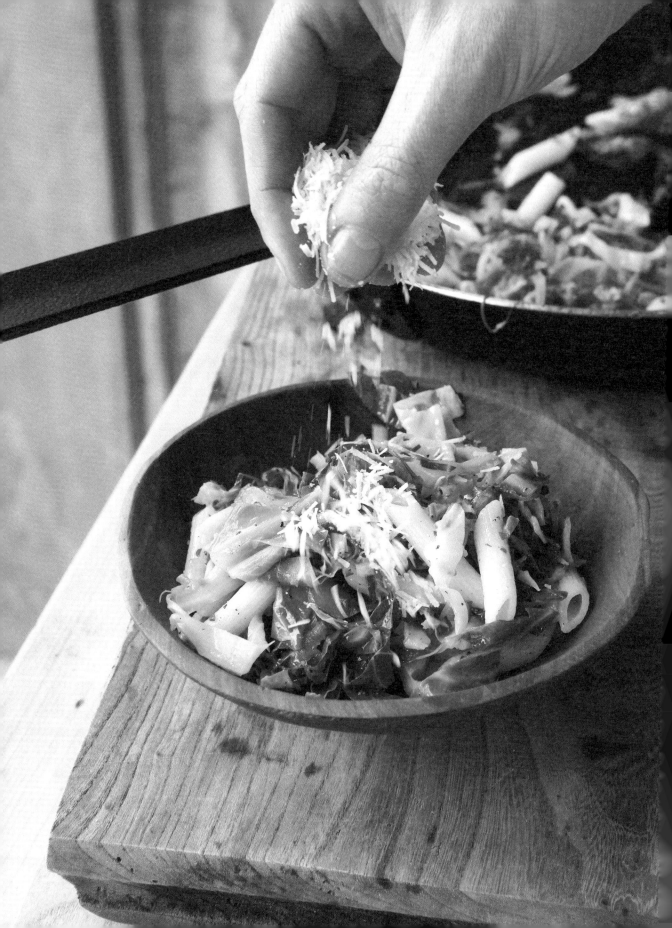

Pasta with greens, garlic and chilli

*Wilted greens combined with a hearty portion of pasta and spiked with garlic
and chilli make a satisfying supper. The following variations on that theme
are equally delicious, sustaining and easy to put together.*

SERVES 4

2–3 heads of spring greens
or kale, or a Savoy cabbage

6 tablespoons olive oil

1 onion, finely sliced

½–1 red chilli, deseeded and
finely chopped, or 2 good
pinches of dried chilli flakes

2 garlic cloves, finely slivered

300g pasta shapes, such
as penne, fusilli, trofie or
strozzapreti

Sea salt and freshly ground
black pepper

TO SERVE

Extra virgin olive oil

Parmesan, pecorino, hard goat's
cheese or other well-flavoured
hard cheese

Put a large pan of well-salted water on to boil, so that you're ready to
cook the pasta while the sauce is coming together. Remove the core
and thick stems from the greens or cabbage and shred the leaves.

Heat the olive oil in a frying pan over a low heat. Add the onion and
cook gently for 10 minutes, or until soft. Add the chilli and garlic and
some salt and pepper, and continue to cook for about 3 minutes.

When the onion is almost cooked, add the pasta to the pan of boiling
water and cook until *al dente*, adding the greens to the pan about
3 minutes before the end of cooking.

Drain the pasta and greens thoroughly and toss with the onion mixture
in the frying pan. Check the seasoning, then serve, with extra virgin
olive oil for trickling and lots of grated cheese.

VARIATIONS

Pasta with broccoli

Use a head of broccoli, cut into small florets, instead of the greens, and
give it a good 5 minutes' cooking with the pasta – it should be well
done so that it starts to break down and cling to the pasta. Omit the
onion, and just warm the oil with the chilli and garlic for a few minutes.

Orecchiette with chickpeas and cavolo nero

Adding chickpeas makes this a more substantial main course dish. Use
250g orecchiette, penne or farfalle pasta (little 'ear' shaped orecchiette
are great with chickpeas, which get stuck in the 'earholes'). You can
use any greens, but it's particularly good with cavolo nero or curly kale,
tough ribs removed, leaves roughly shredded. Gently fry the onion,
chilli and garlic, as above, then add a drained, rinsed 400g tin of
chickpeas with a pinch of ground cumin, and heat through thoroughly
before tossing together with the pasta and greens. Serve trickled with
extra virgin oil, but omit the cheese.

Pasta with fennel, rocket and lemon

This is such a lovely combination of flavours. Use ribbon pasta, linguine, spaghetti or whatever pasta shapes you have to hand – you'll end up with a fantastic summery pasta dish.

SERVES 2

1 large fennel bulb

1 tablespoon rapeseed or olive oil

1 garlic clove, slivered

150g tagliatelle, pappardelle or other pasta

2–3 good handfuls of rocket

Finely grated zest of 1 lemon

3 tablespoons crème fraîche

Sea salt and freshly ground black pepper

Parmesan, hard goat's cheese or other well-flavoured hard cheese, to serve

Put a large pan of well-salted water on to boil, so that you're ready to cook the pasta while the sauce is coming together.

Trim the fennel, removing the tougher outer layer or two, then slice thinly. Heat the oil in a large frying pan over a medium heat. Add the garlic and fennel and sauté gently for about 10 minutes, until the fennel is tender.

When the fennel is almost cooked, add the pasta to the pan of boiling water and cook until *al dente*.

Add the rocket to the fennel and stir until wilted, then add the lemon zest and crème fraîche. Stir well until the crème fraîche coats all the vegetables, then add salt and pepper to taste.

Drain the pasta well, toss with the fennel mixture and serve straight away, with grated cheese.

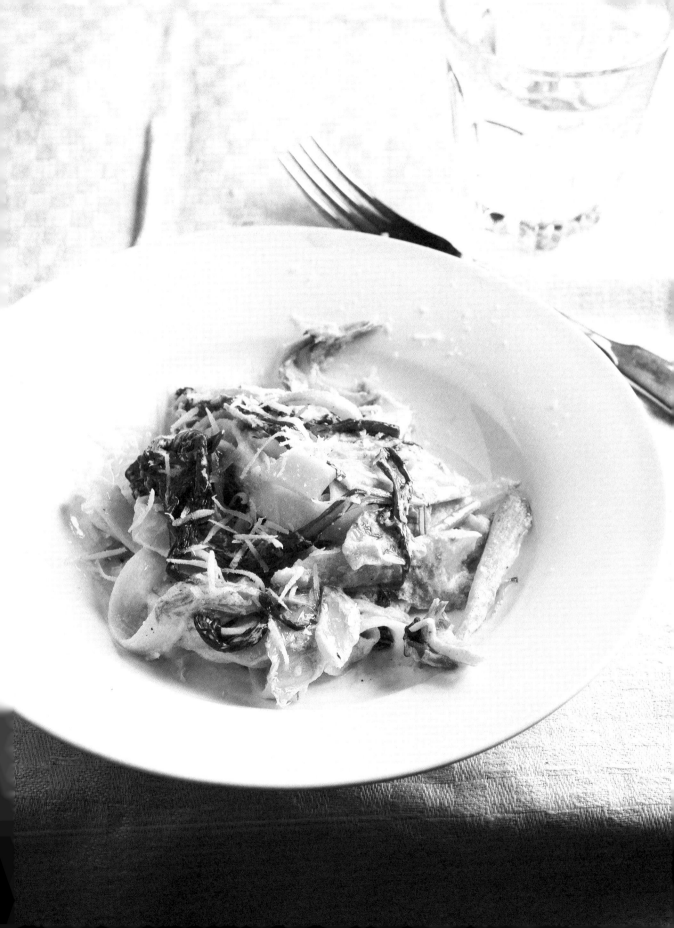

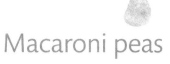

Macaroni peas

Peas and pasta with bacon or ham is a classic combination. In this dish (inspired by a lovely Nigella Lawson risotto recipe), Parmesan gives the desired salty-savoury note. Some of the peas remain whole, to give a pleasing, pop-in-the-mouth texture; the rest are blitzed to form a creamy pea sauce.

SERVES 4

500g peas (fresh or frozen) or petits pois

300g small macaroni, or smallish pasta shapes such as orecchiette or fusilli, or even risoni

50g butter

1 garlic clove, chopped

25g Parmesan, hard goat's cheese or other well-flavoured hard cheese, coarsely grated, plus extra to serve

Sea salt and freshly ground black pepper

Shredded basil or flat-leaf parsley, to serve (optional)

Put a large pan of well-salted water on to boil, so that you're ready to cook the pasta while the sauce is coming together.

Put the peas in a pan, cover with water, bring to the boil and simmer until tender – just a couple of minutes for frozen or very tender fresh peas, longer for older fresh peas.

When the peas are almost cooked, add the pasta to the pan of boiling water and cook until *al dente*.

Meanwhile, melt the butter in a small pan over a low heat and add the garlic. Let it cook gently for just a couple of minutes, without colouring, then remove from the heat.

Drain the peas, reserving the cooking water. Put about half of them in a blender with 6 tablespoons of the cooking water, the butter and garlic, and the grated cheese. Blitz to a smooth, loose purée, adding a little more water if needed. Combine with the whole peas and season with salt and pepper to taste.

Drain the pasta as soon as it is ready and toss immediately with the hot pea sauce. Serve topped with plenty of ground black pepper and more grated Parmesan. Shredded basil or chopped flat-leaf parsley is a good, but by no means essential, finishing touch.

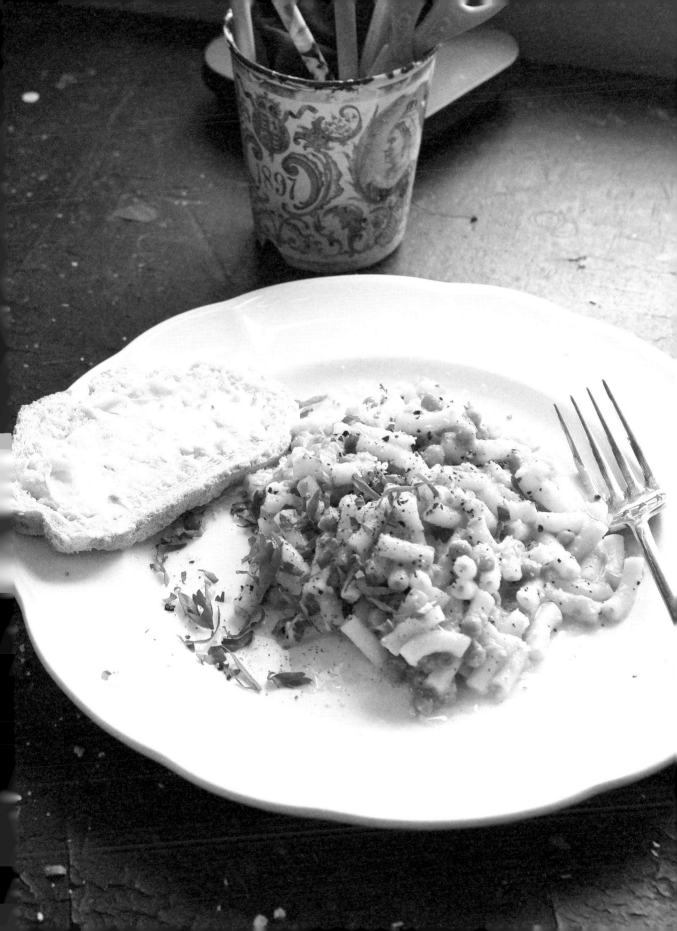

Linguine with mint and almond pesto and tomatoes ᵛ

This light, zesty pesto is perfect for summer pasta. I've always preferred linguine to spaghetti – something about the flat shape makes it more pleasing in the mouth – but of course spaghetti would work here. I make the pesto without cheese, as I often serve the pasta topped with Parmesan or hard goat's cheese. The quirky pesto is versatile: thin it with a little oil and it makes a great salad dressing – try it with crisp Little Gem lettuces and quartered hard-boiled eggs.

SERVES 4

300g linguine or spaghetti

400g tomatoes, cut into wedges

FOR THE MINT PESTO

50g blanched almonds, lightly toasted

A large bunch of mint (about 50g), leaves only

1 garlic clove, chopped

Finely grated zest of 1 lemon, plus a squeeze of juice

½ teaspoon Dijon mustard

A pinch of sugar

About 75ml rapeseed or olive oil

Sea salt and freshly ground black pepper

TO SERVE (OPTIONAL)

Parmesan, hard goat's cheese or other well-flavoured hard cheese

First make the pesto: put the toasted almonds into a food processor, along with the mint, garlic and lemon zest. Blitz until very finely chopped. Add the mustard and sugar then, with the motor running, slowly pour in the oil until you have a thick, sloppy purée. Season with salt, pepper and a good squeeze of lemon juice. This will keep in the fridge for a few days.

Put a large pan of well-salted water on to boil. Add the pasta to the boiling water and cook until *al dente*. Drain well, then toss with the mint pesto and around half of the tomatoes.

Divide between warmed serving bowls or plates and top with the remaining tomatoes. Serve straight away, scattered with cheese shavings if you like.

VARIATIONS
In place of the tomatoes, you could use lightly cooked asparagus, peas or broad beans, or a mixture of summer veg.

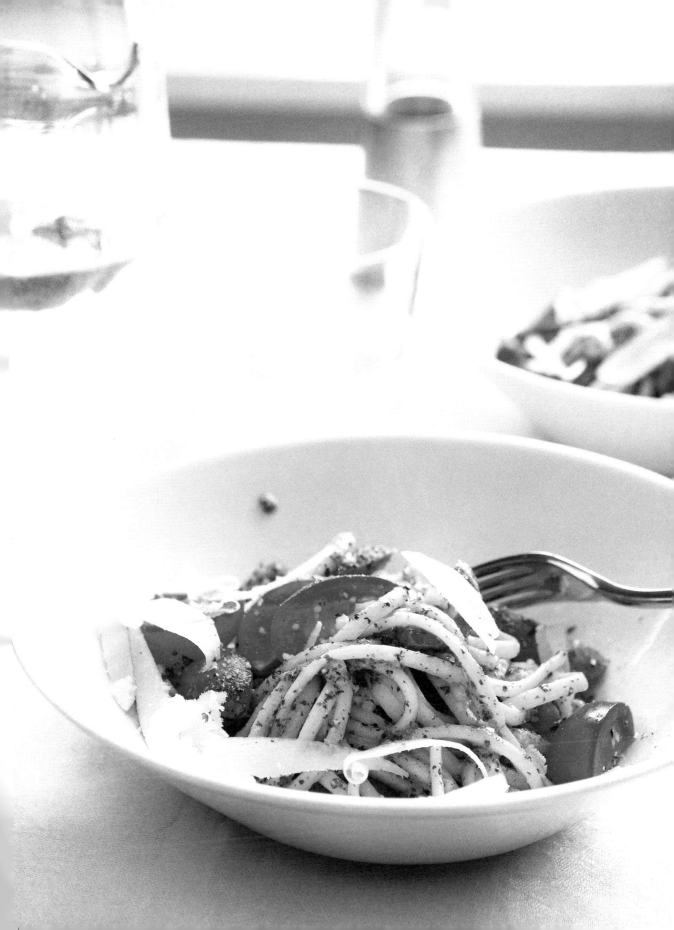

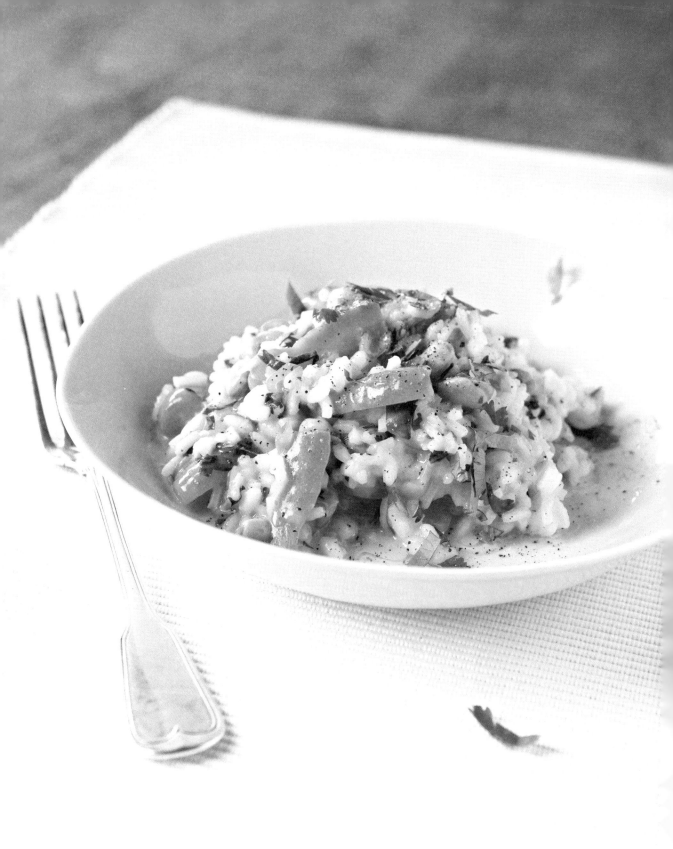

Baby carrot and broad bean risotto

This is a perfect summer supper dish: tender baby carrots and bittersweet broad beans wrapped in a creamy, delicate risotto.

SERVES 4

1 tablespoon rapeseed or olive oil

40g butter

1 large onion, finely chopped

About 800ml vegetable stock

200g risotto rice

100ml dry white wine

250–300g baby carrots, scrubbed and halved or quartered lengthways

150g baby broad beans

20g Parmesan, hard goat's cheese or other well-flavoured hard cheese, finely grated

A handful of flat-leaf parsley, chopped

Sea salt and freshly ground pepper

Rapeseed or extra virgin olive oil, to serve

Heat the oil and 25g butter in a large pan over a medium heat. Add the onion and fry gently for 8–10 minutes, until softened. Meanwhile, bring the stock to a simmer, then keep over a very low heat.

Stir the rice into the onion, and cook for a minute or two, then stir again. Add the wine and bring to a simmer. Cook for a few minutes, stirring from time to time, until the wine is absorbed.

Now add the hot stock, about a quarter at a time, making sure each addition has been absorbed before you add the next. Keep the risotto simmering and stir frequently. It should take 20–25 minutes for the stock to be absorbed and for the rice to be cooked but still *al dente*. Add the carrots when the rice has been cooking for about 12 minutes; put the broad beans in just a couple of minutes before the rice is done.

When the rice and veg are cooked, turn off the heat. Scatter the cheese and dot the remaining butter over the risotto, then cover and leave for a couple of minutes. Now stir the melted cheese and butter into the risotto with most of the parsley and salt and pepper to taste.

Divide the risotto between warmed bowls. Scatter over the remaining parsley, trickle over a little oil and add a grinding of pepper to serve.

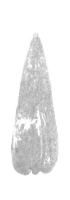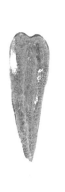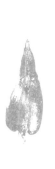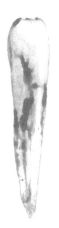

Leek risotto with chestnuts

This creamiest and palest of risottos tastes fantastic with the contrasting chestnuts. Vac-packed, pre-cooked chestnuts are easy to use but if you can roast and peel your own, you'll get that sublime char-grilled flavour too. If you have any risotto left over, use it to make arancini (see below).

SERVES 4

About 75g butter

A little rapeseed or olive oil

3 large leeks (about 500g), trimmed, washed and finely sliced

About 800ml vegetable stock

250g risotto rice

150ml dry white wine

200g cooked, peeled chestnuts, crumbled

Sea salt and freshly ground black pepper

Thyme leaves, to finish

Heat 50g of the butter and a little oil in a large saucepan over a medium heat. As soon as it's foaming, add the leeks, lower the heat and sweat gently, covered, for about 20 minutes until silky, stirring occasionally. Bring the stock to a low simmer in a pan; keep over a very low heat.

Add the rice to the leeks and stir well, then add the wine. Increase the heat a little and let bubble until the liquid has evaporated. Now start adding the hot stock, about a quarter at a time. Stir often, adding more hot stock as it is absorbed. After about 25 minutes, the rice should be cooked, with just a hint of bite to it, and all the stock should be used.

While the risotto is cooking, heat 20g butter and a little oil in a frying pan over a medium heat. Add the chestnuts with a pinch of salt. Turn the heat up a bit and fry, stirring often, for 2 minutes until the chestnuts and butter are browned (don't let either burn). Take off the heat.

When the risotto is cooked, turn off the heat, season with salt and pepper to taste, then dot a little more butter over the surface. Cover the pan and leave for a couple of minutes, then stir the melted butter on the surface in. Serve scattered with the chestnuts and thyme.

VARIATION/LEFTOVERS
Arancini
Cool the risotto quickly (if it's quite sloppy, drain in a sieve), then refrigerate until ready to use. Take a tablespoonful of the rice and squash it into a thick patty. Put a couple of cubes of cheese (mozzarella or a blue, or other nice melting cheese) in the centre and a little dollop of pesto, then add a little more rice on top and mould the rice around the cheese to enclose it. Repeat with all the rice. Dust each rice patty with flour, dip in beaten egg, then roll in fine breadcrumbs. Fry fairly gently in a little oil until golden brown all over and hot right through.

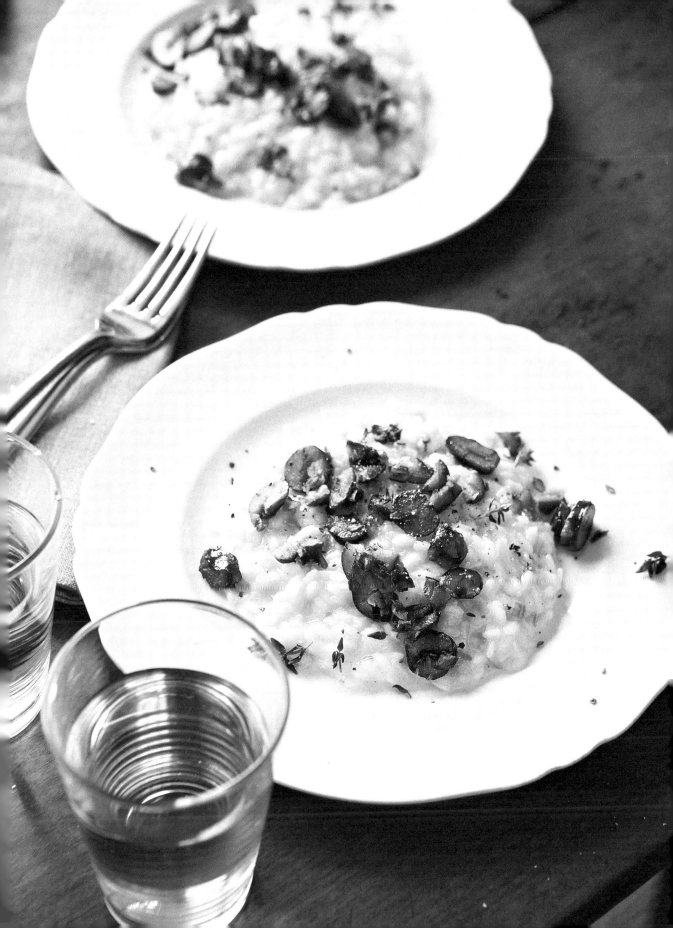

Tomato and mozzarella risotto

As long as you have some roasted tomato sauce to hand, this is one of the easiest risottos you'll ever make. It's soothing and rich, just as risotto should be, and carries a faint evocation of childhood tinned tomato soup – in a good way. You could omit the mozzarella for a cheese-free version.

 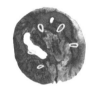   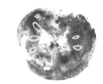

SERVES 4

750ml vegetable stock

A large knob of butter

1 onion, finely chopped

250g risotto rice

About 200ml roasted tomato sauce (see page 366)

1 ball of buffalo mozzarella (100–125g), torn or cut into chunks

Sea salt and freshly ground black pepper

TO SERVE

Extra virgin olive oil

A couple of large handfuls of rocket (optional)

Bring the stock to a low simmer in a small saucepan. Keep over a very low heat.

Heat the butter in a large saucepan over a medium-low heat. Add the onion and sweat for 8–10 minutes, until soft. Add the rice and cook, stirring, for a couple of minutes.

Now start adding the hot stock, about a quarter at a time. Let the risotto cook, stirring often, adding more hot stock as it is absorbed. After 20–25 minutes, the rice should be cooked, with just a hint of chalkiness in the middle, and you should have used up the stock.

Add the tomato sauce and cook for another couple of minutes, until piping hot, then remove from the heat. Stir in some salt and pepper, then add the mozzarella. Leave the risotto, covered, for a minute, then stir through the melting mozzarella, but not too thoroughly – you want to encounter stretchy, melty bits as you eat.

Serve topped with a generous trickle of extra virgin olive oil, with a tangle of rocket on the side, if you like.

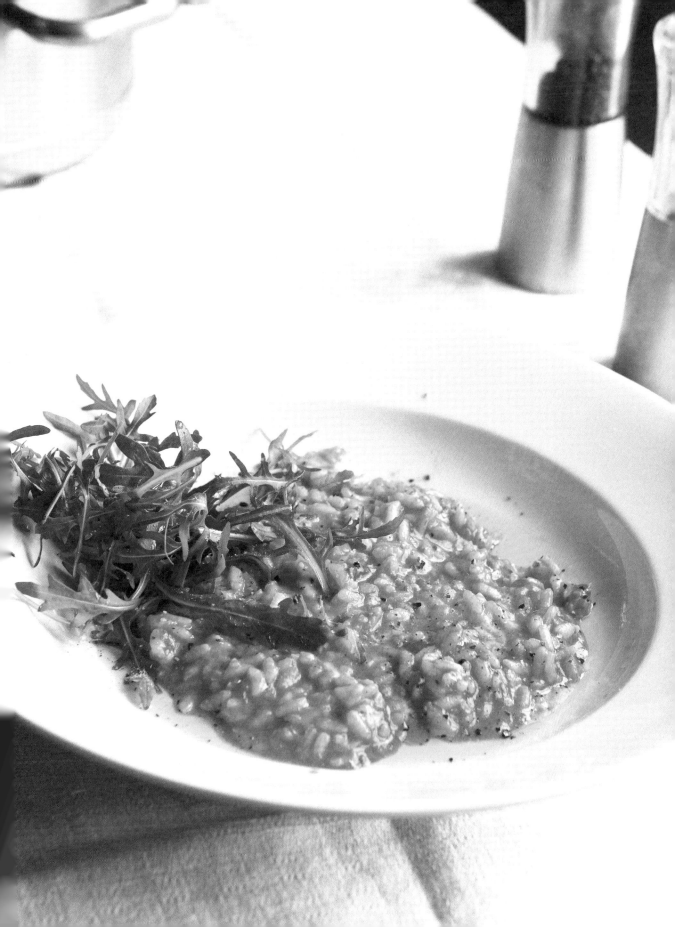

Vegetable biryani ᵛ

For a biryani, the rice and curry are first cooked separately, then together, for a final mingling of textures and flavours. You can cheat by using a biryani (medium-hot) curry powder instead of the individual spices and fresh chilli, but you'll get a more exciting final flavour if you follow this route.

SERVES 6

5 tablespoons sunflower oil

1 bay leaf

3 cardamom pods, bashed

1 teaspoon cumin seeds

5 large onions, finely sliced

2 garlic cloves, crushed

2 teaspoons finely grated ginger

1 large red chilli, finely chopped (deseeded for a milder curry)

1 teaspoon ground cumin

1 teaspoon ground coriander

½ teaspoon ground cinnamon

About 250g carrots, peeled and sliced into thin discs

About 300g waxy potatoes, cut into 1–2cm cubes

200g peas (fresh or frozen and defrosted)

A generous squeeze of lemon juice

50g sultanas

350g basmati rice

A large pinch of saffron strands

Sea salt and freshly ground black pepper

TO SERVE

50g slivered almonds, lightly toasted

Chopped coriander or mint

Heat 2 tablespoons of the oil in a large casserole over a medium-high heat. Add the bay leaf, cardamom pods and cumin seeds and fry for a few minutes. Add 1 sliced onion and fry over a medium heat, stirring often, for about 15 minutes, till golden and soft. Lower the heat and add the garlic, ginger, chilli and ground spices. Cook, stirring, for 2 minutes.

Add the carrots, potatoes and peas and enough water to almost cover the vegetables. Bring to the boil, then reduce to a simmer. Cover and cook, stirring from time to time, for 10–15 minutes, or until the veg are *al dente*. Season with salt and pepper to taste and add a squeeze of lemon juice. Sprinkle the sultanas on top.

Meanwhile, rinse the rice thoroughly in several changes of water. Put into a saucepan with the saffron and a large pinch of salt. Add enough water to cover the rice by 2cm. Bring to the boil, stir once, then simmer very gently until the water is nearly all absorbed (indicated by deep steam holes on the surface). Preheat the oven to 160°C/Gas Mark 3.

Cover the rice pan with a damp tea towel and a tight-fitting lid and turn the heat as low as possible. Cook for 5 minutes. Remove the lid and use a fork to separate the rice grains.

Spoon the rice in a thick layer over the curry in the casserole. Cover the pan with a damp tea towel and put on the lid tightly. Place over a high heat for a few minutes to get the curry bubbling again, then transfer to the oven for 20 minutes. Remove and leave to stand for 10 minutes.

While the biryani is cooking, heat the remaining 3 tablespoons oil in a large frying pan over a medium-high heat and add the rest of the sliced onions. Cook briskly, stirring often, for about 20 minutes, until well browned and reduced down. Season with salt.

Uncover the biryani and scatter over the browned onions, almonds and coriander or mint. Serve with a cooling, yoghurty raita, and/or a spicy chutney (the tamarind raita on page 318 is particularly good).

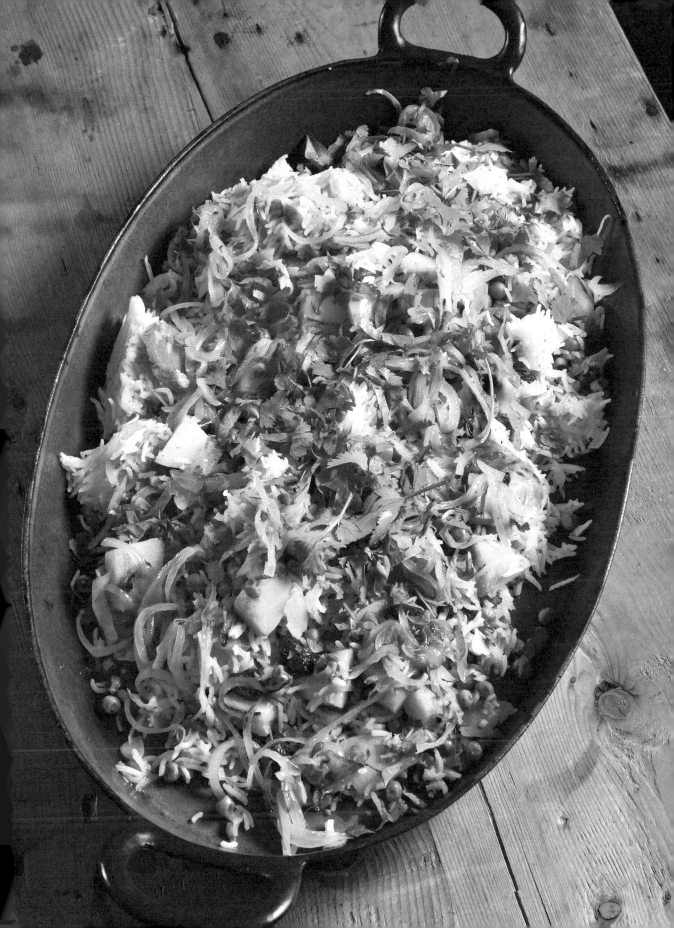

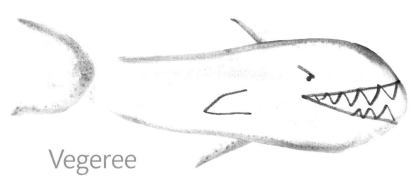

Vegeree

I love a good kedgeree: that incredibly warming, comforting combination of rice, curry spices and smoked fish. I wondered if it would be possible to create a similarly satisfying dish without fish – and, it turns out, it is. Roasted aubergines are the key – smoky and sweet, they certainly hit the spot when combined with all that spicy, ricey goodness. Courgettes and onions, and a few 'soft, hard-boiled' eggs on top, round out the dish nicely. You can make this with just aubergines and onions, but I like the addition of a few courgettes too.

SERVES 4

3 medium onions

1 large aubergine (about 350g)

2 medium courgettes (about 250g), halved lengthways if large

3 tablespoons sunflower oil

1 tablespoon good curry powder

300g basmati rice

4 large eggs, at room temperature

Sea salt and freshly ground black pepper

Preheat the oven to 190°C/Gas Mark 5. Slice the onions from root to tip into eighths, keeping them together at the root end. Quarter the aubergine lengthways, then cut each quarter into 1cm thick slices. Cut the courgettes into 1cm thick slices.

Toss all the veg together in a large roasting tray. Pour over the sunflower oil, sprinkle with the curry powder and add some salt and pepper. Toss together again. Roast for 40 minutes, stirring 2 or 3 times.

Meanwhile, cook the rice. Rinse well in several changes of water, then put into a saucepan, add salt and pour on enough water to cover by 2cm. Bring to the boil, stir once, then simmer until the water is nearly all absorbed (there should be deep steam holes in the surface). Cover the pan with a damp tea towel and a tight-fitting lid and turn the heat as low as possible. Cook for 10 minutes. Then turn off the heat and leave the rice for a further 5 minutes. Remove the lid and use a fork to separate the rice grains.

To cook the eggs, bring a pan of water to the boil, add the eggs and boil for 7 minutes. Run under cold water to stop the cooking and leave until cool. Shell, peel and halve the eggs.

Toss the cooked rice with the roasted spiced vegetables. Taste and add more salt and pepper if you think it is needed. Serve topped with the halved boiled eggs and a grinding of black pepper.

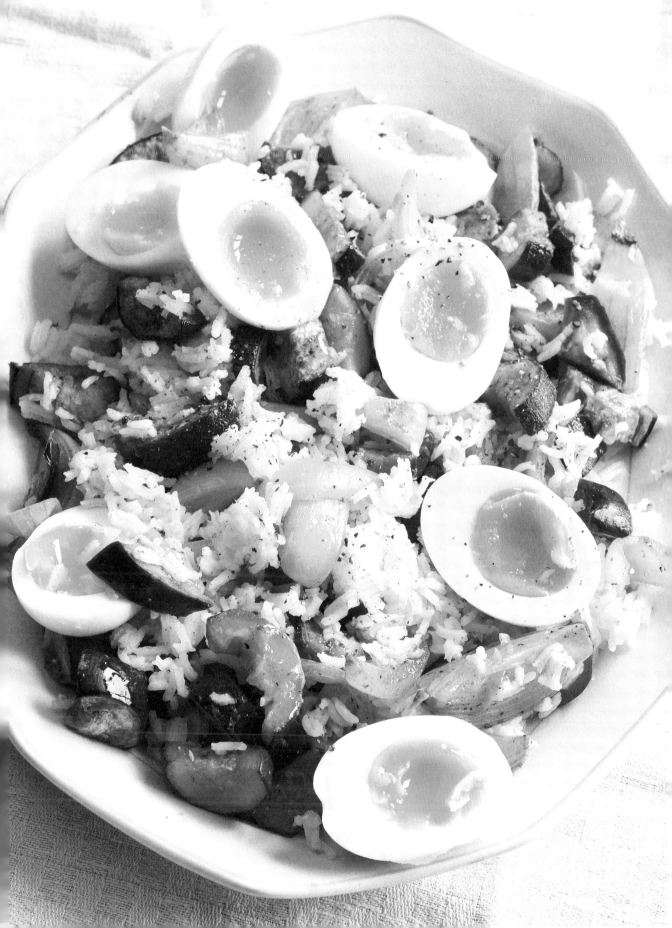

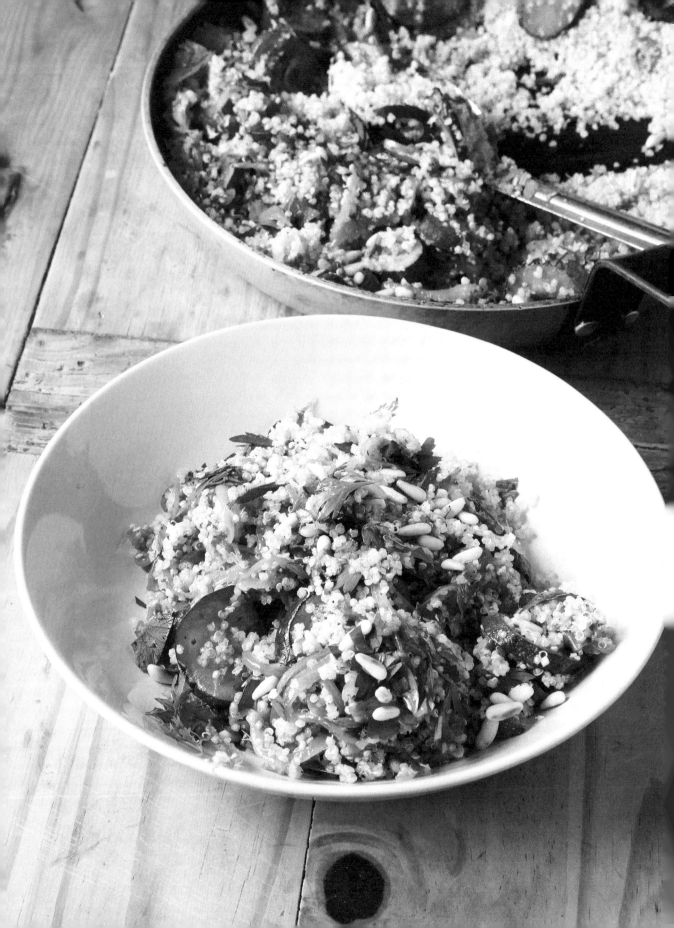

Quinoa with courgettes and onions

Quinoa is a highly nutritious little seed that makes a nice alternative to rice or couscous (in fact, you can substitute it for those ingredients in all manner of recipes). I love it with tender courgettes, sweet onions and crunchy pine nuts in this simple supper dish. The more wintry leek and squash version below is a real favourite too.

SERVES 4

800g courgettes

A knob of butter

2 tablespoons rapeseed or olive oil

3 onions, halved and finely sliced

A few sprigs of thyme, leaves only

3 garlic cloves, finely chopped

200g quinoa

A good handful of flat-leaf parsley, roughly chopped

A squeeze of lemon juice

50g pine nuts, lightly toasted

Sea salt and freshly ground black pepper

Cut the courgettes on the diagonal into 5mm thick slices. Melt the butter with the oil in a large frying pan over a medium heat. Add the onions, courgettes, thyme and some salt and pepper. Cook for 20–25 minutes, stirring from time to time, until the courgettes are tender and starting to turn golden. Add the garlic and fry for another couple of minutes.

Meanwhile, rinse the quinoa well in several changes of cold water. Put into a saucepan with a pinch of salt and cover with plenty of cold water. Bring to the boil, reduce the heat and simmer for about 12 minutes, or until the quinoa is tender but still slightly nutty, and the long white kernels are coming away from the seeds. Tip into a sieve and leave to drain and steam a little to drive off excess moisture.

Add the drained quinoa to the courgettes, along with the chopped parsley and lemon juice. Stir well, then taste and add more salt and pepper if needed. Serve topped with the toasted pine nuts.

VARIATION

Quinoa with leeks and squash

Replace the courgettes and onions with 500–600g squash or pumpkin and 3 trimmed medium leeks. Peel and deseed the squash and cut into 1cm dice. Cut the leeks into roughly 1cm slices. Heat the butter and oil in a large pan, add the squash, leeks, thyme and some salt and pepper, cover the pan and sweat for 20–25 minutes, stirring from time to time, until the leeks and squash are tender. Cook the quinoa as above. Add the drained quinoa to the squash and leeks. Stir well and check the seasoning. Serve topped with the pine nuts.

Kale speltotto with goat's cheese

This is very similar to a risotto, but based on nutty grains of pearled spelt, rather than rice. We serve this lovely wintry dish in the River Cottage Canteen, and enrich it with Quickes hard goat's cheese – but any tasty, hard goat's cheese would be good, or Parmesan. If you prefer, you can finish the dish with some slices of soft, rinded goat's cheese, as shown.

SERVES 4

1 litre vegetable stock

50g butter

2 tablespoons olive or rapeseed oil, plus a trickle to finish

1 onion, finely chopped

1 garlic clove, finely chopped

A few sprigs of thyme, leaves only, chopped

2–3 medium leeks, trimmed and washed

About 150g kale or spring greens

300g pearled spelt (or pearl barley)

125ml dry white wine

50g hard goat's cheese, Parmesan, or other well-flavoured hard cheese, grated, plus extra to serve

Sea salt and freshly ground black pepper

Heat the stock in a saucepan and keep it at a low simmer over a very low heat.

Heat about half the butter and 1 tablespoon oil in a large saucepan over a medium heat. Add the onion, garlic and thyme and sweat gently for about 10 minutes, until the onion is soft.

In the meantime, cut the leeks on the diagonal into 2cm thick slices. Remove the tough stems from the kale or greens and shred the leaves.

Stir the spelt (or barley) through the softened onions and cook gently for a minute or two. Add the wine and let it bubble until all the liquid is absorbed.

Now start adding the stock, about a quarter at a time, as you would for a risotto, stirring often and letting each addition be absorbed before you add the next. It should take about 25 minutes for the spelt (or a bit longer for barley) to cook to a tender texture with a hint of bite still in the grains.

While the spelt (or barley) is cooking, sweat the leeks in the remaining oil and butter in a small frying pan over a medium heat, tossing and stirring occasionally, until tender, but retaining a slight bite. Lightly steam the kale or greens, or wilt in a saucepan with a little water, for 3–4 minutes, until just tender. Drain if necessary.

Take the finished speltotto off the heat and stir through the leeks, kale or greens and grated cheese. Add salt and pepper to taste. Serve topped with extra cheese, a grinding of black pepper and a final trickle of oil.

VARIATION

Nettle speltotto
Instead of the kale, use tender young nettle tops. Wash thoroughly (wear rubber gloves for this!) and then wilt in a pan of salted water for 5–6 minutes, until tender. Drain in a sieve, pressing out the water, then chop fairly finely. Stir through the finished speltotto with the leeks and cheese, then serve.

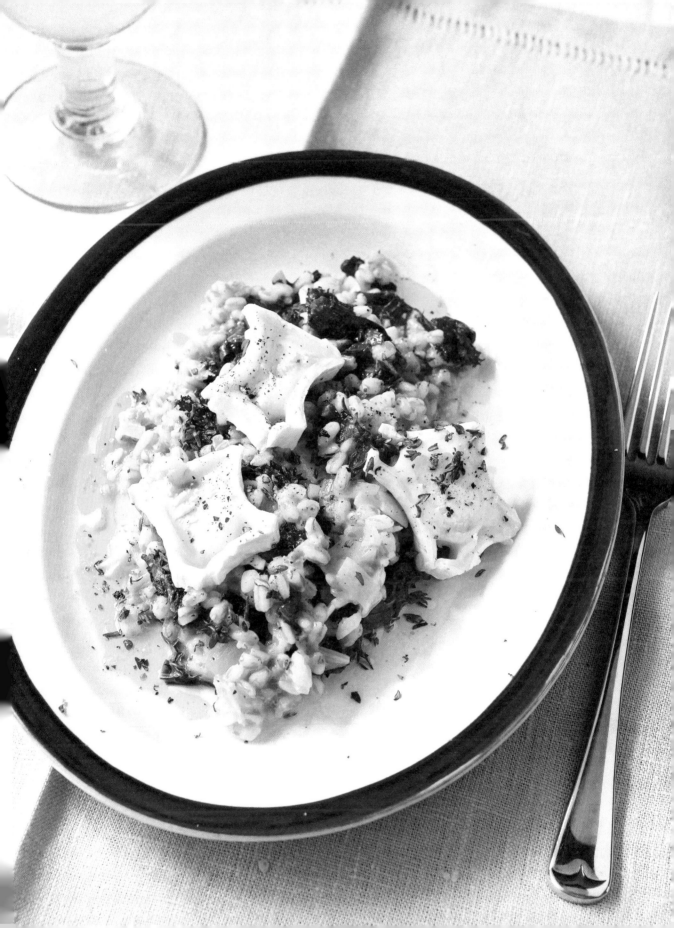

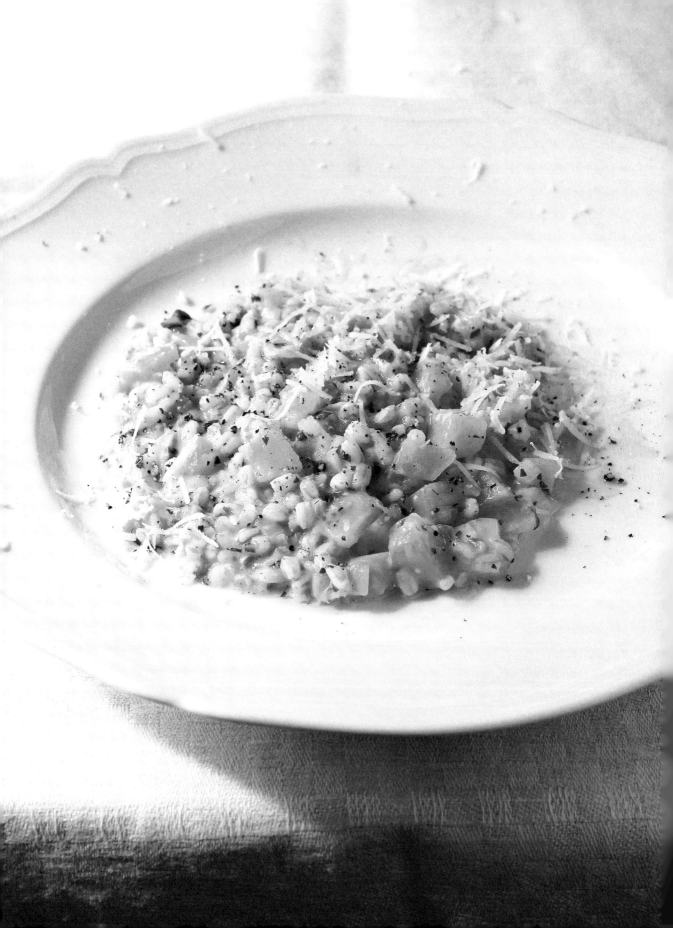

Swede speltotto

Spelt has a nutty flavour that goes very well with earthy root vegetables. Roasted wedges of pumpkin or beetroot work brilliantly in place of the swede, but instead of adding at the beginning, stir in the diced flesh of the roasted veg just a minute or two before the speltotto is finished.

SERVES 4

1 litre vegetable stock

20g butter

2 tablespoons rapeseed or olive oil

2 medium onions, chopped

1 garlic clove, finely chopped

350g swede, peeled and cut into 1cm dice

300g pearled spelt (or pearl barley)

A good handful of parsley, finely chopped

50g Parmesan, hard goat's cheese or other well-flavoured hard cheese, grated, plus extra to serve

A few gratings of nutmeg

Salt and freshly ground black pepper

Bring the stock to a low simmer in a small pan and keep over a very low heat.

Heat the butter and oil in a large saucepan over a medium-low heat. Add the onions and sweat gently, stirring, for about 10 minutes, until soft. Add the garlic and swede and stir for a couple of minutes.

Add the spelt (or barley) to the pan and stir for a couple of minutes, making sure all the grains are well coated with butter and oil.

Now start adding the stock, about a quarter at a time, as you would for a risotto, stirring often and letting each addition be absorbed before you add the next. It should take about 25 minutes for spelt (or a bit longer for barley) to cook to a tender texture with a hint of bite still in the grains. By this time the swede will be completely tender too.

Stir in the chopped parsley and grated cheese. Add salt, plenty of black pepper and a few gratings of nutmeg. Serve, topped with more grated cheese. A crisp green salad is the ideal accompaniment.

New potato gnocchi

Gnocchi – little savoury potato dumplings that beg to be smothered in a rich sauce, pesto, or just lots of butter and cheese – may be the ultimate comfort food. And these may well be the easiest gnocchi you'll ever make.

SERVES 4

500g new potatoes

100g soft goat's cheese, crumbled

200g plain flour

1 large egg, lightly beaten

Sea salt and freshly ground black pepper

TO SERVE

Roasted tomato sauce (see page 366) or pesto (see page 256), or butter/olive oil

A handful of parsley and/ or chives, finely chopped (optional)

Parmesan, hard goat's cheese or other well-flavoured hard cheese (optional)

Scrape or scrub all the skin from the potatoes, removing any blemishes, bruises or 'eyes', then cut the potatoes into similar-sized chunks. Put them in a pan, cover with water, salt well and bring to the boil. Lower the heat and simmer for 8–12 minutes, until tender, then drain well.

Mash the potatoes but not too thoroughly – the gnocchi should have a little texture to them. Transfer to a bowl and let cool until tepid, then add the goat's cheese, flour, egg and some salt and pepper. Using a wooden spoon or your hands, mix thoroughly and bring together to a firm dough. Knead gently for a few minutes, then roll the dough into sausages, about 1.5cm in diameter. Cut each one into 2.5–3cm lengths.

Bring a large pan of water to a gentle simmer. Cook the gnocchi, in batches, for a minute or two. As they rise to the surface, scoop them out with a slotted spoon and transfer to a lightly buttered warm dish.

Serve with roasted tomato sauce or pesto, or just butter or olive oil and plenty of black pepper. Finish with a scattering of chopped herbs and/ or grated or finely shaved cheese, if you like.

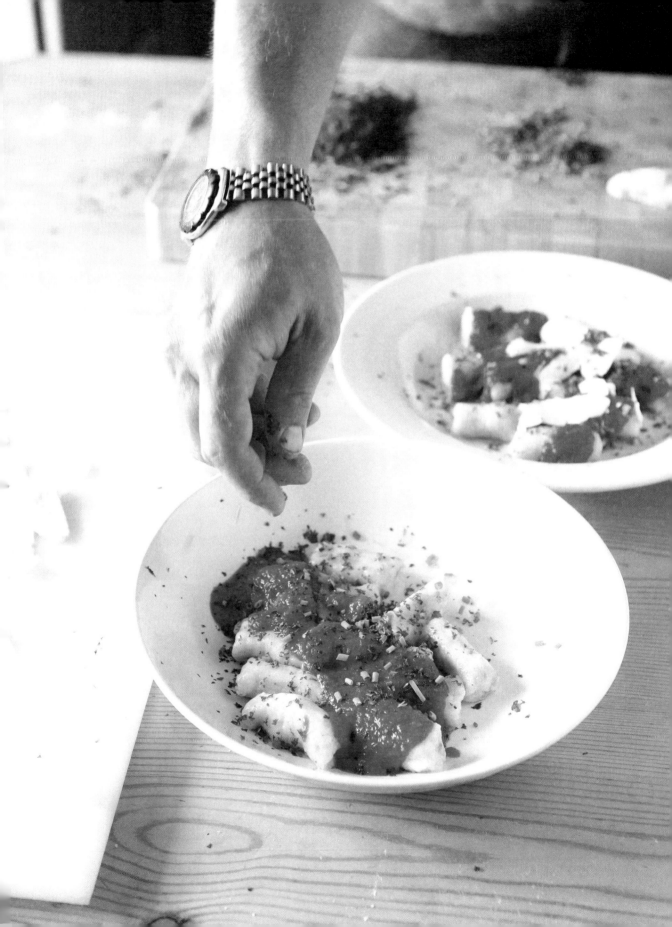

Summer stir-fry with egg-fried rice

It's best to prepare all the ingredients for this lovely, green dish before you start cooking. Once the wok is on the go, it's all ready in a matter of minutes. You don't have to serve the stir-fry with the egg-fried rice – plain, steamed rice or a couple of nests of quick-cook noodles will do.

SERVES 2

1 medium courgette
(about 125g)

A few spring onions, trimmed

A good handful of young spinach, rocket, mizuna, pak choi or any other tender green leaf (about 50g)

About 75g mangetout

About 75g small fresh peas or defrosted petits pois

1 tablespoon rapeseed or sunflower oil

2cm piece of ginger, peeled and finely grated

1 garlic clove, crushed

1 green chilli, deseeded and chopped

A dash of soy sauce

A dash of toasted sesame oil

A handful of mint, finely shredded

1 tablespoon lightly toasted sesame seeds

FOR THE EGG-FRIED RICE

1 tablespoon rapeseed or sunflower oil

150g freshly cooked basmati or fragrant Thai rice

1 teaspoon soy sauce

1 egg, beaten

TO SERVE

Soy sauce

Toasted sesame oil

Prepare the veg first: halve the courgette lengthways, then slice thinly on the diagonal. Slice the spring onions on the diagonal. Trim the spinach or other greens of any tough stalks and roughly shred the leaves. Set aside with the other veg, keeping them separate.

Heat a large wok over a medium-high heat and add the oil. When it's hot, add the mangetout and stir-fry for about 2 minutes, until starting to soften. You now need to add the courgette, peas, onions and greens, one at a time, giving each vegetable a minute or so of stir-frying before you add the next. Keep the heat fairly high so the moisture is driven off and the mixture doesn't start to simmer, and keep everything moving so nothing starts to catch and burn.

When you've added the greens and they've wilted down, throw in the ginger, garlic and chilli. Stir-fry for another 2 minutes, then remove from the heat. Transfer to a hot serving dish and scatter with soy sauce and sesame oil. Finally add the mint and the sesame seeds.

Now quickly cook the egg-fried rice: wipe out the wok with a wad of kitchen paper. Add the oil and place over a medium-high heat. When the oil is hot, add the rice and stir-fry over a fairly high heat until the grains are coated in oil and the rice is piping hot. Create a bit of space on the base of the pan. Mix the soy sauce into the beaten egg and pour into the space. As the egg starts to cook, scrape it up and stir it into the rice. Keep going until the egg is completely cooked and distributed throughout the rice.

Serve the egg-fried rice immediately, topped with the stir-fry. Have some more soy sauce and sesame oil on the table.

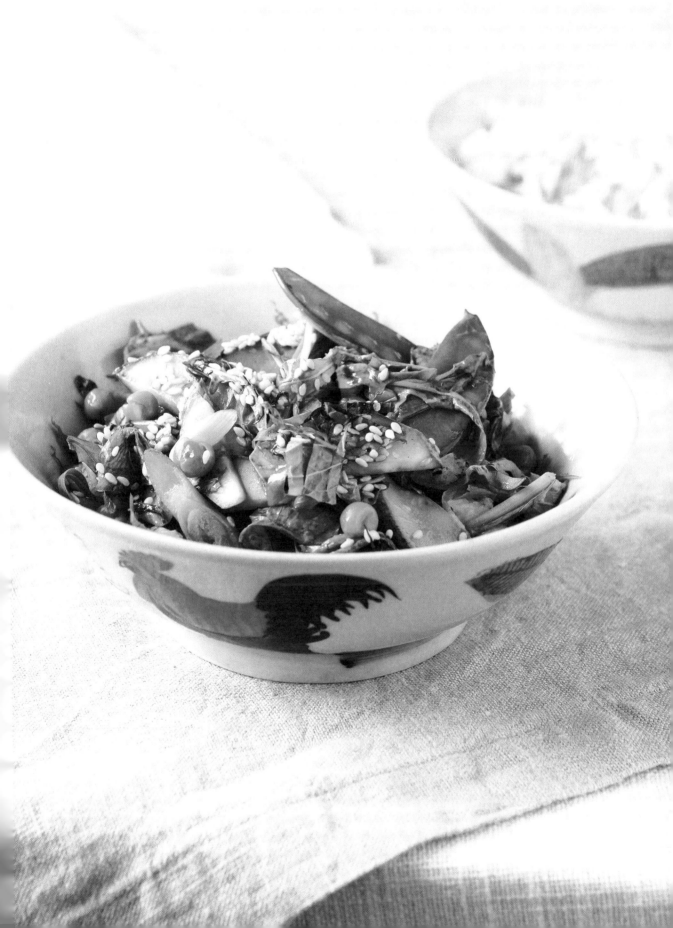

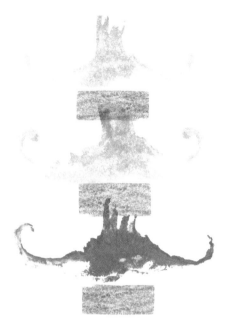

Winter stir-fry with chinese five-spice

The warming hint of star anise within Chinese five-spice powder gives this dish character. You can chop and change the vegetables a little depending on what you have to hand – celeriac instead of parsnip, for instance, or shredded cabbage rather than sprouts – but I do think this is a particularly fun way of using Brussels sprouts.

SERVES 2

1 large carrot, peeled

1 small parsnip, peeled

About 100g shiitake, chestnut or firm button mushrooms, trimmed

About 100g Brussels sprouts, trimmed

2 nests of fine, quick-cook egg noodles (about 50g)

2 tablespoons sunflower oil

3 shallots, or 1 medium onion, finely sliced

½–1 medium-hot red chilli, deseeded and finely chopped

1 garlic clove, finely chopped

A good pinch of sugar

2 tablespoons soy sauce

2 tablespoons rice wine

½ teaspoon Chinese five-spice powder

A good squeeze of lime juice

Sea salt and freshly ground black pepper

Prepare the veg first: cut the carrot into thin batons and the parsnip into thin discs; finely slice the mushrooms; finely shred the Brussels sprouts.

Cook the egg noodles according to the packet instructions.

Meanwhile, heat the sunflower oil in a wok over a high heat. Add the shallots or onion and chilli and stir-fry for 1 minute. Add the carrot and parsnip and cook for 2 minutes, then add the mushrooms and garlic and stir-fry for a couple more minutes.

Finally, add the Brussels sprouts and cook for another couple of minutes until wilted. Season well with salt, pepper and a good pinch of sugar and scoop out of the wok.

Drain the noodles. Reduce the heat under the wok and add the soy sauce, rice wine, five-spice powder and noodles. Cook, stirring for a couple of minutes, then return the vegetables and toss the lot together over the heat.

Heap the stir-fry into warmed serving bowls and finish with a good squeeze of lime juice.

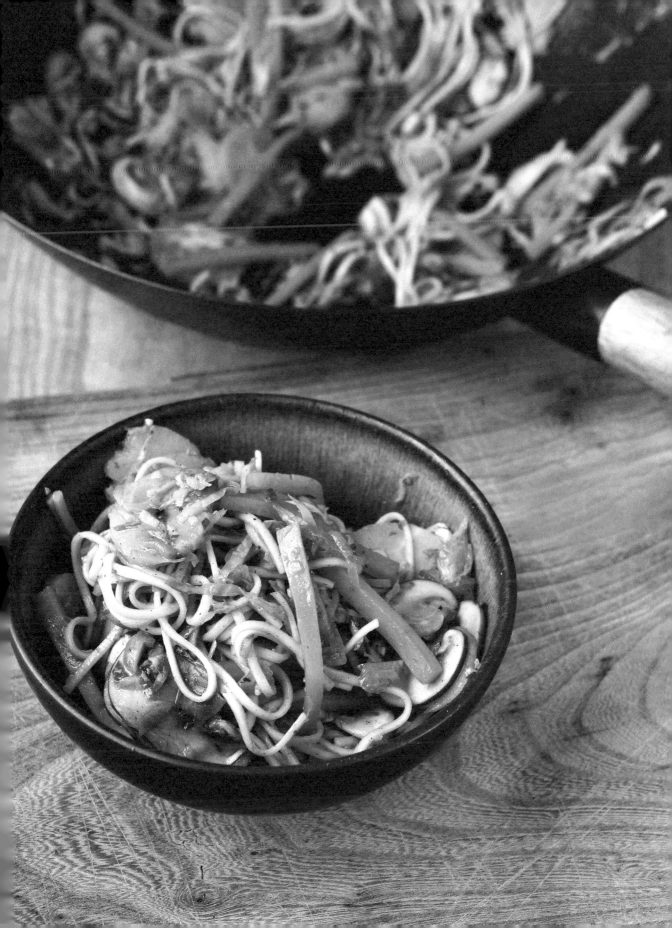

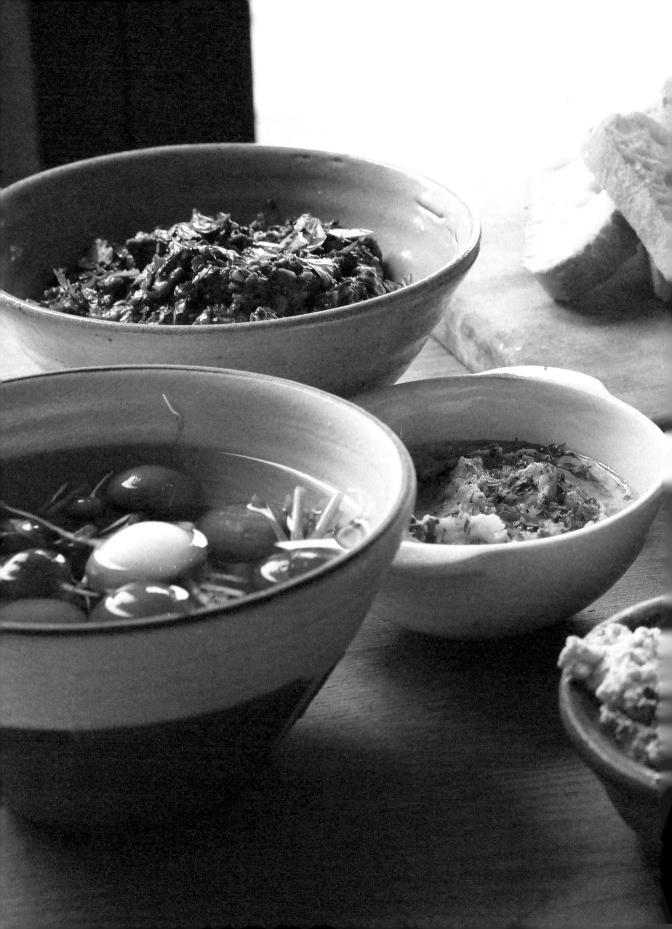

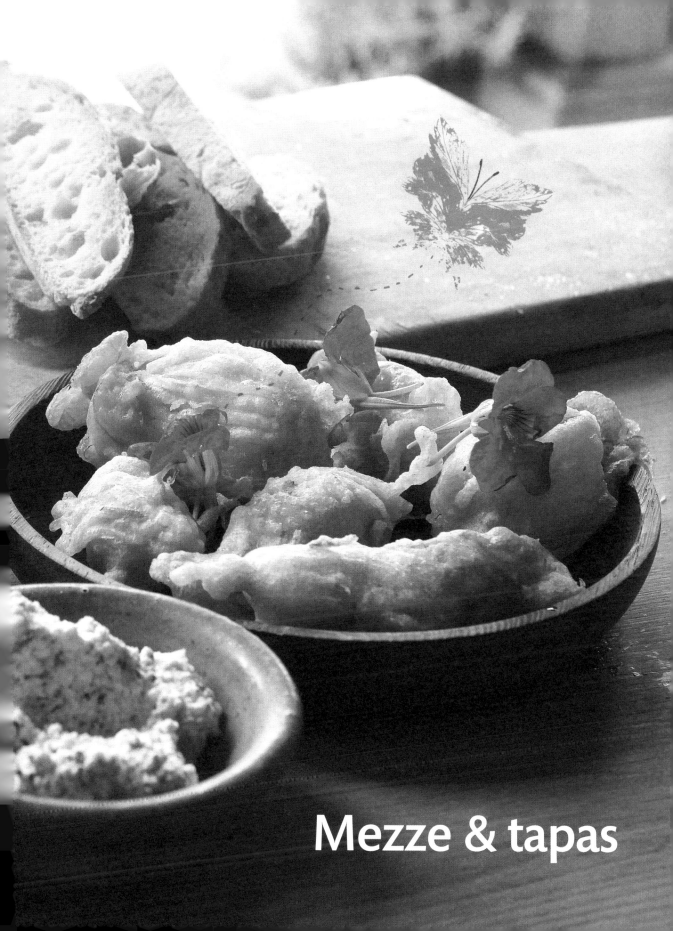

Mezze & tapas

This is as much a plea for a way of eating as it is an

introduction to a batch of recipes. It's important to me personally as, over the last couple of years, it has become increasingly the style in which we choose to eat together as a family. It's also how we like to feed our extended family and friends. Of course it isn't always a meat-free table. But it often is.

It's all about sharing. We're sitting down at the table to a kind of indoor picnic – a range of dishes in bowls and on platters that are passed around, put down, grazed, picked up and passed around again. It's the kind of cooking and eating that makes me rub my hands with glee – not just because of the way it shows off the fantastic ingredients that have gone into it, but also because it heightens the anticipation of sharing a really wonderful table of food with people I love.

I've said before, there is a wonderful democracy to cooking without meat, because so often you are putting a range of dishes on the table of roughly equal weight and importance. These are all, in a sense, 'little' dishes – but I don't mean this in a derogatory sense. They might not, alone, have quite enough substance for a meal, but they support and enhance each other, so that just a few of them together will give you and your fellow diners the feeling that you're sitting down to a feast.

There are not many dishes in this book that do not lend themselves to this 'indoor picnic' approach. But the recipes corralled in this chapter are particularly designed for it – some of them by me, others, over generations, by the cultures they have evolved in. They represent what I see as the very exciting end of mixed-spread eating. There are some real favourites of mine here, from the delicious roasted carrot hummus (see page 296) and vibrant beetroot and walnut hummus (see page 300) to the lovely stuffed courgette flowers (see page 313) and spicy cauliflower pakoras (see page 318). So many of these can be rustled together without a great deal of effort, then placed on the table, maybe just two or three together, with some salad and bread, to produce a really generous spread.

If you choose to embrace this way of eating, then I hope you will go beyond this chapter, and pick and mix from all over the book – and indeed from other books and from all over your culinary repertoire. But the chapters perhaps most complementary to this one are Roast, grill and barbecue (pages 328–67) and Side dishes (pages 368–99).

I'm sure you can see how a tray of roasted pumpkin wedges or a few big, juicy baked mushrooms might fit delightfully into this scheme.

Presenting a patchwork of dishes in this way is something that other cultures do much better than us. Middle Eastern mezze, Spanish tapas, Italian antipasti, the Scandinavian smorgasbord – all are perfect examples of the relaxed relish to be had in a collection of 'little' dishes. It's such a civilised, and civilising, way of eating – particularly shared eating. I think we have much to gain by exploring it ourselves, using the beautiful, seasonal, fresh ingredients that our climate and countryside bestow on us. We will be international mezze magpies, for sure, thieving recipes from here and there and mixing them up and re-working them in ways that might distress a purist. But frankly, that's what British cooks do best – it's *our* national culinary characteristic, and we may as well flaunt it.

If the thought of a meal based around several dishes fills you with a fear of overwork, then take a second look. It's true that preparing ten or so of these recipes from scratch for a big celebration meal would take some time (spectacular though the result would be). But you really don't need that many for a family meal, and in any case a simple hunk of good bread and a salad of ripe cherry tomatoes, say, or a pile of scrubbed raw carrots will be just as much appreciated as a dish that requires chopping, cooking and mixing. Preparing a bowl of simply dressed lentils takes mere minutes. The vast majority of these things can be made ahead and left to marinate happily in the fridge or larder.

In my house, food like this tends to be prepared and consumed in a sort of rolling relay, from meal to meal. I might make a fresh salad for supper, then eat it with the leftovers of a caponata, or a frittata, or a dish that doesn't even end in 'ata', that I made at the weekend. Some leftover roast beetroot might get hummussed in the blender, a tin of chickpeas might get the merguez spice treatment, and some green beans fresh from the garden, lightly steamed, might get tossed with a few chopped olives. None of these preparations need be arduous.

This should be a genuinely relaxing way of cooking and eating. In fact, in my experience, the resulting spread always looks like far more work than it actually was. And that's a good way to make any cook feel relaxed.

Pistachio dukka

This traditional Persian combination of nuts, seeds and spices is usually served in a small dish, alongside a bowl of olive oil. You dip a piece of bread in the oil, then into the dukka, capturing every last, delicious crumb. I sometimes use rapeseed oil for a change. Dukka has other uses too – try scattering it over grilled vegetables, or over a simple salad of lettuce and soft, hard-boiled eggs.

If you can only find roasted, salted pistachios, skip the roasting bit and perhaps rub off some of the salt. And you can use other nuts – almonds and cashews are particularly good.

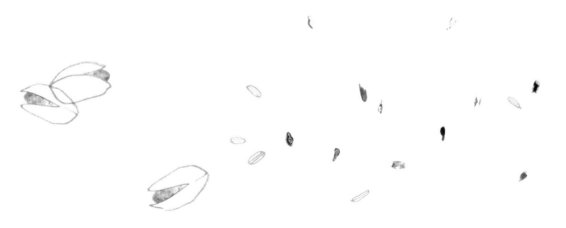

MAKES 125g

120g shelled, unsalted pistachios

1 tablespoon cumin seeds

1 tablespoon coriander seeds

3 tablespoons sesame seeds

A good sprig of mint, leaves only, chopped (optional)

1 teaspoon dried chilli flakes

1 teaspoon flaky sea salt

Preheat the oven to 200°C/Gas Mark 6. Scatter the pistachio kernels on a baking tray and roast in the oven for about 5 minutes, until just starting to turn golden. Cool, then chop them roughly.

In a small pan over a medium heat, warm the cumin and coriander seeds until they begin to release their aroma. Transfer to a mortar and bash with the pestle until broken up, but not too fine. In the same pan, lightly toast the sesame seeds.

Add the roughly chopped nuts to the mortar, and bash until they are broken up into smallish pieces. Stir in the sesame seeds, mint if using, chilli flakes and salt and transfer to a serving bowl.

The dukka will keep for a couple of weeks in a screw-topped jar.

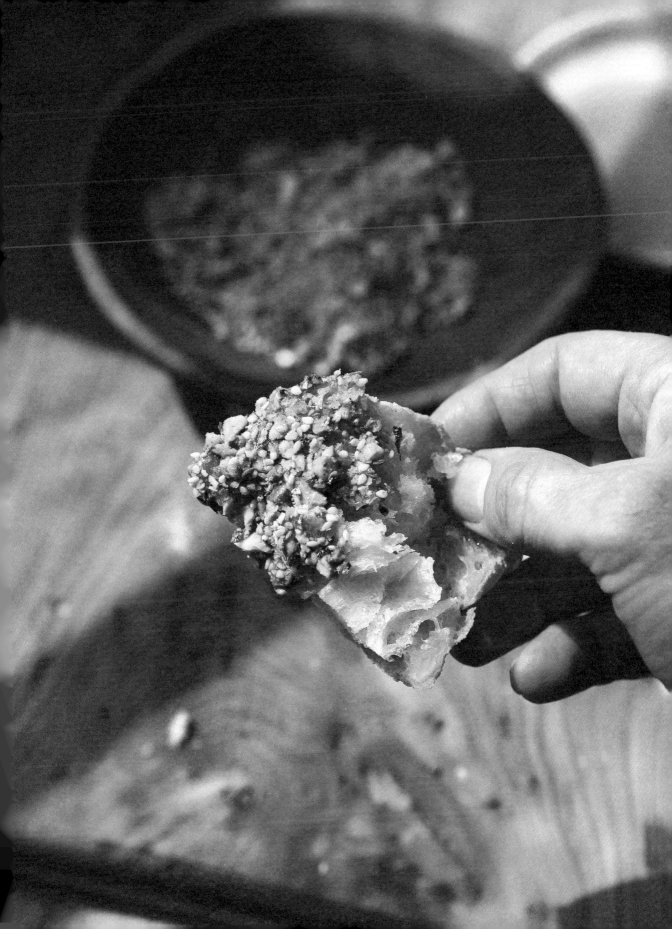

Lemony guacamole ᵛ

A good guacamole is creamy and comforting, and peppy and invigorating at the same time. This one is great with triangles of hot garlicky flatbread (see page 176), or stuffed into a sandwich or wrap.

SERVES 4

½–1 small red chilli, deseeded and finely chopped

2 tablespoons finely chopped coriander

Juice of 1 lemon, or ½ lemon and 1 lime

2 large, ripe avocados

1 tablespoon rapeseed oil

Sea salt and freshly ground black pepper

½–1 tablespoon plain (full-fat) yoghurt (optional)

Put the chilli, coriander and lemon (or lemon and lime) juice into a bowl. Halve, stone and peel the avocados, then cut into chunks and drop into the bowl. Add the oil and plenty of salt and pepper.

Now mash the lot together – you can keep it a bit rough and lumpy if you like, or keep mashing until smooth. And you can make it even smoother and saucier (ideal for dressing wraps, kebabs and foldovers) by whisking in a little yoghurt. Check the seasoning and serve.

Carrot hummus

Another delicious member of the ever-expanding family of River Cottage hummi. It's lovely with crudités, warm garlicky flatbreads (see page 176) or pitta and salad leaves, and I often serve it as part of a mezze-style spread, as shown on pages 6–7.

SERVES 4

1 teaspoon cumin seeds

1 teaspoon coriander seeds

6 tablespoons olive or rapeseed oil

1 teaspoon clear honey

500g carrots, peeled

3 large garlic cloves, bashed

Juice of ½ lemon

Juice of 1 orange

3 tablespoons tahini (or smooth peanut butter)

Flaky sea salt and freshly ground black pepper

Preheat the oven to 200°C/Gas Mark 6. In a dry frying pan, toast the cumin and coriander seeds for about a minute until just fragrant. Grind to a fine-ish powder using a pestle and mortar. In a large bowl, whisk 4 tablespoons of the oil with the honey and toasted spices.

Cut the carrots into 4–5cm chunks and add to the dressing with the garlic. Toss to coat and season with salt and pepper. Tip into a small roasting tin and roast, turning once, until the carrots are tender and just starting to char slightly around the edges, about 35 minutes.

Allow to cool slightly, then scrape everything into a food processor, slipping the garlic cloves out of their skins as you do so. Add the lemon and orange juices, tahini (or peanut butter) and remaining oil and pulse to a purée. Adjust the seasoning if necessary and serve.

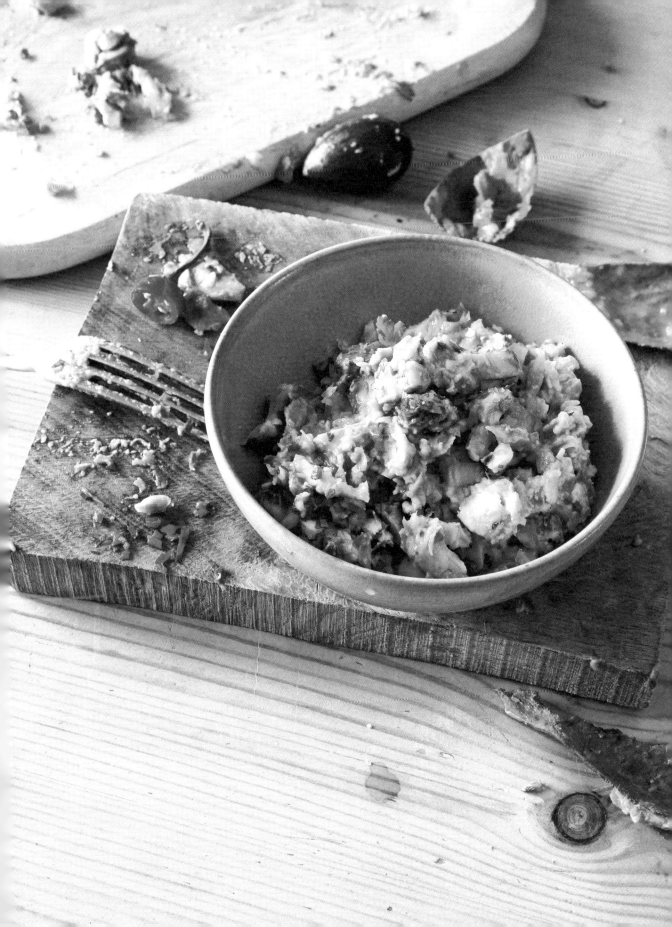

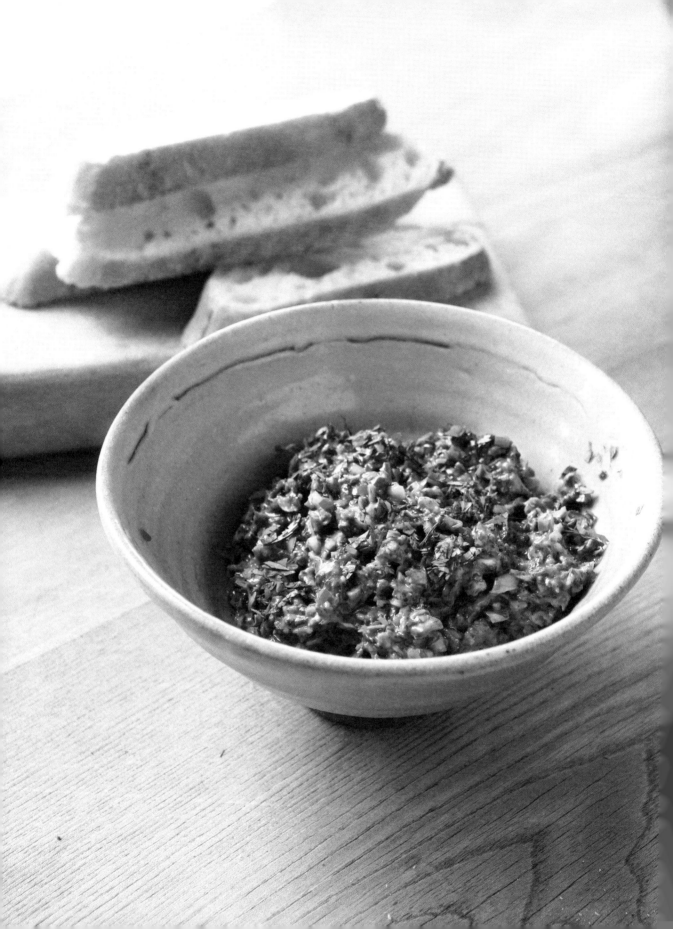

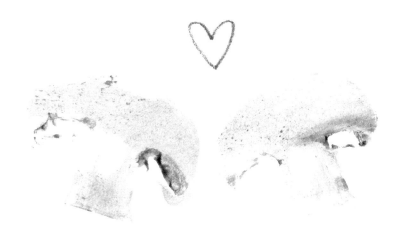

Cambodian wedding day dip ^v

*This is my version of a delicious, easy dish shown to me by David Bailey,
formerly head chef of the lovely vegetarian restaurant Saf, and now
running his own catering company. As well as presenting it as part of
a spread, you can make a meal of it by serving it hot with rice and maybe
some garlicky greens (see page 372). A good teaspoon of chilli and garlic
paste from a jar can be used instead of the fresh garlic and chilli.*

SERVES 8

500g chestnut or cup
mushrooms, or a combination

1 tablespoon sunflower oil

½ small, hot chilli, such as bird's
eye (with seeds), finely chopped

3 garlic cloves, crushed

1 tablespoon curry powder
or mild curry paste

2 tablespoons crunchy peanut
butter

400ml tin coconut milk

Juice of ½ lime

A dash of soy sauce

Finely chopped coriander,
to finish (optional)

Finely dice the mushrooms into 3–4mm pieces. Alternatively, chop
them in a food processor – but don't blitz them too fine.

Heat the sunflower oil in a wok or large frying pan over a high heat.
Add the mushrooms and cook briskly, stirring often, until all the liquid
they release has evaporated. Add the chilli and garlic and fry for
another 1 minute.

Add the curry powder or paste and peanut butter, stir in thoroughly
and then stir in the coconut milk. Let it all bubble rapidly, stirring
occasionally to make sure it doesn't burn, until thick and reduced –
up to half an hour. Add the lime juice and soy sauce to taste.

Scoop the dip into a bowl. Scatter, if you like, with chopped coriander,
and serve warm or at room temperature. Flatbreads - or any good
bread - as well as fresh veg crudités are ideal accompaniments.

Beetroot and walnut hummus🌱

I make no apology for including this recipe – tweaked from its River Cottage
Every Day *incarnation. It's such a great way to use beetroot, and superb as a
starter, dip or lunchbox treat. I love it with hot garlicky flatbreads (see page 176).*

SERVES 4

50g walnuts

1 tablespoon cumin seeds

15g stale bread, crusts removed
and torn into chunks

200g cooked beetroot (not
pickled), cut into cubes

1 tablespoon tahini
(or smooth peanut butter)

1 large garlic clove, crushed

Juice of 1 lemon

A little rapeseed or olive oil

Sea salt and freshly ground
black pepper

Preheat the oven to 180°C/Gas Mark 4. Toast the walnuts on a baking
tray in the oven for 5–7 minutes, until fragrant. Leave to cool.

Warm a small frying pan over a medium heat and dry-fry the cumin
seeds, shaking the pan, until they start to darken and release their
aroma – this should take less than a minute; don't burn them. Crush
the still-warm seeds with a pestle and mortar or spice grinder.

Put the bread and toasted nuts into a food processor or blender and
blitz to fine crumbs. Add the beetroot, tahini (or peanut butter), most
of the garlic and cumin, the juice of ½ lemon, ½ tablespoon oil, a little
salt and a grinding of pepper. Blend to a thick paste. Taste and adjust
by adding a little more cumin, garlic, lemon, salt and/or pepper,
blending again. Loosen with a dash more oil if required. Refrigerate
until required (it'll keep for a few days). Serve at room temperature.

Cannellini bean hummus🌱

*Perfect with warm pitta or garlicky flatbreads (page 176), this is also
delicious with roasted leeks (see page 336).*

SERVES 4

400g tin cannellini or other
white beans, drained and rinsed

½ garlic clove

1 tablespoon tahini

2 tablespoons extra virgin
olive oil

A good squeeze of lemon juice

A sprig of thyme, leaves only

Sea salt and freshly ground black
pepper

FOR THE PAPRIKA OIL

1 tablespoon rapeseed or olive oil

½ teaspoon paprika (smoked
or sweet)

Put the beans in a food processor. Crush the garlic with a little salt and
add about half of it to the processor, along with the tahini, extra virgin
olive oil, lemon juice, thyme leaves, 1 tablespoon water and some salt
and pepper. Process to a purée. Taste and adjust the flavour by adding
more garlic, lemon juice, salt and/or pepper, if you like. Transfer to a
serving dish.

For the paprika oil, warm the oil and paprika very gently for a couple
of minutes to infuse; let cool. Trickle over the hummus to serve.

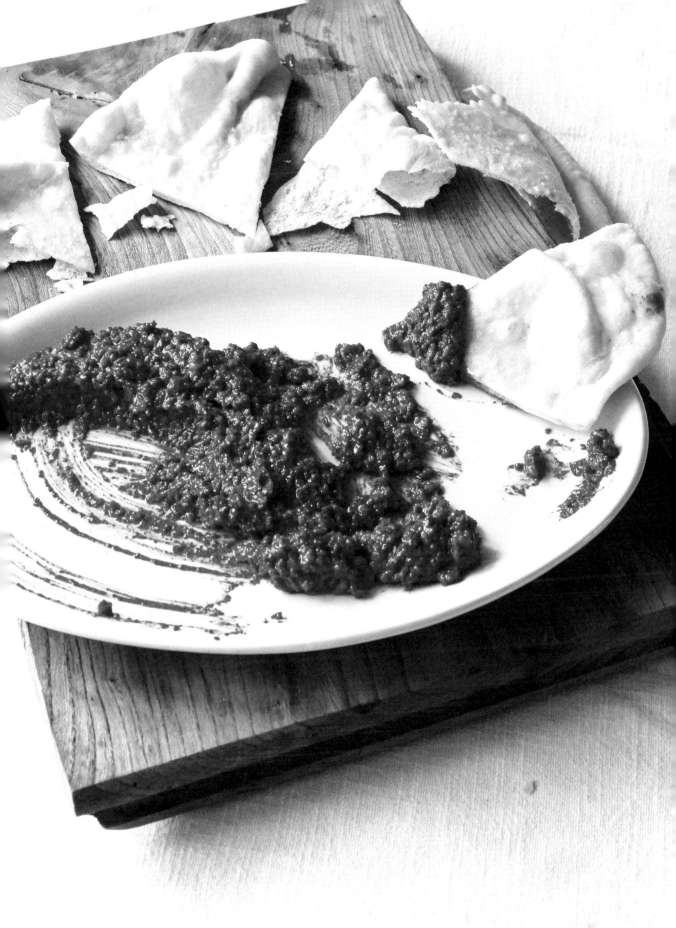

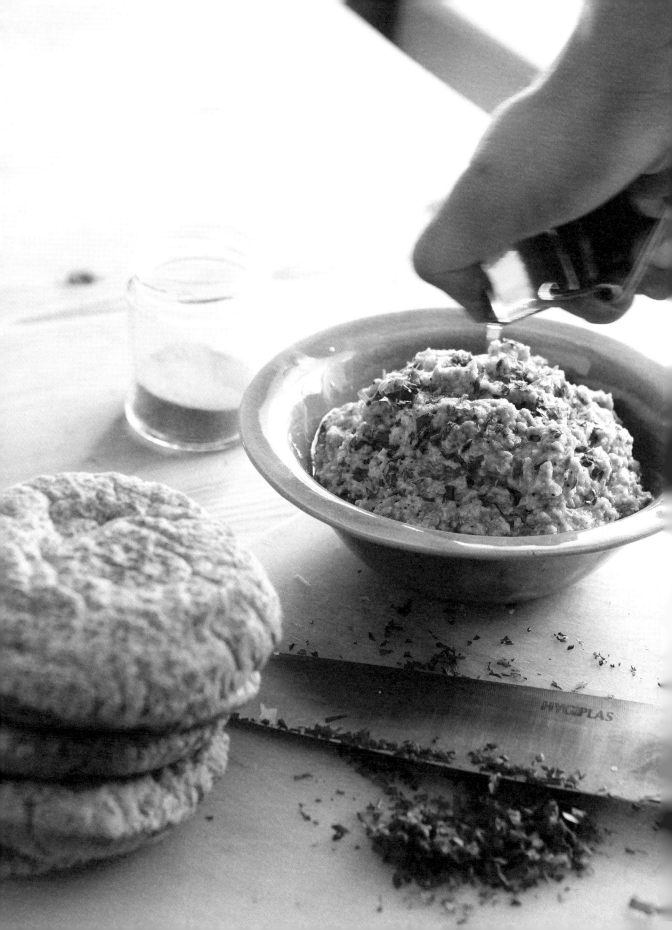

Baba ganoush 🌱

This classic, smoky purée is still one of the best things you can do with an aubergine. Serve it as a dip, or cram into pitta bread or soft tortillas, along with some chopped tomatoes, cucumber, spring onion and/or peppery salad leaves.

SERVES 4

4 medium aubergines (about 1kg)

1 large garlic clove, crushed

2 tablespoons tahini (or smooth peanut or cashew nut butter)

A good squeeze of lemon juice

Sea salt and freshly ground black pepper

TO FINISH

A handful of parsley, chopped

Rapeseed or extra virgin olive oil, to trickle

1–2 teaspoons ground cumin

Preheat your grill to high. Prick the aubergines once or twice with a fork. Lay them on a foil-lined tray and grill, turning often, for at least 10 minutes, until the skin is blackened all over and the flesh beneath is tender. Leave until cool enough to handle, then peel off the skin. Put the aubergine flesh into a colander and roughly chop it, using a small, sharp knife. Leave to drain, until completely cool.

Tip the aubergine into a food processor and add the garlic, tahini (or nut butter), lemon juice and plenty of salt and pepper. Process to a purée. Taste for seasoning and add more lemon juice if you like.

Serve scattered with chopped parsley, trickled with oil and dusted generously with cumin. To use as a sandwich filling, stir the oil, cumin and parsley into the purée.

Artichoke and white bean dip

This rich, creamy, deeply savoury dip is wonderful with crudités, or dolloped on to a warm flatbread. It also works well served on some crisp lettuce, as a salad.

SERVES 4–6

2 tablespoons olive oil

1 small onion, chopped

200g artichoke hearts in olive oil, drained, oil reserved

3 garlic cloves, finely chopped

A few sprigs of oregano, leaves only, finely chopped

400g tin cannellini beans, drained and rinsed

Juice of ½ lemon

½ teaspoon dried chilli flakes

2 tablespoons thick, plain (full-fat) yoghurt

25g walnuts, toasted (optional)

Sea salt and freshly ground black pepper

Heat 1 tablespoon olive oil in a frying pan over a medium-low heat and sauté the onion for about 10 minutes, until soft and translucent. Meanwhile, roughly chop the artichoke hearts.

Add the garlic to the pan and stir for another couple of minutes. Tip in the oregano, cannellini beans and artichokes and cook, stirring, for a couple of minutes, until everything is heated through.

Tip the mixture into a food processor and add the lemon juice, chilli flakes and yoghurt. Blend to a coarse purée. Add salt and pepper to taste and thin with a couple of tablespoons or so of the olive oil from the artichokes, until you have the texture you like.

Serve the dip warm or cold, trickled with olive oil, and scattered with toasted walnuts if you like.

Oven-dried tomatoes ^v

I find commercially produced 'sun-dried' tomatoes are often lip-pursingly intense, sharp and sometimes a little leathery. Home-dried ones are altogether different. The beauty of drying your own is that you can control their plumpness, sweetness and chewiness. Here I'm aiming for a semi-dried state – intense but still a touch juicy.

This is also, I must concede, a good way to use out-of-season or less-full-flavoured tomatoes, as the seasoning and drying will bring out the best in them. Dried tomatoes are delicious stirred into salads, pasta or couscous, or just served as a piquant nibble with a selection of other dishes. Try them also in a sandwich with goat's cheese, in a frittata with potatoes and onions, or even stirred into scrambled eggs.

SERVES 4-6

1kg tomatoes

½ teaspoon sugar

A few sprigs of thyme, broken up

3 bay leaves, each snipped into 2 or 3 pieces

2–3 tablespoons olive oil, plus extra for storage

Fine sea salt and freshly ground black pepper

Halve the tomatoes, or quarter particularly large ones. Scoop out and discard the seeds, if you prefer. Stand a wire rack over a double sheet of newspaper.

Combine the sugar with ½ teaspoon fine salt in a small bowl. Sprinkle a tiny pinch of this mixture over the inside of each tomato half, then put the tomatoes upside down on the rack. Leave for 1 hour for the juices to drip.

Preheat the oven to very low, about 100°C/Gas Mark ¼. Transfer the tomatoes, turning them cut side up, to a large baking tray. Scatter with the thyme, bay, some black pepper and the olive oil and place in the oven. Check after an hour or two – just in case your oven is hotter than it says! It should take 4–5 hours to get the tomatoes 'semi-dried': ie considerably reduced but still quite tender and plump. This is how I like them. However, you can leave them in the oven for 7–8 hours – to become much more like commercial 'sun-dried' tomatoes.

Tossed in a generous amount of olive oil, these oven-dried tomatoes will keep for a few days in the fridge. You'll find endless uses for them.

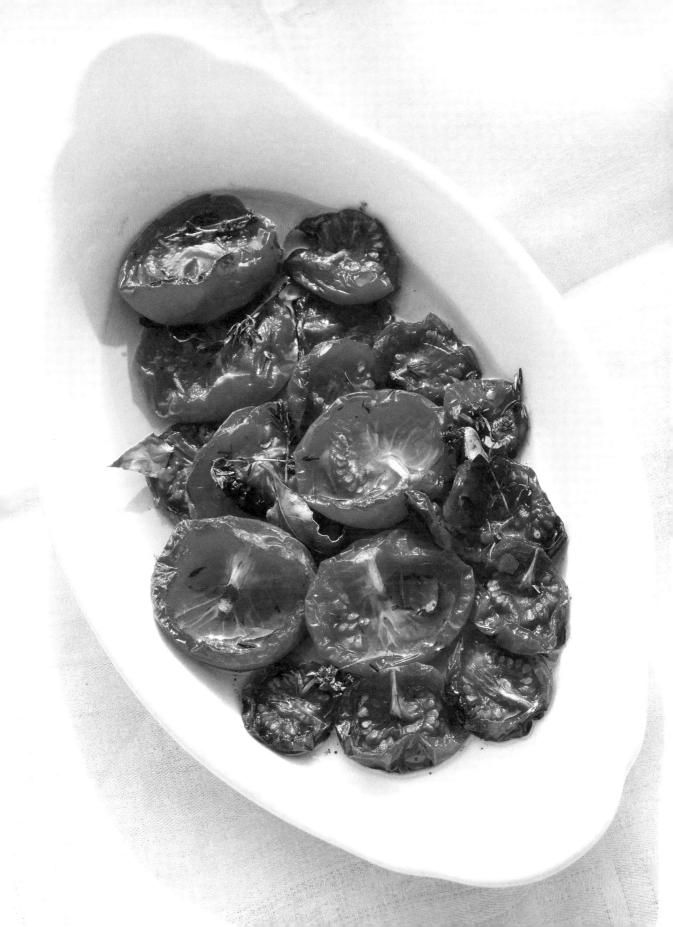

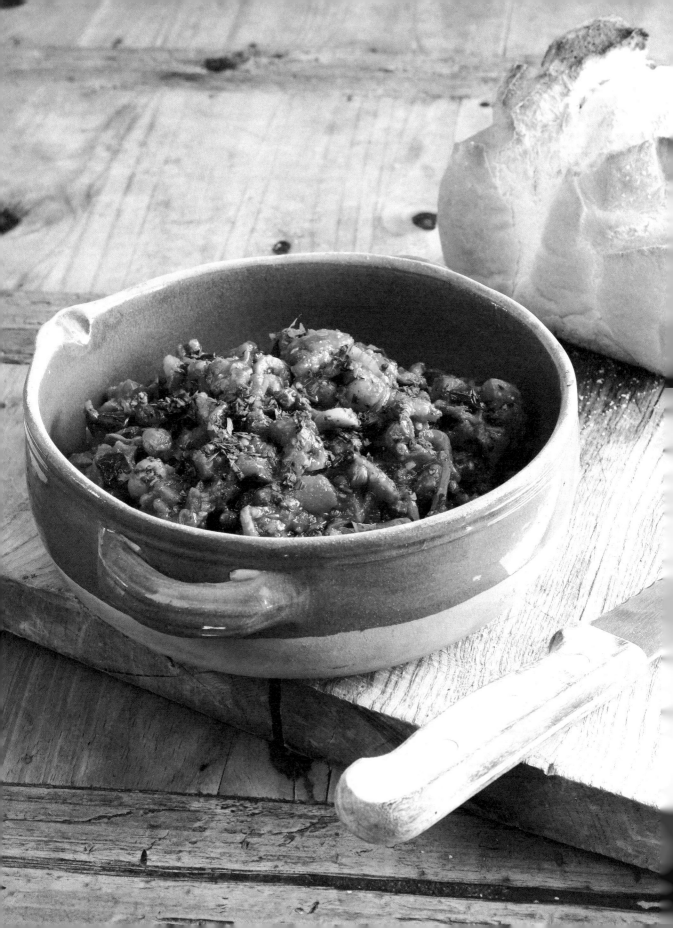

Caponata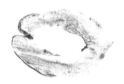

As well as being a lovely element in a spread of vegetable dishes, this classic, sweet-sour aubergine stew makes a fabulous crostini topping (see page 178). It's also a very good accompaniment to barbecued foods.

SERVES 4

2 medium aubergines (about 500g), cut into 1cm cubes

2 tablespoons olive oil

1 onion, finely chopped

2 inner celery stalks, finely sliced

1 garlic clove, chopped

6 large plum or other ripe tomatoes, peeled, deseeded and chopped, OR a 400g tin plum tomatoes, chopped, any stalky ends and skin removed

2 tablespoons balsamic vinegar

1 tablespoon soft brown sugar

1 tablespoon finely grated dark chocolate (optional)

50g sultanas

2 tablespoons baby capers, rinsed

50g stoned green olives, sliced

Sea salt and freshly ground black pepper

A good handful of flat-leaf parsley or mint, chopped, to finish

Put the aubergine cubes into a large colander and sprinkle with 2 teaspoons salt. Toss together and then leave to draw out the juices for about half an hour. Rinse the aubergine and pat/squeeze dry with a tea towel.

While the aubergine is salting, heat 1 tablespoon olive oil in a large saucepan. Add the onion, celery and garlic and fry over a fairly low heat for about 10 minutes until tender and golden. Add the tomatoes with their juice and simmer for 5 minutes to reduce a little.

Now add the balsamic vinegar, sugar, chocolate if using, sultanas, capers and olives to the pan. Simmer for another 5–10 minutes, stirring often, then turn off the heat.

In a large frying pan, heat another 1 tablespoon oil over a medium-high heat. When hot, fry the aubergine cubes for about 5 minutes, until golden and tender. Tip them into the tomato sauce mixture.

Return to a simmer again and cook for another 10 minutes, then remove from the heat, cover and leave until completely cold. Taste and adjust the seasoning.

You can serve the caponata straight away or leave it in the fridge or a very cool place for a day or two to allow the flavours to deepen even further, bringing it to room temperature before serving. Sprinkle with plenty of chopped parsley or mint just before serving.

Vegetable tempura with chilli dipping sauce ♥

All kinds of vegetables are excellent deep-fried within a crisp, light coating of tempura batter. But I'm not averse to doing this with one type of veg only, as in the picture. It may sound extravagant but it's actually a brilliant way of serving asparagus.

The easy chilli sauce will keep sealed in a jar for a week if you have any left over. It's the perfect thing to perk up all manner of dressings and marinades.

SERVES 4-6

A selection from:

Asparagus spears

Courgette slices (cut on the diagonal, 2–3mm thick)

Broccoli or cauliflower florets

Strips of pepper or aubergine

Spring onions or thin wedges of red onion

Sliced large mushrooms

Wide ribbons of kale (stalks removed)

Sunflower oil, for deep-frying

FOR THE TEMPURA BATTER

100g plain flour

40g cornflour

½ teaspoon baking powder

½ teaspoon salt

200–225ml ice-cold sparkling mineral water

FOR THE DIPPING SAUCE

6 tablespoons redcurrant or crab apple jelly

2 tablespoons cider vinegar

2 teaspoons soy sauce

2 red chillies, deseeded and very finely chopped

2 garlic cloves, very finely chopped

A few twists of black pepper

A good handful of coriander, finely chopped (optional)

Make the dipping sauce first. Tip all of the ingredients except the coriander into a small saucepan and stir over a very low heat until the fruit jelly has dissolved and you are left with a silky syrup. Bring it to a simmer and bubble gently for a few minutes – this will mellow the harshness of the garlic. Set aside to cool to room temperature. If the sauce re-sets to a jelly when it's cooled, simply whisk in a splash of warm water. If using the coriander, stir in just before serving.

Have all the veg prepared and ready. Just before you're about to cook them, make the batter. Sift the flour, cornflour, baking powder and salt into a bowl. Begin whisking in the water, ideally with an ice cube or two, until you have a batter the thickness of single cream. Be careful not to over-mix and don't worry if there are a few lumps.

While you prepare the batter, heat about a 5cm depth of oil in a large, deep, heavy-based saucepan until a cube of white bread dropped in turns golden brown in about 50 seconds.

You will need to fry the prepared veg in batches. Begin dipping them in the batter, one piece at a time, transferring them to the hot oil as soon as they are coated; don't overcrowd the pan. Fry until they are crisp and a light golden colour.

Remove carefully with tongs or a slotted spoon. Drain on kitchen paper and serve immediately with the dipping sauce. Eat with fingers or chopsticks!

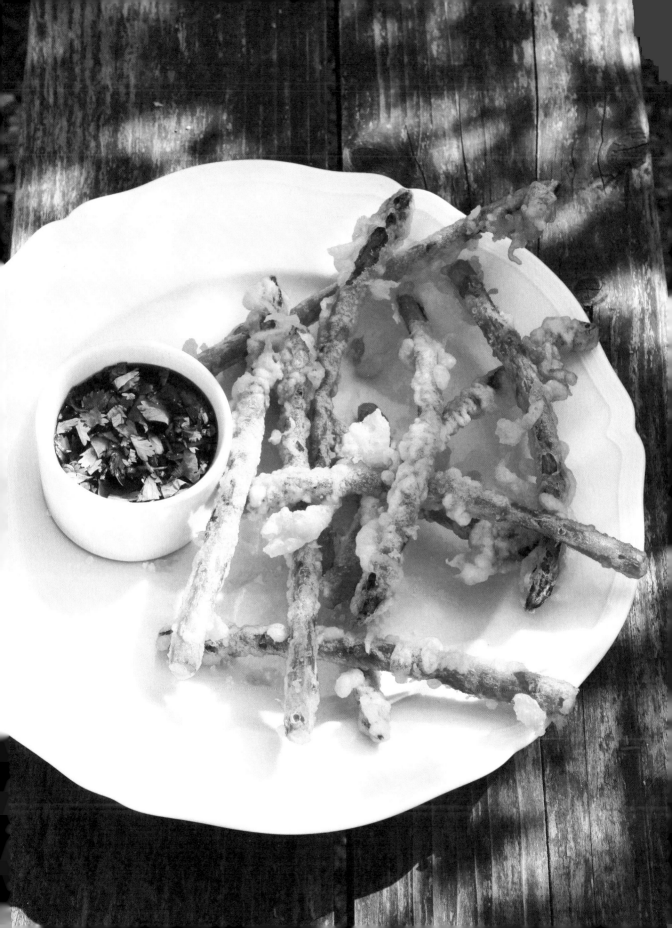

Simple globe artichokes ᵛ

This is more a veg starter or preamble than a mezze-style dish, but I love globe artichokes so much that I want to encourage everyone to eat them. Preparing them can seem fiddly at first, but it's actually pretty straightforward and they make one of the most enjoyable of all summer starters.

SERVES 6

6 medium/large
globe artichokes
A squeeze of lemon juice
Sea salt

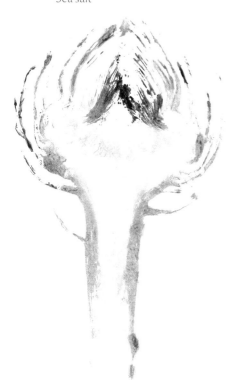

Remove the toughest leaves from close to the base of each artichoke and trim the stem to about 3cm long (or, on good-sized ones, remove the stem completely, so the artichoke will sit flat on its base).

Place in a saucepan of lightly salted boiling water with a squeeze of lemon juice, or in a steamer, and cook for 15–30 minutes, depending on size and freshness. Just-cut artichokes will need less cooking. If you grow your own, you'll find that cooking them within minutes of cutting reduces the cooking time dramatically – to just 7–8 minutes for a small one. An artichoke is cooked when a leaf from the middle pulls away easily and the heart is tender when pierced with a knife.

To eat, pull off the outer leaves, dipping them in your chosen sauce and scraping away the tender part with your teeth. Work your way down to the tiny, papery leaves near the base, discarding these. Remove the hairy part of the choke with a spoon, then tuck into the delicious heart.

HOW TO SERVE YOUR ARTICHOKES

• Enjoy them simply, with melted butter and a squeeze of lemon to dip the leaves into.

• Make a cheaty hollandaise: melt 150g butter and whisk it, a little at a time, into an egg yolk until it has a loose consistency, like mayonnaise. Whisk in a generous squeeze of lemon juice and season with a pinch of salt and some pepper.

• Make a simple vinaigrette: put a crushed garlic clove, 1 teaspoon mustard, some salt and pepper, 2 tablespoons cider vinegar and 6 tablespoons olive or rapeseed oil in a screw-topped jar and shake to emulsify. Add 1 tablespoon finely chopped capers too, if you like.

• Try barbecued artichokes: boil or steam, as above, then slice them in half lengthways, tip to base. Brush with some olive oil and grill them, cut side down, on the barbecue for a couple of minutes. Eat each half as above, relishing that intense, smoky flavour.

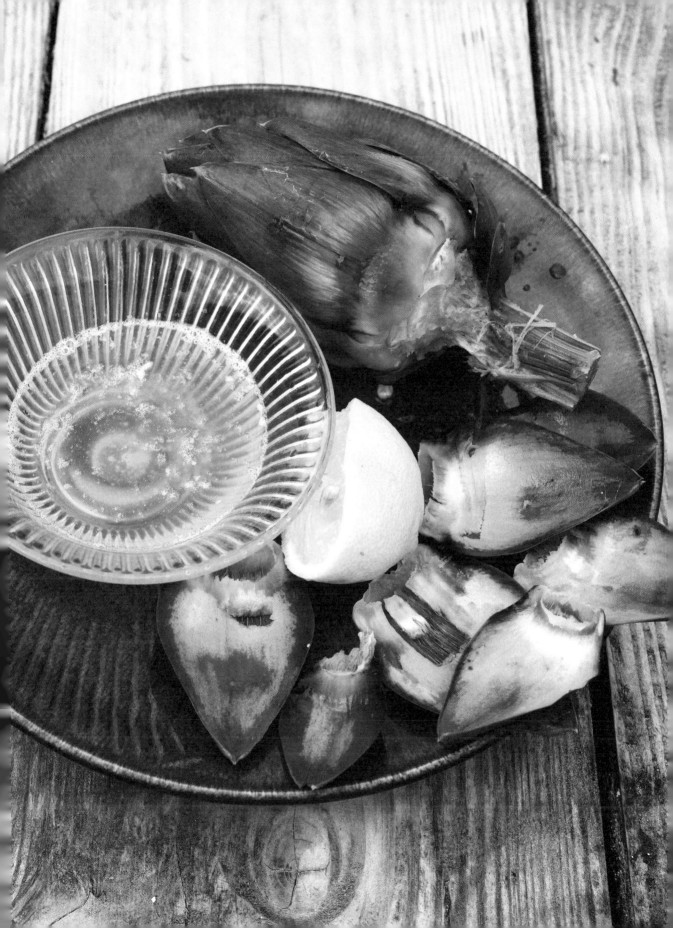

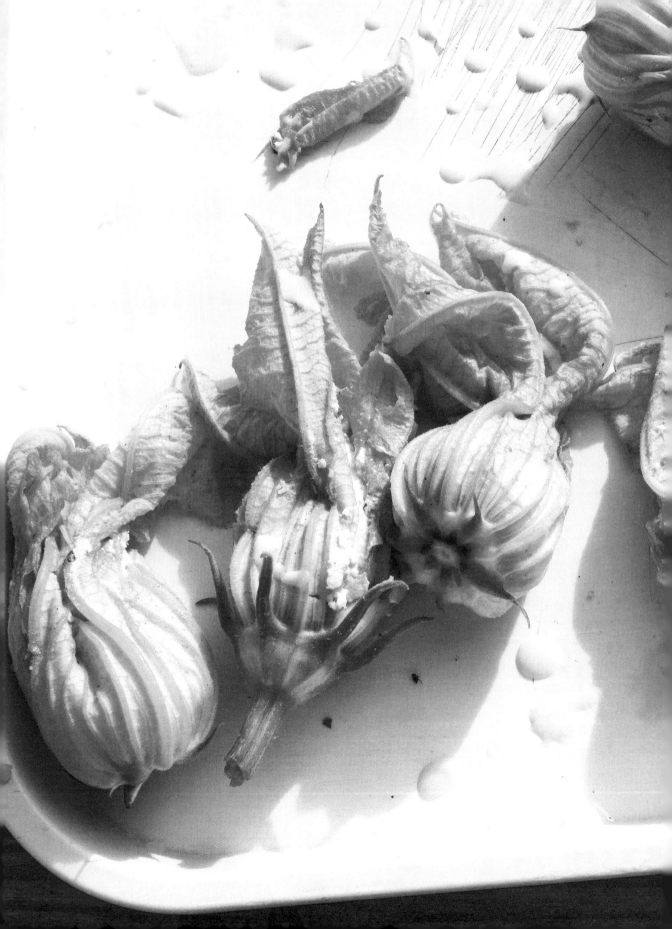

Deep-fried courgette flowers stuffed with ricotta and herbs

This has got to rank as one of the most exquisite and delicious vegetable treats ever – it's certainly among my all-time favourites. You can vary the stuffing – or even leave it out altogether – and the dish will still be fantastic.

SERVES 4

8–12 courgette flowers

Sunflower oil, for deep-frying

FOR THE FILLING

100g ricotta

2 good tablespoons grated Parmesan, hard goat's cheese or other well-flavoured hard cheese

A large handful of mixed herbs, such as parsley and chives with a little marjoram or thyme, or parsley and a little mint, finely chopped

Sea salt and freshly ground black pepper

FOR THE BATTER

100g plain flour

40g cornflour

½ teaspoon baking powder

½ teaspoon sea salt

200–225ml ice-cold sparkling mineral water

TO FINISH

Flaky sea salt

Nasturtiums or other edible flowers (optional)

For the filling, beat the ricotta until soft and smooth, then stir in the cheese, herbs and some salt and pepper. Carefully scoop the filling into the courgette flowers: you should get 2–4 teaspoons in each one, depending on size. Twist the petals gently to enclose the mixture.

Just before you're ready to cook, prepare the batter. Sift the flour, cornflour, baking powder and salt into a bowl. Begin whisking in the water, until you have a batter the thickness of single cream. Be careful not to over-mix and don't worry if there are a few lumps.

Meanwhile, heat about a 6cm depth of oil in a deep-fat fryer or deep, heavy saucepan (to come no more than a third of the way up the pan), till a cube of bread dropped in turns golden brown in about 1 minute.

Dip one stuffed courgette flower into the batter and immediately lower into the hot oil. Repeat with a couple more; do not cook more than 3 or 4 at a time. Cook for 1–2 minutes, until puffed up, crisp and golden brown. Drain on kitchen paper while you cook the remaining flowers. Serve as soon as possible, sprinkled with a little flaky sea salt and decorated, if you like, with other edible flowers.

VARIATIONS

Courgette and goat's cheese stuffed flowers
Use goat's cheese in place of the ricotta and the soft courgette mix from the bruschetta on page 200, mixing them together before stuffing the flowers. Continue as above.

Risotto stuffed courgette flowers
Stuff the flowers with leftover risotto (see pages 269-73). As the risotto will have been chilled, you'll need to fry the flowers for a little longer.

Courgette flowers stuffed with mozzarella
Slip a thick slice of good buffalo mozzarella, lightly seasoned with pepper, inside the courgette flower, along with a couple of basil leaves. Dip in the batter and deep-fry as above. I've even managed to stuff a whole bocconcino (mini mozzarella) inside a large courgette flower. As you'd expect, the cheese comes out lovely and melty.

Marinated courgettes with mozzarella

If you can make this with a mixture of green and yellow courgettes it is particularly attractive, but just one type looks – and tastes – pretty good too.

SERVES 2

4 medium courgettes
(about 500g)

5 tablespoons extra virgin
olive or rapeseed oil

1 large garlic clove,
finely slivered

Finely grated zest of 1 lemon,
plus a little juice

A handful of mint or basil,
roughly torn

1 ball of buffalo mozzarella
(about 125g), or other mild,
soft cheese, sliced or roughly
torn

Sea salt and freshly ground
black pepper

Top and tail the courgettes, then cut them lengthways into thin slices, 1–2mm thick. Put them in a bowl with 2 tablespoons of the oil and use a pastry brush to get them all lightly coated.

Heat a large non-stick frying pan over a fairly high heat. Working in batches, sear the courgette slices for about 2 minutes on each side until tender and golden. Transfer them to a shallow dish.

Take the frying pan off the heat and let it cool down a bit. Add the remaining 3 tablespoons oil, the garlic and lemon zest. Heat very gently for a few minutes – the residual heat in the pan may be enough – you just want to take the raw edge off the garlic and infuse the flavours into the oil.

Pour the infused oil over the courgettes. Add some salt and pepper, a little squeeze of lemon juice and the mint or basil. Toss together, cover and leave for 1 hour at room temperature.

Strew with mozzarella and serve with good bread or, better still, warm flatbreads (see page 176).

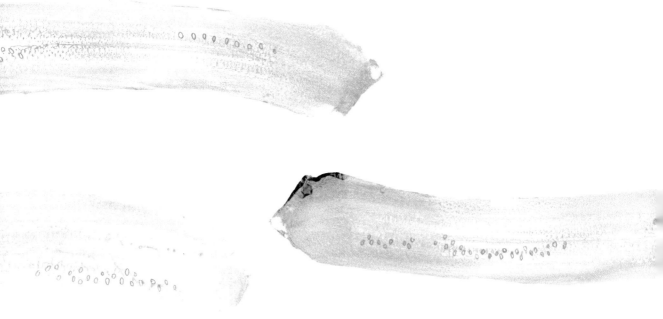

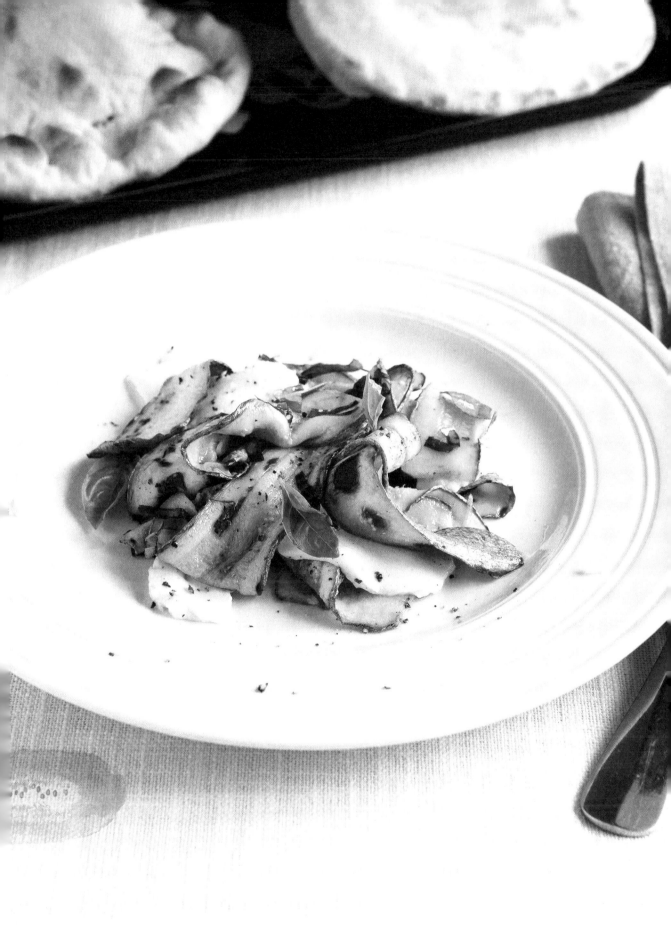

Broad beans with herbed goat's cheese

*This is wonderful as part of a spread of small tapas-style dishes. It is also
a great starter or lunch, served with a hunk of bread or wedge of oily toast,
or folded into a wrap for a lunchbox or picnic basket.*

SERVES 4–6

400–500g young podded broad beans (about 1.5kg unpodded)

FOR THE HERBED GOAT'S CHEESE

125g soft, mild goat's cheese

4–5 tablespoons plain (full-fat) yoghurt

A good handful of mixed herbs, such as parsley, chives, tarragon and thyme, chopped

A scrap of garlic, crushed

Sea salt and freshly ground black pepper

Bring a large pan of water to the boil and drop in the broad beans. Return to a simmer and cook until the beans are tender. For very small, tender beans, this will be only a minute. Larger beans may take 2–3 minutes, but I wouldn't recommend using older, bigger beans that need any longer. Drain well and slip larger beans out of their skins; tender babies are fine as they are. Leave to cool completely.

Beat the goat's cheese with the yoghurt until reasonably smooth. Mix in the chopped herbs, garlic and some salt and pepper.

Fold the cooled beans into the goat's cheese mixture. Taste and adjust the seasoning if necessary before serving.

Broccoli salad with asian-style dressing ♥

*This simple salad is full of aromatic Eastern flavours, all beautifully carried
by the crunchy broccoli.*

SERVES 4

1 large head of broccoli (about 500g)

½ garlic clove

1 teaspoon freshly grated ginger

A pinch of sugar

1 tablespoon rice vinegar or cider vinegar

2 teaspoons soy sauce

1 tablespoon toasted sesame oil

2 teaspoons sesame seeds

2–3 spring onions, trimmed and finely sliced

Sea salt and freshly ground black pepper

Cut the broccoli into small florets and steam, or cook it in some lightly salted boiling water, until just tender but still a bit crunchy – about 4–5 minutes.

Meanwhile, crush the garlic and ginger with the sugar and some salt and pepper to a paste, using a pestle and mortar. Combine with the vinegar, soy sauce and sesame oil.

As soon as the broccoli is cooked, drain it in a colander and leave for a few minutes so all the moisture can steam off. While still hot, toss with the dressing and put into a serving dish. Set aside to cool.

Lightly toast the sesame seeds in a dry frying pan until fragrant. When the broccoli has cooled to room temperature, scatter over the spring onions and sesame seeds, and serve.

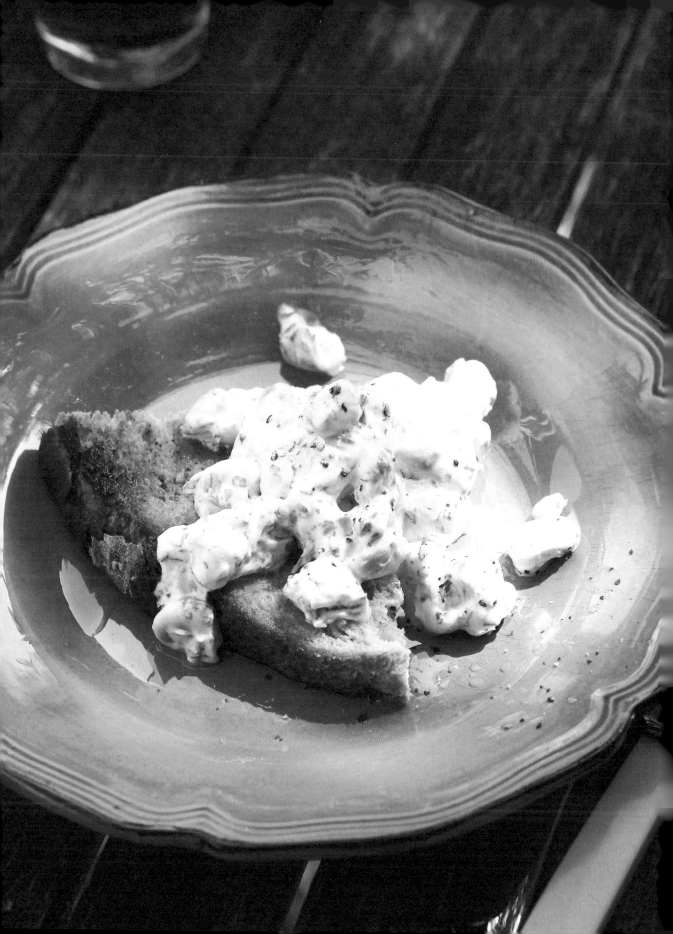

Cauliflower pakoras with tamarind raita

These irresistible morsels make a great canapé, but they are also very good alongside or before a curry. Eat them with your fingers, as soon as they're cool enough to pick up: the contrast between the hot, spicy pakoras and the cold, slightly sour yoghurt is delicious. If tamarind paste is not to hand, use mango chutney, or any spicy-sweet fruit chutney, instead.

SERVES 6-8

1 medium-large cauliflower (about 800g), trimmed

Sunflower oil, for frying

FOR THE BATTER

150g gram flour (chickpea flour)

½ teaspoon baking powder

2 teaspoons ground cumin

2 teaspoons ground coriander

½ teaspoon ground turmeric

A good shake of cayenne pepper

½ teaspoon fine sea salt

FOR THE TAMARIND RAITA

6 heaped tablespoons plain (full-fat) yoghurt

A large handful of coriander, chopped (optional)

2 teaspoons tamarind paste or mango chutney

Sea salt and freshly ground black pepper

For the raita, mix all the ingredients together, seasoning with salt and pepper to taste. Set aside.

Cut the cauliflower into small florets, no more than 2cm across in any direction, discarding nearly all the stalk.

For the batter, put the gram flour, baking powder, ground spices and salt into a large bowl. Whisk to combine and get rid of any lumps. Slowly whisk in 175ml cold water, which should give you a smooth batter with a similar consistency to double cream. Add a little more water if necessary – different brands of gram flour will vary in how much they absorb.

Add the cauliflower florets to the batter and turn them, making sure they are all thoroughly coated.

Heat about a 1cm depth of oil in a heavy-based pan over a medium-high heat. When the oil is hot enough to turn a cube of white bread light golden brown in 30–40 seconds, start cooking the pakoras, a few at a time so you don't crowd the pan. Place spoonfuls of battered cauliflower – just a few florets per spoonful – into the hot oil. Cook for about 2 minutes, until crisp and golden brown on the base, then turn over and cook for another minute or two.

Drain the pakoras on kitchen paper, then serve piping hot with the raita for dipping.

VARIATION

Flat onion bhajis

Make the batter as above, but use 3 medium onions or 2 dozen spring onions instead of the cauliflower. Slice the onions fairly thinly and stir into the batter, making sure they're well coated. Heat the oil as above and fry spoonfuls of the onions in batches, being careful not to crowd the pan, for about 4 minutes, turning halfway through, until crisp and golden. Serve immediately, with the raita.

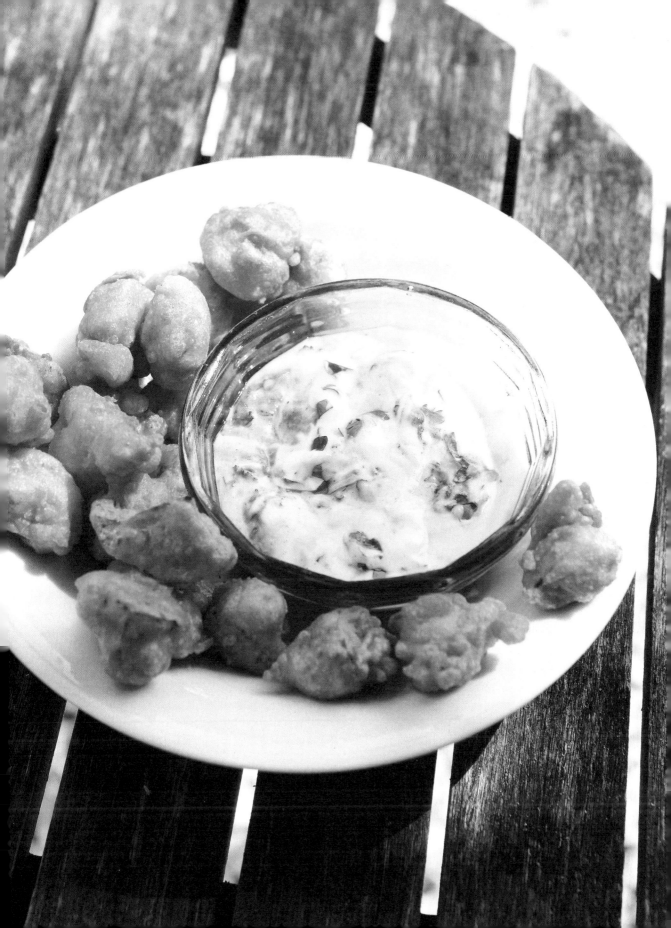

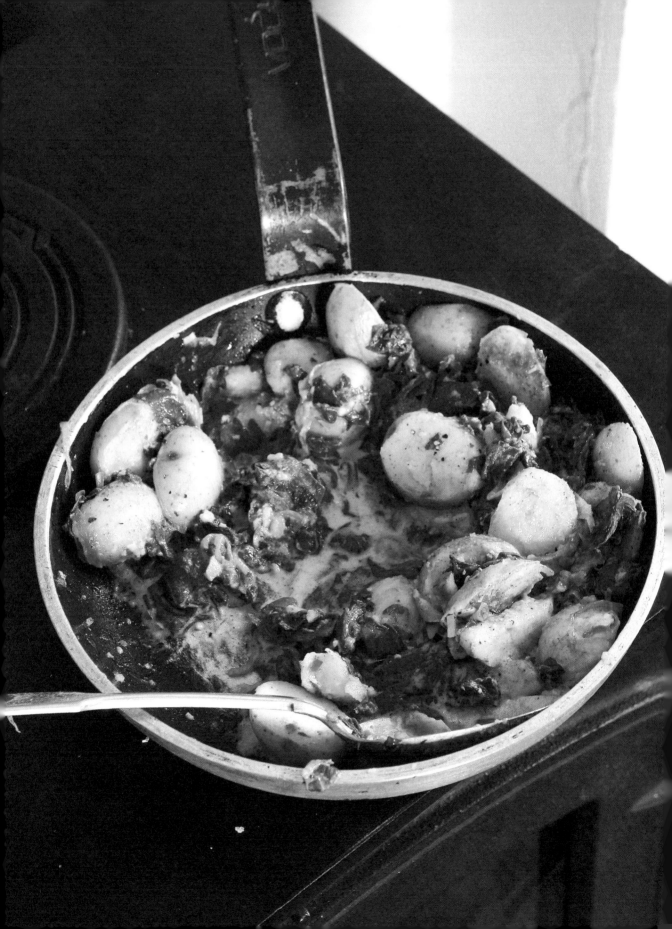

Spiced spinach and potatoes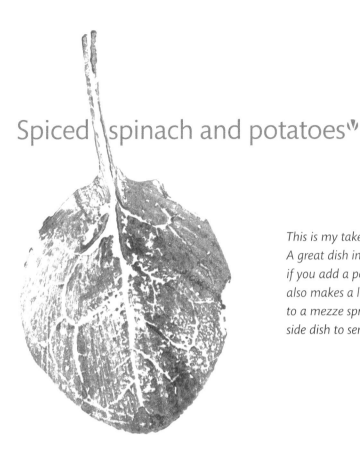

This is my take on saag aloo. A great dish in itself (especially if you add a poached egg), it also makes a lovely addition to a mezze spread or a tasty side dish to serve with curries.

SERVES 4

400g waxy or new potatoes

400g spinach, stripped of any coarse stems

2 tablespoons rapeseed or sunflower oil

1 onion, thinly sliced

1 garlic clove, finely chopped

1 red chilli, deseeded and finely chopped

1 good teaspoon freshly grated ginger

2 teaspoons garam masala

2–3 tablespoons double cream or coconut cream (optional)

Sea salt and freshly ground black pepper

Halve or quarter larger potatoes so that all the pieces are roughly the same size. Put into a saucepan, cover with water, add salt and bring to the boil. Simmer for 8–12 minutes, until tender. Drain. (You can use leftover cooked potatoes for this dish too.)

Wash the spinach thoroughly, then pack it, with just the water that clings to it, into a saucepan. Cover and put over a medium heat until the spinach has wilted in its own liquid – just a few minutes. Drain and leave in a colander until cool enough to handle, then squeeze out as much liquid as you can with your hands. Chop the spinach roughly.

Heat the oil in a frying pan and gently sweat the onion for 10 minutes or so, until soft. Add the garlic, chilli, ginger and garam masala. Cook for a couple of minutes more, then thickly slice the potatoes into the pan. Cook for a couple of minutes.

Now add the chopped spinach and cook briefly to warm through. The dish is lovely like this, or you can make it a little richer and more luxurious by stirring in the double cream or coconut cream with the spinach. Either way, season with salt and pepper, and serve.

Patatas bravas ᵛ

This is a classic Spanish tapa that works beautifully with a selection of other little dishes – chunks of frittata, simple salads, olives, dips etc – but it also makes a great starter in its own right. Add an extra chilli if you want more heat. And if you have any sauce left over, save it to toss through hot pasta.

SERVES 4–6

1kg waxy or new potatoes, cut into 3cm cubes

5 tablespoons olive or rapeseed oil

Flaky sea salt

FOR THE SPICY TOMATO SAUCE

2 tablespoons olive or rapeseed oil

1 onion, finely chopped

A handful of thyme sprigs, leaves only, chopped

3 garlic cloves, finely chopped

1 small, fairly hot red chilli, deseeded and finely chopped

400g tin plum tomatoes, chopped, any stalky ends and skin removed

2 teaspoons sweet paprika

A pinch of sugar

Sea salt and freshly ground black pepper

TO FINISH

A handful of parsley, roughly chopped

First make the sauce. Heat the 2 tablespoons oil in a saucepan over a medium-low heat. Add the onion with the thyme and sweat until softened and translucent, about 10 minutes. Add the garlic and chilli and cook, stirring, for a minute.

Now add the tomatoes with their juice, paprika, sugar and some salt and pepper. Simmer for about 10 minutes, stirring occasionally and breaking up the tomatoes with a wooden spoon, until you have a nice, rich, piquant tomato sauce. Taste and adjust the seasoning if necessary and keep the sauce warm.

Bring a large pan of water to the boil, salt well and add the potatoes. Bring back to the boil and cook for 5–8 minutes, until on the firm side of tender; ie not quite done. Drain in a colander and leave to steam for a few minutes. Gently tip on to a clean tea towel and pat dry.

Warm the 5 tablespoons oil in a large frying pan over a medium-high heat and sauté the potatoes for 10–15 minutes, until crisp and golden. Drain on kitchen paper, tip into a warmed dish and season with a scattering of sea salt.

Check the consistency of the tomato sauce and thin it with a splash of hot water if necessary, then pour over the potatoes. Scatter with chopped parsley and serve warm.

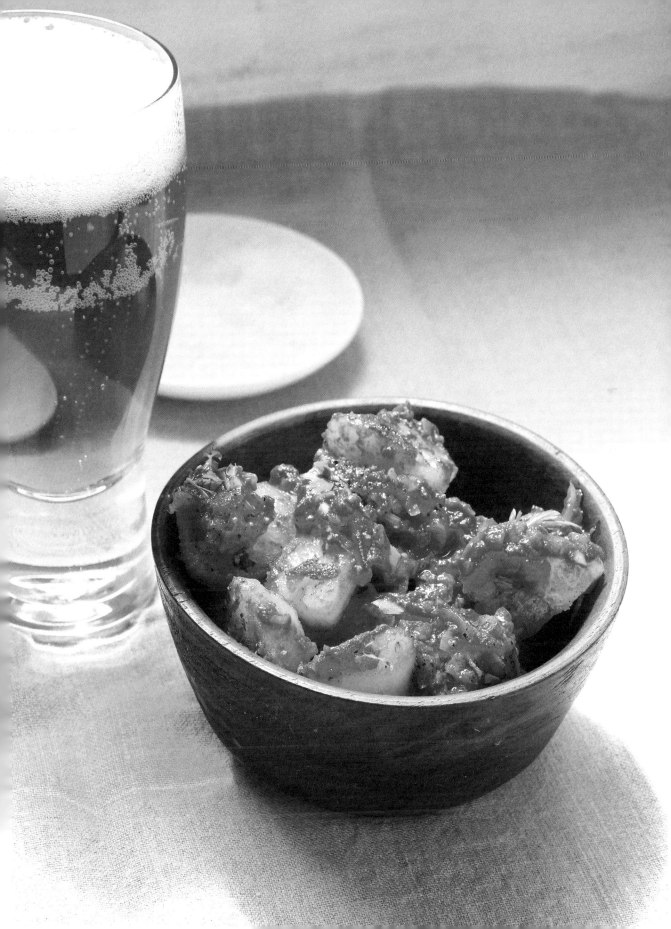

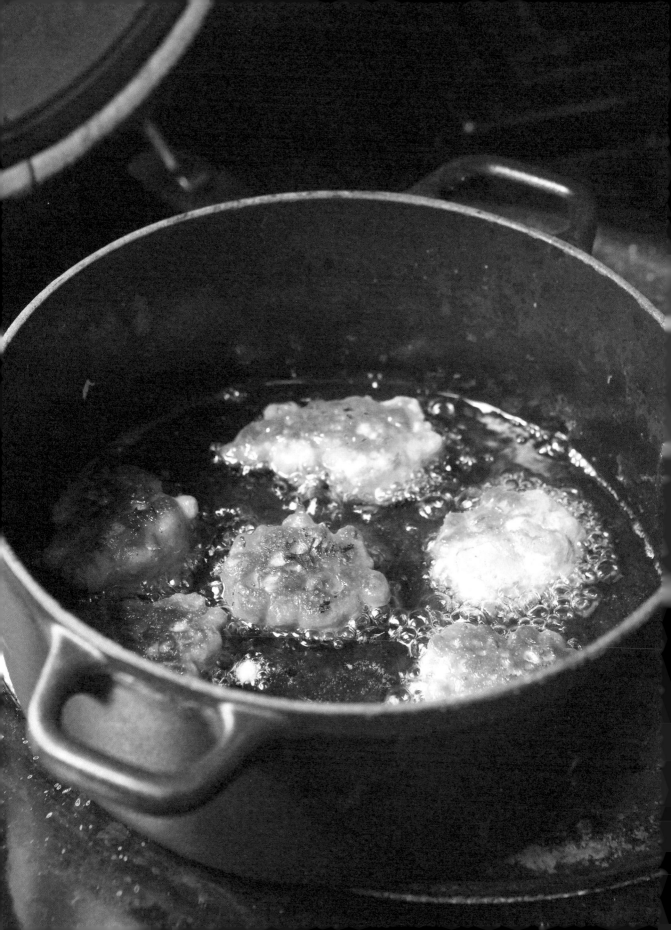

Sweetcorn fritters with coriander or mint raita

Sweet kernels of corn combine wonderfully with the earthy, fiery spices in these fritters. Serve small fritters as a mezze/nibble, larger ones with a salad or two as a meal in themselves. The recipe makes 12 large or 24 canapé-sized fritters.

SERVES 4

120g gram flour (chickpea flour)

½ teaspoon baking powder

2 teaspoons ground cumin

2 teaspoons ground coriander

½ teaspoon ground turmeric

A shake of cayenne pepper

½ teaspoon fine salt

200g fresh or frozen sweetcorn kernels (no need to defrost if using frozen)

3 spring onions, trimmed and finely chopped

A big handful of coriander, roughly chopped

½–1 small green chilli, deseeded and finely chopped (optional)

160ml whole milk or water

Sunflower or rapeseed oil, for frying

FOR THE CORIANDER/MINT RAITA

200g thick, plain (full-fat) yoghurt (plus an extra 75g if not using goat's cheese)

About 75g fresh, very soft goat's cheese (optional)

A small bunch of coriander or mint, roughly chopped

Flaky sea salt and freshly ground black pepper

First make the raita. Stir together the yoghurt and goat's cheese, if using. Add the chopped coriander or mint and season with salt and pepper to taste.

For the fritter batter, sift together all the dry ingredients into a bowl. Mix in the sweetcorn, spring onions, coriander and chilli, if using. Slowly whisk in the milk or water until everything is well combined and there are no floury lumps.

Heat about a 1cm depth of oil in a heavy-based frying pan over a medium-high heat until a cube of white bread dropped into the oil turns light golden brown in 30–40 seconds. You will need to cook the fritters in batches. Drop spoonfuls of the batter (soup spoonfuls for large ones, heaped teaspoons for canapé sized) into the oil, spacing them well apart; don't overcrowd the pan. Cook for about 3 minutes on each side, turning once. Remove and drain on kitchen paper.

Keep the sweetcorn fritters warm while you cook the rest. Serve with the coriander or mint raita.

Spinach and thyme pasties

These tasty little parcels are very good still warm from the oven, but let them cool down and they'll pack a real punch for a picnic, a party or a lunchbox. If using ricotta, it's a good idea to add in the Parmesan, but if you're using a fairly strong goat's cheese you won't need it.

MAKES 6

FOR THE PASTRY

250g plain flour

A pinch of sea salt

125g chilled unsalted butter, cut into small cubes

About 75ml cold milk

FOR THE FILLING

350g spinach, any tough stalks removed

1 tablespoon rapeseed or olive oil

1 medium onion, finely chopped

1 garlic clove, finely chopped

125g soft goat's cheese or ricotta

50g Parmesan, finely grated (optional)

A pinch of freshly grated nutmeg

A handful of thyme sprigs (lemon thyme is particularly good), chopped

1 teaspoon finely grated lemon zest (optional)

1 egg, lightly beaten

Sea salt and freshly ground black pepper

To make the pastry, sift the flour and salt together, or give them a quick blitz in a food processor. Add the butter and rub in with your fingertips, or blitz in the food processor, until the mixture resembles fine breadcrumbs. Mix in the cold milk, little by little, until the pastry just comes together, then turn out on to a work surface and knead briefly to bring it into a ball. Wrap and chill for 30 minutes.

Preheat the oven to 180°C/Gas Mark 4. Line a baking sheet with baking parchment or a non-stick liner.

For the filling, wash the spinach thoroughly, then pack it, with just the water that clings to it, into a saucepan. Cover and put over a medium heat until the spinach has wilted in its own steam. Drain in a colander. When the spinach is cool enough to handle, squeeze out as much moisture as you possibly can with your hands, then chop roughly.

Meanwhile, heat the oil in a frying pan over a medium heat and sweat the onion and garlic for about 10 minutes, until soft and translucent. Stir in the chopped spinach and leave to cool.

Tip the spinach mix into a bowl and add the goat's cheese or ricotta, Parmesan if using, nutmeg, thyme, lemon zest if using, about half the beaten egg and plenty of salt and pepper. Mash together thoroughly.

Roll out the pastry to a 26 x 39cm rectangle, about 3mm thick, and cut into six 13cm squares. Brush the rim of each square with a little water. Divide the spinach mixture between the squares, then fold the pastry diagonally to enclose the filling and crimp the edges well to seal. Brush with the remaining beaten egg and make a hole in the top of each with a small, sharp knife.

Transfer the parcels to the prepared baking sheet and bake for about 25–30 minutes or until golden brown. Eat the pasties warm or cold.

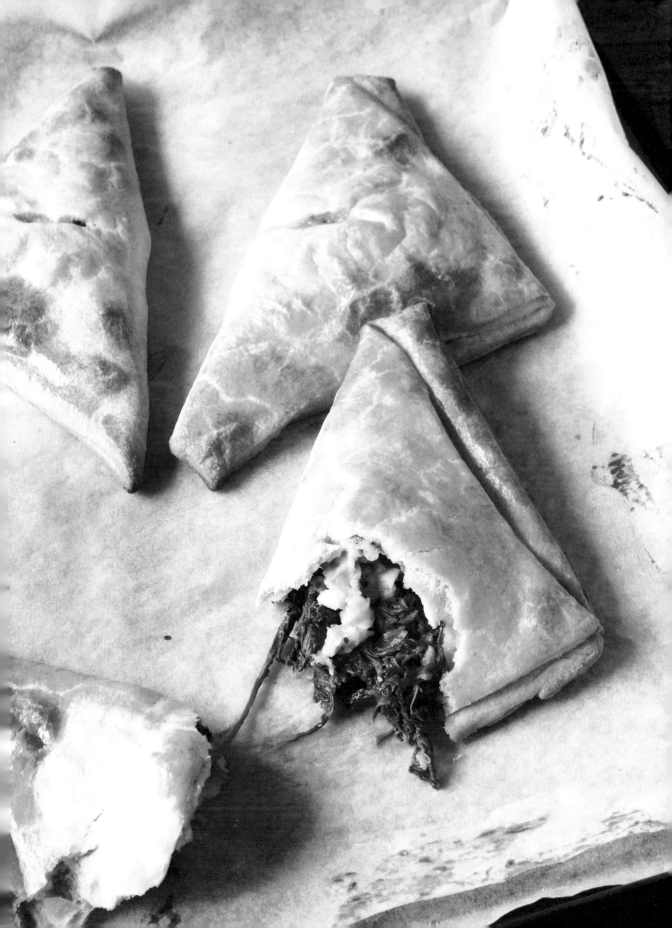

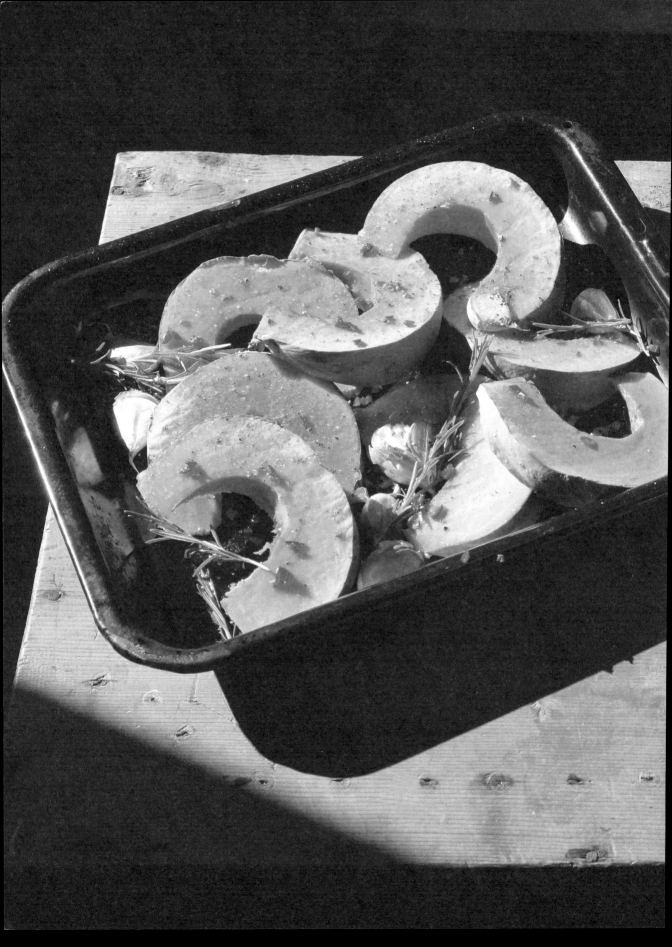

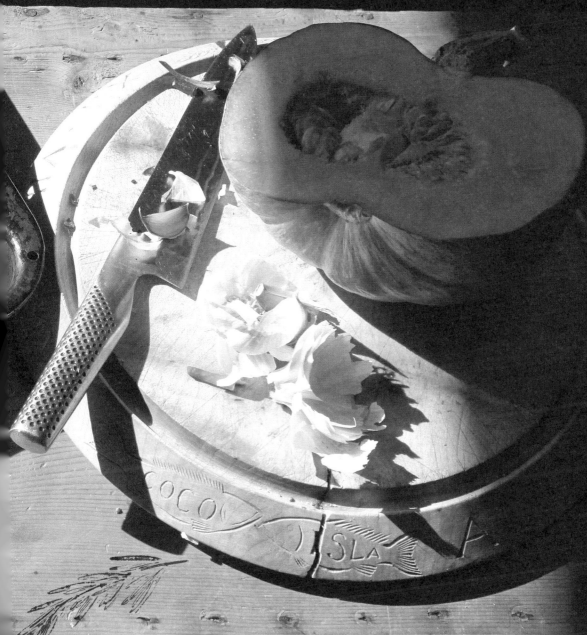

Roast, grill & barbecue

I look to roasting, grilling and barbecuing to add whole

new layers of flavour to vegetables. These methods, of controlled burning if you like, caramelise the rich supply of natural sugars that most vegetables possess, giving them a resonance and character that simple boiling or steaming – useful techniques though these are – cannot.

We all know that the effect of roasting and grilling on meat is to give it a fantastic, deep, smoky-sweet taste, which comes from that browning and crisping of the exterior. What is perhaps not so widely recognised is that much the same transformation takes place when you char vegetables. Put a courgette on the barbecue, get it really well cooked so the edges are almost burnt, the flesh striped with a thin layer of 'vegetable charcoal', and you will create a delicious taste that simply wasn't there before. It's a pretty magical moment. It even has a name, if you want to get all scientific about it: the 'Maillard reaction', which describes the chemical change that occurs when sugars react, in the presence of heat, with other substances in a food, creating new molecules and thereby a new range of complex and highly appealing tastes and smells.

Vegetable cookery makes use of this flavour-generating technique all the time – when you fry and lightly brown an onion, or roast some spuds for Sunday lunch, you are pursuing just this aim – but the recipes in this chapter really bring it to the fore. And here's the big news: because the range of textures and flavours in the vegetable kingdom is so much wider than that of the animal kingdom, the charring of veg offers a far greater variety of novel tastes than the charring of meat.

I roast vegetables several times a week. The technique is so simple and so forgiving, and I've not yet met a vegetable that didn't respond well to it. (Lettuce, maybe...) Indeed, I hope this chapter will have you roasting things you never would have considered before: not just potatoes, parsnips and peppers, but squash, carrots, beetroot, even cauliflower and Brussels sprouts.

Once you've got the hang of the taste-transforming alchemy, you can develop it – with the addition of spices, perhaps some garlic and chilli. What goes into the oven as a simple assembly of veg, oil and seasoning becomes something else entirely: a glorious dish full of complexities and different flavour notes. The beautiful colours of browned veg shouldn't be overlooked either – this is food that tends to look incredibly appetising.

Roast veg is not only delicious but wonderfully versatile. It's good hot, of course –
but I frequently eat the leftovers cold, in a salad, or blitzed with some stock and maybe
some herbs or spices to make a soup that I can then reheat. A blended soup made with
roast veg has deeper and more resonant flavours than one made with boiled. In short,
a hot oven is often, for me, the most obvious tool to use when I want to rustle up some
delicious veg with very little effort.

Grilling and griddling use the same application of high heat to brown and sweeten
veg, but these techniques are even more direct and controlled, especially when the
contact is with hot metal, rather than hot air. I use the overhead grill to turn out things
like tomatoes on toast or tender, smoky aubergine slices, but the ridged grill pan is my
favourite tool here. This heavy-based, corrugated pan is essentially a sort of indoor
barbecue. Its main marketing pitch may be the promise of those alluring char lines
on your home-cooked steak, but it delivers them just as effectively to veg, producing
zebra stripes of irresistible flavour on aubergines, courgettes, beetroot... you name it.

Of course, if it's full-on, freshly fired smokiness you're after, it's really hard to beat
the barbecue. It can work wonders on everything from fennel to asparagus, sweet
potato to spring onion. It's true that this is something of a seasonal cooking method –
but include an umbrella as well as a sun hat in your barbecuing kit, and you should be
able to get good results for at least six months of the year. (If it's truly torrential, you can
always default indoors to the aforementioned ridged grill.)

A platter of roasted, grilled or barbecued veg, of just one kind or several, is welcome
on any table. Some of the recipes you'll find in the following pages, such as caramelised
carrots with gremolata (see page 355) and roast parsnip chips (see page 357) are
definitely more side dish than centrepiece: perfect when combined with other roasted
veg and/or salads, good bread and some kind of dressing, even if it's just a trickle of
good oil and a squeeze of lemon. However, others such as halloumi, new potato and
tomato kebabs (see page 334) stand as dishes in their own right, where that alluring,
almost-burnt flavour can really steal the show.

One of the greatest challenges to which I've risen while exploring a life with less
meat has undoubtedly been the veg-only barbecue. Thanks to some of these recipes,
it was also one of the most rewarding.

Chargrilled summer veg🌱

I learned the joy of chargrilling veg over 20 years ago when I was working at the River Cafe. I still come back to it every summer. Vary the vegetables as you like here, bumping up the courgettes if you have lots in the garden, or adding some quartered peppers, aubergine sticks or slices of red onion. I like to toss the veg with chopped herbs, though they are very good just as they are. They're also delicious trickled with the tahini dressing on page 74.

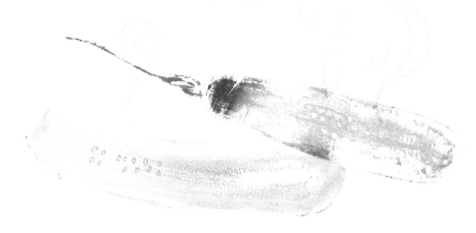

SERVES 2

4 courgettes

2 fennel bulbs, trimmed

A generous bunch of spring onions, trimmed

4–6 tablespoons olive oil

1 garlic clove, very finely sliced

Juice of 1 lemon

A small bunch of parsley or basil, plus a few sprigs of chervil, tarragon or thyme, chopped fairly finely (optional)

Sea salt and freshly ground black pepper

20g Parmesan, hard goat's cheese or other well-flavoured hard cheese, to finish (optional)

Light the barbecue well in advance if you are cooking the veg outside. If cooking indoors, heat the griddle or grill until hot.

Cut the courgettes and fennel lengthways into 5mm slices and set aside with the whole spring onions.

In a small bowl, lightly mix together the olive oil, garlic and lemon juice with some salt and pepper.

Cook the vegetables in batches. Brush them lightly with a little of the olive oil mixture (try not to get any bits of garlic on the veg at this stage, as it will burn on the grill). Cook on a medium-hot barbecue or griddle pan, or under the grill, until marked with scorch lines on the outside and tender right through. Courgettes and fennel should take 3–5 minutes per side, spring onions 1–2 minutes per side, but be vigilant as a hot barbecue can burn them very quickly. As you bring each batch off the grill or griddle, put into a large serving dish and toss with a little more of the seasoned lemon and oil dressing.

When everything is cooked, toss it together with the chopped herbs, if using, and finish with cheese shavings if you like. Serve either warm or at room temperature.

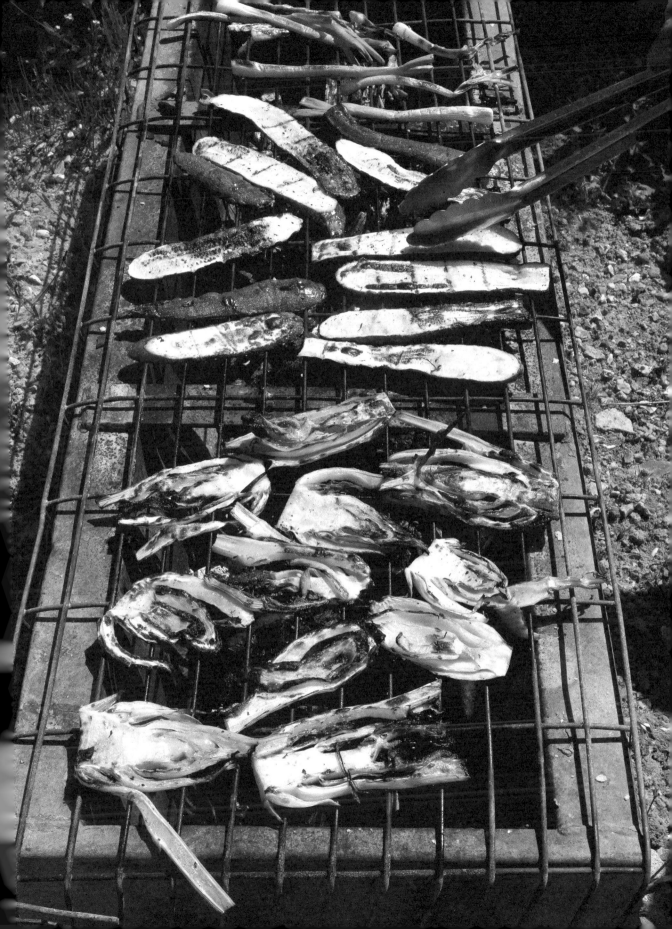

Halloumi, new potato and tomato kebabs

Salty, chewy halloumi cheese is great with all kinds of grilled summer vegetables. You can adapt this recipe as you like, using courgettes, aubergines and peppers as well as, or instead of, the potatoes and tomatoes.

SERVES 4

250g small, waxy new potatoes, such as Ratte, Anya, Charlotte or Pink Fir Apple

450g halloumi cheese

200g cherry tomatoes

A handful of bay leaves

FOR THE MARINADE

3 tablespoons olive oil

A handful of thyme sprigs, leaves only, finely chopped

A handful of mint, finely chopped

1 teaspoon clear honey

½ teaspoon dried chilli flakes

TO SERVE

Plain (full-fat) yoghurt

A few mint leaves, chopped

Hummus (optional)

A little extra virgin olive oil

A squeeze of lemon juice

Light the barbecue, if using – to allow time for the flames to die down and the coals to develop an even cooking heat. If you're using wooden skewers, soak them in cold water at least 30 minutes ahead of cooking.

Put the new potatoes in a pan, cover with water, add salt and bring to the boil. Simmer for 8–10 minutes, until almost tender – just a shade underdone. Drain and leave to cool slightly.

Whisk together the ingredients for the marinade. Cut larger potatoes into halves or quarters. Cut the halloumi into 2–3cm cubes and add to the marinade with the potatoes and tomatoes. Turn to coat well and leave to marinate for 10 minutes.

Thread the potatoes, tomatoes and halloumi cubes on to the skewers, interspersing a few bay leaves with the veg on each one. If you are cooking indoors, preheat the grill to high. If cooking on a barbecue, you need a medium heat – you should be able to hold the palm of your hand about 15cm above the coals for 5–6 seconds.

Put the skewers on the barbecue or under the grill and cook for about 10 minutes, turning from time to time, until the cheese and veg are hot and starting to blister on the outside.

For the full 'kebab-style' presentation, serve with yoghurt flavoured with some chopped mint, and hummus loosened with a little extra virgin olive oil and a squeeze of lemon. (Or try the cannellini bean hummus and paprika oil on page 300.) Accompany with warm, soft flatbreads (see page 176) or pitta.

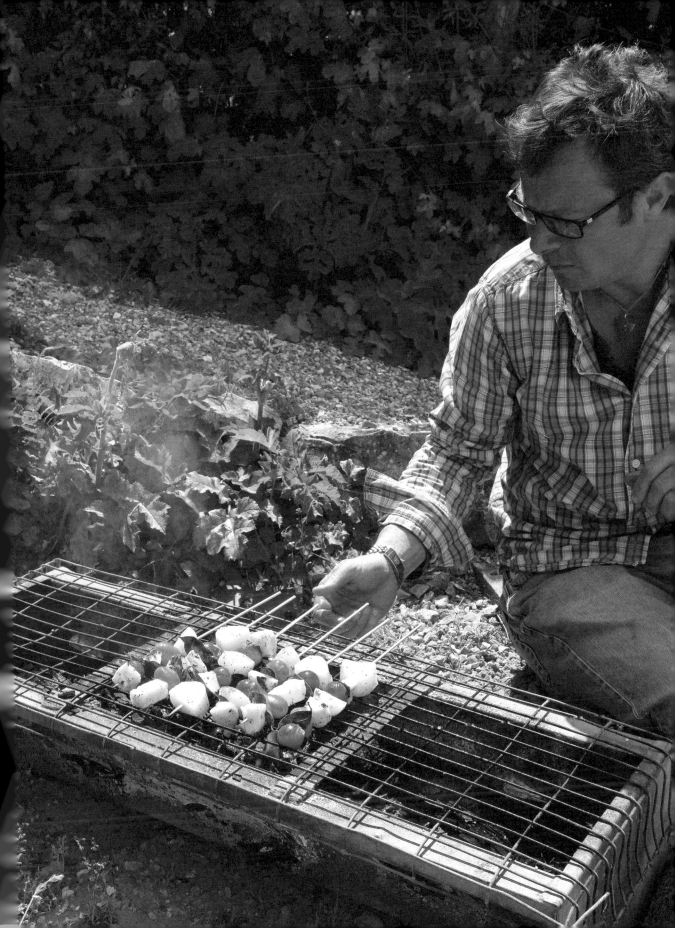

Charred baby leeks with romesco 🌱

*Romesco, a brick-orange blend of garlic, nuts, tomatoes and chillies, is
a Catalan sauce traditionally served with grilled calçots (somewhere between
a fat spring onion and a leek). However, it's great with pretty much any
grilled or barbecued vegetable – certainly courgettes, aubergines and fennel.*

SERVES 4 AS A STARTER

About 400g baby leeks, or
large spring onions

1 tablespoon olive oil

FOR THE ROMESCO

1 large or 2 medium red chillies
(hot, but not too fiery)

3–4 large plum or other large
ripe tomatoes (about 300g)

½ red pepper (optional)

1 slice of sourdough or other
robust bread (about 50g),
crusts removed

100ml olive oil

2 fat garlic cloves, peeled
and halved

50g hazelnuts, lightly toasted

1 tablespoon red wine vinegar

½ teaspoon sweet smoked
paprika

Sea salt and freshly ground
black pepper

Light the barbecue well in advance if you are cooking the veg outside. To make the sauce, on the barbecue, cast-iron grill pan, or foil-lined tray under a hot grill, char the chilli(es), tomatoes and red pepper, if using, until blackened all over. (Or roast at 200°C/Gas Mark 6, for 25–30 minutes, but you'll have less of the charred flavour). Leave to cool, then peel off the skins. Cut out the stem end from the tomatoes. Remove the seeds and stalk from the chilli and pepper. Put the chilli, tomatoes and red pepper in a food processor.

Cut the bread into chunks. Heat the olive oil gently in a small frying pan. Add the halved garlic cloves and fry gently for a few minutes until they are just turning golden. Scoop out and add to the food processor. Add the bread cubes to the pan and fry for a few minutes until golden. Leave to cool a little, then add to the processor with the toasted nuts, wine vinegar, paprika and some salt and pepper. Blend to a chunky purée. Taste and adjust the seasoning. If the sauce seems overly thick, you can let it down with a little more oil and/or a dash of hot water.

Very slender baby leeks or spring onions won't need pre-cooking but leeks more than 1cm thick will benefit from being blanched before barbecuing. Add to a pan of boiling water and blanch for 1-2 minutes, then drain and refresh under cold running water. Drain and pat dry.

Toss the leeks with the olive oil and some salt and pepper. Cook on a medium-hot barbecue or under a hot grill for a few minutes, turning from time to time, until lightly charred and tender right through to the middle. Serve with the warm sauce.

VARIATION

Roasted leeks with romesco or cannellini bean hummus 🌱
Trim 4 medium leeks, removing the outer layer, wash and cut into 3–4cm lengths. Toss in a roasting dish with 2 tablespoons rapeseed or olive oil and plenty of salt and pepper. Cover with foil and roast at 180°C/Gas Mark 4 for 30 minutes, until tender. Uncover and roast for a further 10 minutes. Let stand for a few minutes. Serve warm, with romesco or cannellini bean hummus and paprika oil (see page 300).

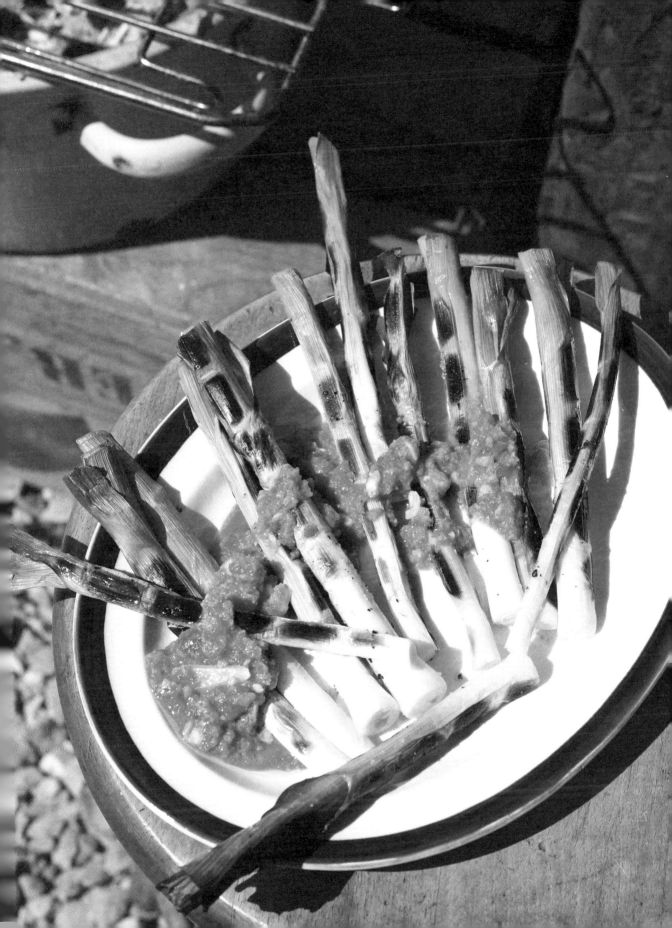

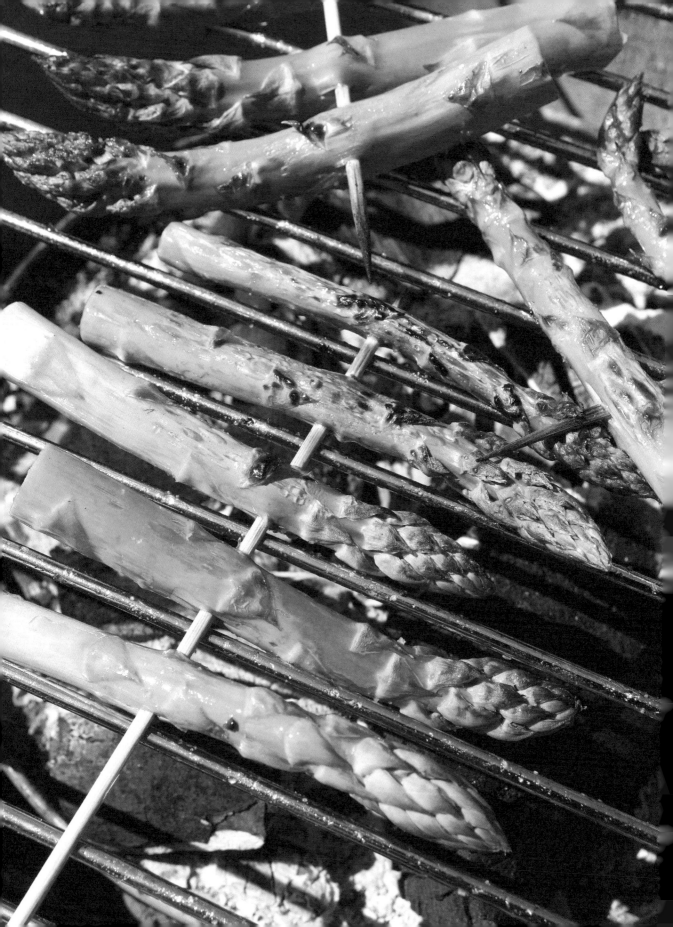

Griddled asparagus spears with lemon dressing ◊

These can be done on a barbie outdoors, or on a ridged cast-iron griddle in the kitchen, or even, at a pinch, under a grill. When barbecuing, threading the asparagus spears onto skewers makes it easier to turn and cook them without losing them through the bars of the grill.

SERVES 4

20–30 asparagus spears, trimmed

4 tablespoons olive or rapeseed oil

Juice of ½ lemon

6–10 mint leaves, finely shredded

Flaky sea salt and freshly ground black pepper

Parmesan, pecorino or hard goat's cheese, to serve (optional)

Light the barbecue well in advance if you are cooking the asparagus outside. Soak 8 wooden barbecue skewers in water for 30 minutes.

If the asparagus spears are pretty thick – more than 5mm across the middle of the stem – or perhaps not so freshly cut, it's best to blanch them first. Add to a pan of boiling water, blanch for 1 minute, then drain and refresh in cold water. Drain well and pat dry.

Thread the asparagus on to the skewers, about 5 or 6 to a skewer – you can mount several of them on a single skewer, pushing it through the middle of the spears. Brush the asparagus with some of the oil and season with salt and pepper.

If cooking indoors, heat the griddle or grill until hot, then place the asparagus skewers on the griddle or under the grill about 10cm from the heat. If using a barbecue, you want it medium-hot, rather than super-fierce – you should be able to hold your palm about 15cm above the coals for a few seconds. Grill the asparagus spears for about 3 minutes on each side, depending on thickness, until tender in the centre and lightly charred on the outside.

Whisk about 2 tablespoons oil with the lemon juice, some pepper and the mint to make a dressing. Remove the asparagus from the skewers, arrange on a plate and trickle the dressing over them. Sprinkle with flaky salt and shave some cheese over the top, if you like.

Grilled aubergines with chilli and honey

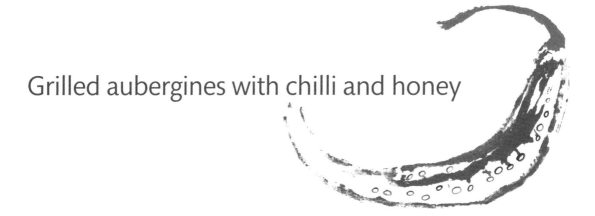

Well-oiled aubergine slices – grilled until really soft and yielding – make a delicious, velvety sponge for the flavours of honey, lemon, chilli and thyme. Other herbs would work well here too, giving the dish a subtly different character – try parsley, basil, mint or coriander.

SERVES 4

3 medium aubergines (about 750g), trimmed

Olive oil, for brushing

1 red chilli, deseeded and finely chopped

A few sprigs of thyme, leaves only

A little clear honey, to trickle

A little lemon juice

Sea salt and freshly ground black pepper

Preheat the grill to medium-high. Slice the skin off the aubergines, then cut across into 1cm slices. Place on a foil-lined grill tray. Brush liberally with oil and sprinkle with salt and pepper. Grill until golden brown on one side, then flip the slices over, brush with more oil and season with more salt and pepper. Keep grilling until the slices are a deep golden brown all over and very tender, flipping them again if you need to. This will take around 15–20 minutes.

Transfer the grilled aubergine slices to a plate or dish, layering them if you need to and sprinkling each layer with chopped chilli and thyme leaves. Trickle with a little honey and lemon juice. Leave for at least 10 minutes until tepid or, even better, 30 minutes until cool, by which time the juices will have run and mingled a little.

Add more salt and pepper if you think it necessary, then serve as a starter, with bread, or as part of a mezze spread.

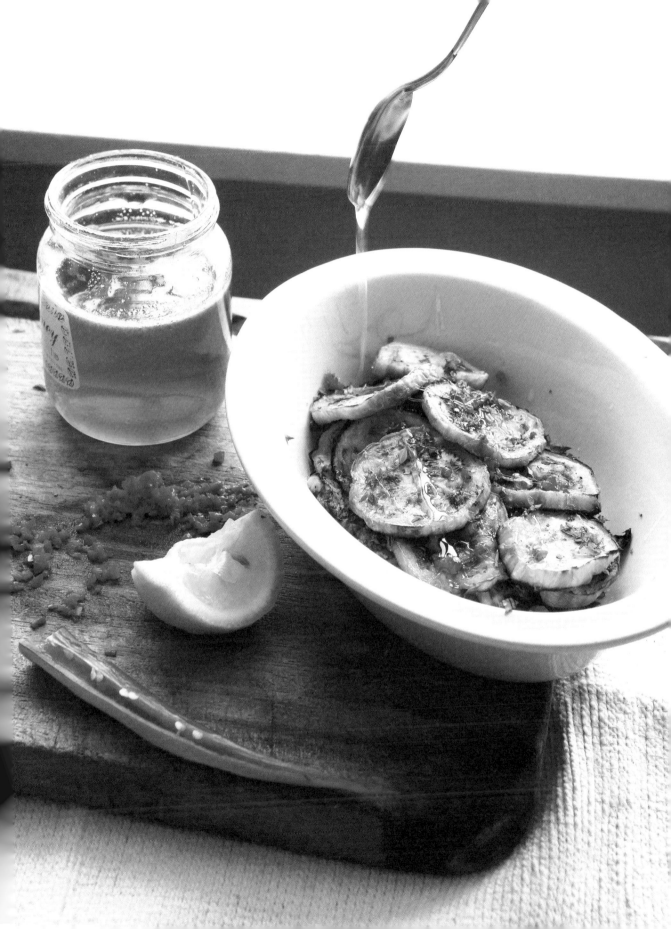

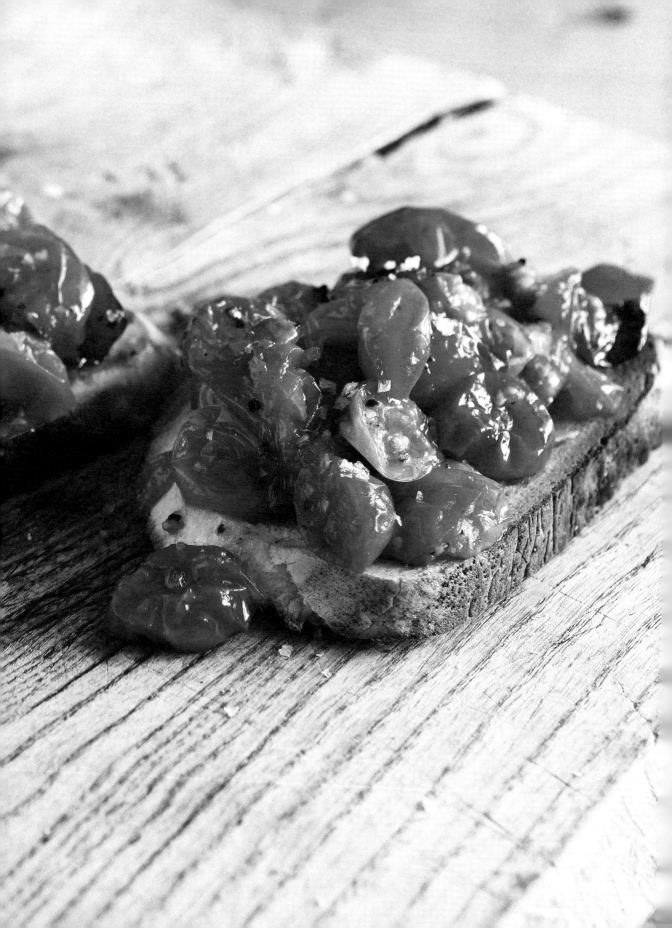

Honey roasted cherry tomatoes

*These gorgeously sweet and tangy, juicy and sticky tomatoes are fantastic
served on top of a simple, saffron-infused risotto. You can also serve them
as a complement to almost any other grilled or roasted veg, but I particularly
like them piled on toast with a sprinkling of flaky sea salt on top.*

SERVES 4

500g cherry tomatoes

2 garlic cloves

1 tablespoon clear honey

3 tablespoons olive oil

Flaky sea salt and freshly ground
black pepper

Preheat the oven to 190°C/Gas Mark 5. Lightly oil a medium roasting
dish. Halve the tomatoes and place them, cut side up, in the dish.
They should fit snugly with little or no space between them.

Crush the garlic with a pinch of salt, then beat it with the honey, olive
oil and a good grinding of pepper. Spoon this sticky, garlicky mixture
over the cherry tomatoes. Roast for about 30 minutes, until golden,
juicy and bubbling.

Seared chicory with blue cheese

*The combination of hot, tender, wilted, bittersweet chicory with some bubbling,
salty blue cheese is a love it or hate it thing. No prizes for guessing which way I go.*

SERVES 4

4 small or 2 large heads
of chicory

3 tablespoons rapeseed
or olive oil

125g blue cheese, thinly sliced

Sea salt and freshly ground
black pepper

Extra virgin olive oil, to finish

Cut each head of chicory in half lengthways, keeping them joined
at the root end. Put them into a large bowl, trickle over the oil and
add plenty of salt and pepper. Work the oil and seasoning all over
the chicory with your hands.

Preheat the grill to medium-high. Put a large, non-stick frying pan
or a ridged griddle pan over a fairly high heat. When hot, add the
chicory, cut side down. Cook for about 2 minutes, until golden brown
and wilted on the base, then turn the chicory halves over and cook
for another minute or two.

Lay the sliced cheese over the chicory and put under the grill for
a minute or two until melted and bubbling. Trickle over some extra
virgin olive oil and serve straight away, with bread.

Roasted aubergine 'boats'

This is a really simple but delicious way to cook aubergines. Usually I serve them with fresh mint and yoghurt, but I've also tried smearing them with a little home-made pesto, which is lovely. To make a meal of them, serve alongside a simple couscous salad, or just a green salad and some hot flatbreads (see page 176).

SERVES 2-4

2 large aubergines (about 700g)

3 garlic cloves, finely chopped

2–3 pinches dried chilli flakes or ½–1 large red chilli, deseeded and finely chopped

4–5 tablespoons olive oil

Sea salt and freshly ground black pepper

TO SERVE

4–6 tablespoons thick, plain (full-fat) yoghurt, plus about 8 mint leaves, shredded
OR
2–3 tablespoons pesto (see page 256)

Preheat the oven to 190°C/Gas Mark 5. Cut the aubergines in half lengthways. Using a small, sharp knife, make a series of deep slashes diagonally across the flesh, going about two-thirds of the way into the flesh, but not right through to the skin. You want to end up with 6–10 slashes, 1–2cm apart, depending on the size of your aubergines.

Mix the garlic and chilli with 3 tablespoons of the olive oil. Hold one aubergine half in your hand and squeeze it from side to side so the slashes open up a little. Spoon some of the garlic and chilli oil over the aubergine with a teaspoon, using the back of the spoon to work the oil down into the slashes. Repeat with the other halves.

Put the aubergine halves, flesh side up, in a roasting dish. Sprinkle with salt and pepper, then trickle over a little more olive oil – there should be little or no un-oiled flesh showing on each aubergine half. Roast in the oven for about 50 minutes, or until a deep golden brown and considerably reduced in size.

Leave the aubergines to cool slightly. Serve them hot or warm, either dabbed with yoghurt and sprinkled with mint and a touch more salt, or smeared with a little pesto.

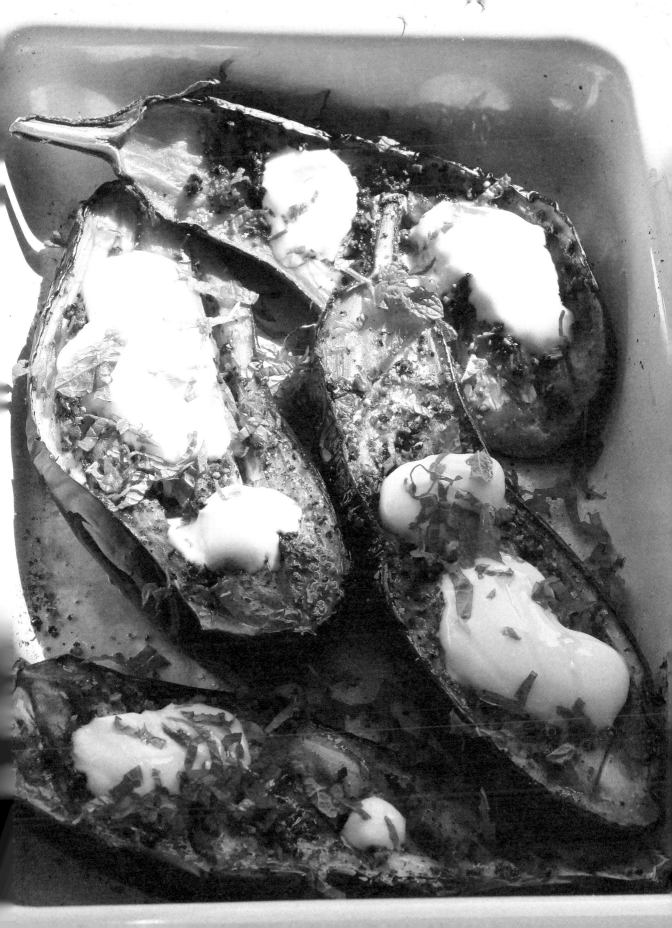

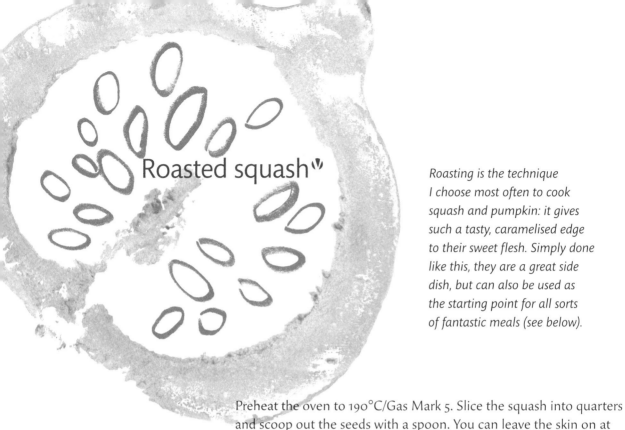

Roasted squash ♥

Roasting is the technique I choose most often to cook squash and pumpkin: it gives such a tasty, caramelised edge to their sweet flesh. Simply done like this, they are a great side dish, but can also be used as the starting point for all sorts of fantastic meals (see below).

SERVES 6

1 large Crown Prince squash (about 1kg), or the equivalent weight of acorn, butternut or other squash or pumpkin

6–8 fat garlic cloves, skin on, lightly squashed

4–5 tablespoons rapeseed or olive oil

Sea salt and freshly ground black pepper

OPTIONAL EXTRAS

Used alone or in combination:

A few sprigs of rosemary

A few sprigs of thyme

1 red chilli, finely chopped, or a good pinch of dried chilli flakes

Preheat the oven to 190°C/Gas Mark 5. Slice the squash into quarters and scoop out the seeds with a spoon. You can leave the skin on at this stage, or peel it off if you prefer. Cut the squash into wedges or large chunks and put them in a small roasting tin. Add the garlic, with any of the optional extras you fancy, and some salt and pepper.

Trickle over the oil and toss the lot together. Roast for 40–55 minutes, turning once or twice during cooking, until the squash is completely soft and starting to caramelise on the corners and edges.

THINGS TO DO WITH YOUR ROASTED SQUASH

• Toss with toasted walnuts, pine nuts or hazelnuts, or a scattering of pistachio dukka (see page 294), trickle over a little more oil and squeeze over some lemon juice before serving with a green salad.

• Combine with roasted red onion wedges, couscous, grated lemon zest and juice, lots of chopped parsley, a generous trickle of oil and plenty of salt and pepper.

• Add to a risotto or a 'speltotto' (see page 283), towards the end of cooking. Finish with some chopped sage.

• Blitz roasted squash in a food processor to make a delicious purée, or do so with some stock for a fast and satisfying soup. Finish the soup with a scattering of toasted pumpkin seeds if you like.

• Add chunks of roasted squash to vegetable curries.

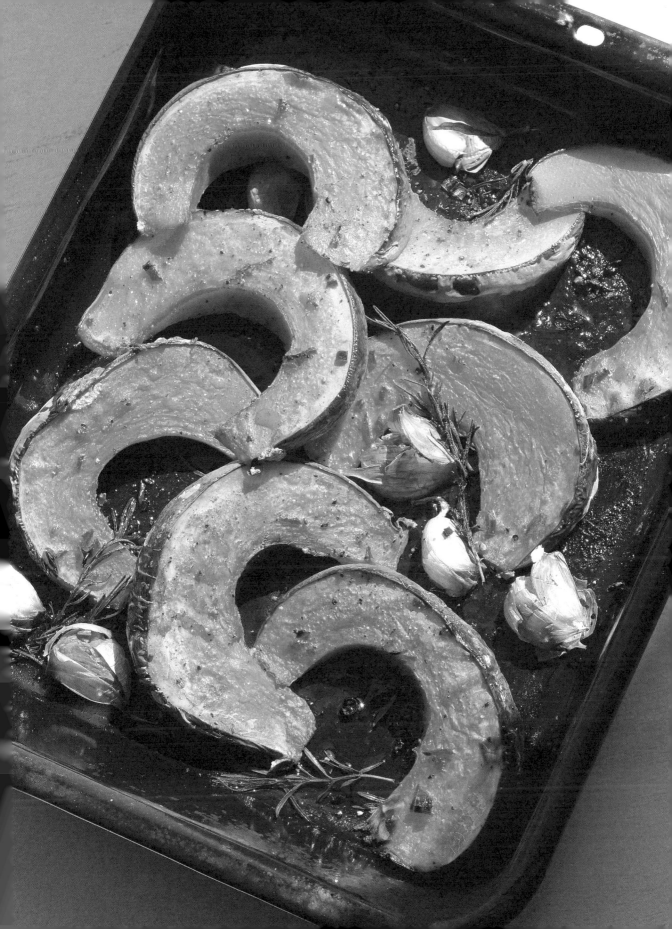

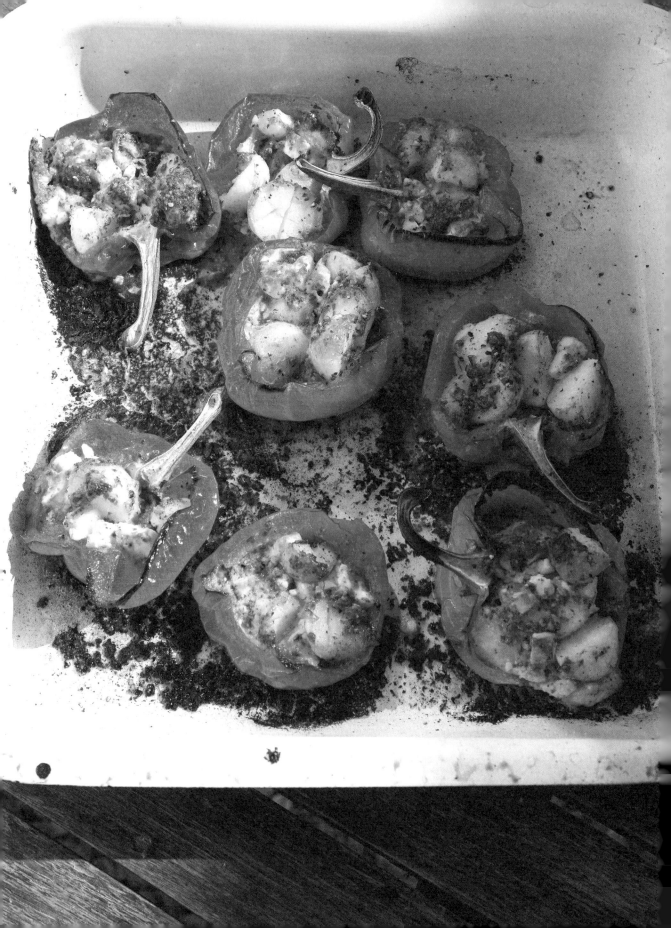

Stuffed peppers with new potatoes, feta and pesto

This is a lovely, simple way to enjoy the smoky taste of roasted peppers without any of the bother of peeling them. The potatoes, meanwhile, make this a pleasingly substantial dish. You could use a good shop-bought pesto but a home-made one will be better.

SERVES 4

200g small new potatoes

4 red peppers

1 tablespoon olive oil

200g feta cheese

4 tablespoons pesto
(see page 256)

Sea salt and freshly ground
black pepper

A small handful of basil leaves,
shredded, to finish (optional)

Preheat the oven to 200°C/Gas Mark 6. Bring a pan of salted water to the boil, add the new potatoes and boil for 8–12 minutes, until just tender. Drain and cool slightly.

Halve the peppers lengthways and remove the seeds and pith. Brush the outsides with olive oil, then place on a baking tray lined with baking parchment.

Halve or quarter the new potatoes and place in a bowl. Cut the feta into 1cm cubes and add to the potatoes. Toss both with the pesto until well combined.

Spoon the filling into the halved peppers and bake for 40–45 minutes until browned on the top. If using shredded basil, scatter over the top before serving.

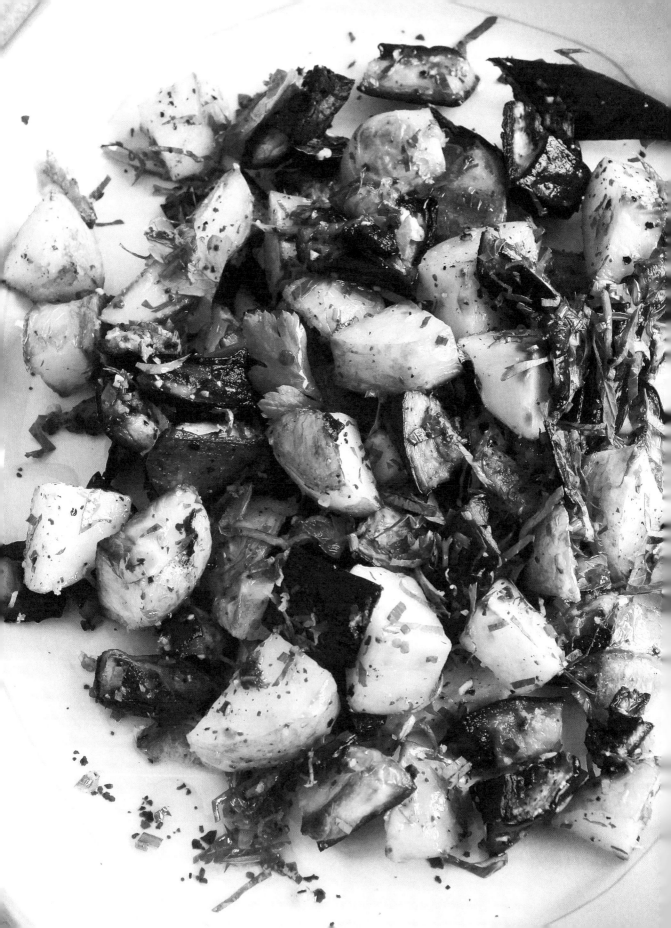

Roasted potatoes and aubergines ❥

This is a very simple dish and one that doesn't take long to cook. You can serve it alongside a rich stew, or as part of a spread of mezze-type dishes. There are various ways to finish it, which subtly alter its character: stir in the finely grated zest of a lemon when it comes out of the oven, or dust with hot smoked paprika for a patatas bravas effect. Leftovers are great in an omelette or frittata.

SERVES 4

4 tablespoons rapeseed or olive oil

2 medium aubergines (about 500g)

About 500g potatoes (any type will do), unpeeled

2 garlic cloves, sliced

Lemon juice

Sea salt and freshly ground black pepper

TO FINISH (OPTIONAL)

Finely grated lemon zest, hot smoked paprika or chopped herbs

Preheat the oven to 200°C/Gas Mark 6. Put the oil in a large, non-stick roasting dish and heat in the oven for a good 10 minutes, until the oil is sizzling hot.

Meanwhile, cut the aubergines and potatoes into 2cm cubes, tip into a bowl and season with salt and pepper. Take the roasting dish from the oven and place on a stable, heatproof surface. Add the aubergines and potatoes and turn to coat in the oil, being careful not to splash yourself. Roast for about 30 minutes, stirring halfway.

Take out the dish, stir in the garlic and roast for another 10–15 minutes, until the veg are golden brown all over. Add a squeeze of lemon juice, a little more salt and pepper if needed, and any finishing touches you fancy. Serve warm or at room temperature.

VARIATION

Roasted spiced aubergines with chickpeas ❥

Replace the potatoes with 3 medium aubergines (about 750g). Toss the cubed aubergine with ¼ teaspoon ground cumin, ¼ teaspoon ground coriander and a small red chilli, finely chopped (or a good pinch of cayenne). After the initial 30 minutes' roasting time, add a drained and rinsed 400g tin chickpeas, along with the sliced garlic, and return to the oven for 10 minutes. Season with salt, pepper and lemon juice, and add the grated zest of a small lemon and lots of chopped parsley and coriander. Serve warm or at room temperature.

Roasted brussels sprouts with shallots❦

This is a dish to convert sprout shirkers – it's a delicious, easy way to serve sprouts, and one that's likely to encourage you to dish them up more often. For a change, try a sprinkling of cumin or caraway seeds instead of thyme.

SERVES 4

400g Brussels sprouts, trimmed and halved (or whole if small)

350g shallots, peeled and halved, or small onions, peeled and halved or quartered

3 tablespoons rapeseed oil

Several sprigs of thyme

A squeeze of lemon juice

Sea salt and freshly ground black pepper

Preheat the oven to 190°C/Gas Mark 5. Put the Brussels sprouts and shallots or onions into a large roasting dish, trickle over the oil, season with salt and pepper and toss to coat, then tuck in the thyme sprigs.

Roast for about 35 minutes, giving a good stir halfway through, until everything is a bit crispy, brown and caramelised.

Squeeze some lemon juice over the roasted sprouts, along with a sprinkling of fresh thyme if you like, and serve.

Roasted cauliflower with lemon and paprika❦

Another 'veg-you-wouldn't-think-of-roasting', this makes a great nibble to go with drinks but it is also very good as part of a spread of tapas-type dishes. Its smoky, caramelised flavour has been known to win over even the most cauliflower-sceptical.

SERVES 4

1 medium-large cauliflower (750–800g), trimmed

2 lemons

3 tablespoons olive oil

½ teaspoon hot smoked paprika

Flaky sea salt and freshly ground black pepper

Preheat the oven to 220°C/Gas Mark 7. Cut the cauliflower into medium florets and rinse, leaving some of the water clinging to the florets. Put them in a large roasting tray, squeeze over the juice from one of the lemons, trickle over the olive oil, add the paprika and some salt and pepper and toss the whole lot together.

Cut the remaining lemon into 6 segments and scatter these in the tray. Roast for 25–30 minutes, turning once, until the florets are slightly caramelised at the edges.

Squeeze the juice from the roasted lemon segments over the roasted cauliflower and serve at once, scattered with a little flaky sea salt.

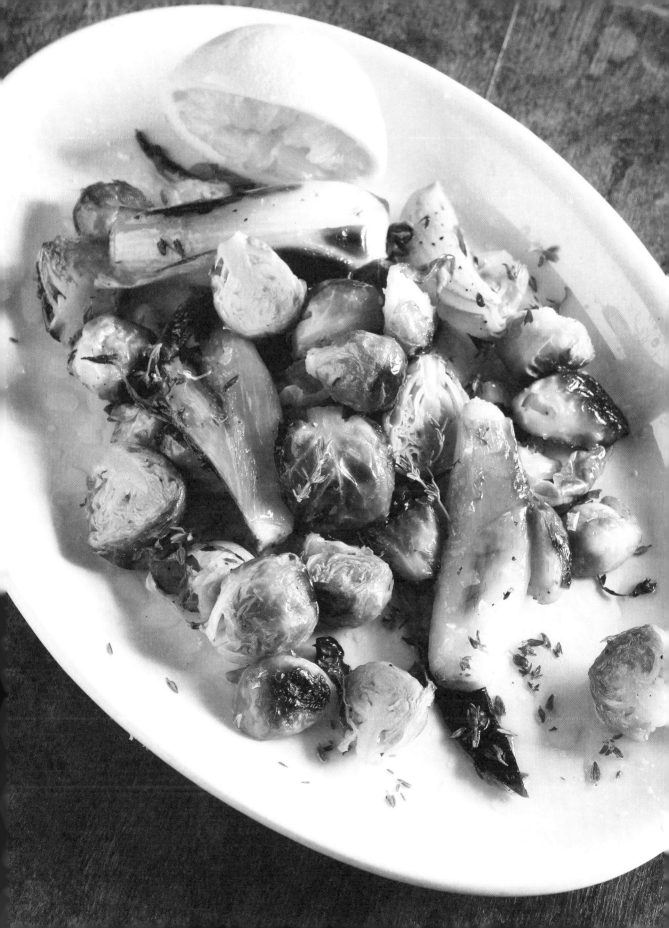

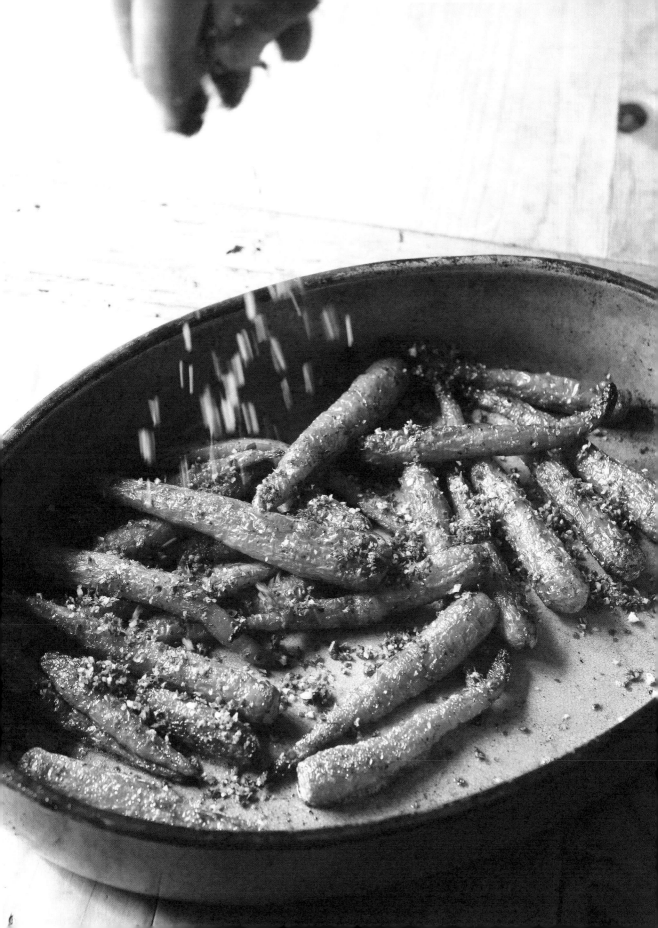

Caramelised carrots with gremolata

The contrast of sweet, caramelised carrots and zesty gremolata is brilliant – and it looks great too. But, if you fancy ringing the changes, try tossing the cooked carrots instead with my pistachio dukka (see page 294). I like to do this with young, small summer carrots, but you can use bigger winter ones if you cut them into long, thin batons.

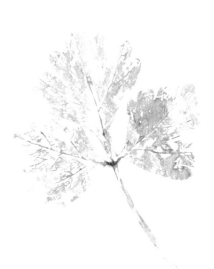

SERVES 4

1 tablespoon rapeseed or olive oil

30g butter

500g young carrots, larger ones halved lengthways

Sea salt and freshly ground black pepper

FOR THE GREMOLATA

½ garlic clove

A small bunch of flat-leaf parsley, leaves only

Finely grated zest of 1 lemon

Preheat the oven to 180°C/Gas Mark 4. Put the oil and butter in a large roasting dish and place in the oven until the butter melts. Add the carrots, season generously with salt and pepper and toss well. Cover with foil and roast in the oven for 30–40 minutes, until the carrots are tender.

Take the dish out of the oven, remove the foil and give the carrots a stir. Roast, uncovered, for 20–30 minutes, until they start to brown and caramelise.

While the carrots are in the oven, make the gremolata. Roughly chop the garlic on a large board, then add the parsley and lemon zest. Use a large, sharp knife to chop and mix the three ingredients together until very fine and well mixed.

As soon as the carrots are ready, toss them with the gremolata and serve straight away.

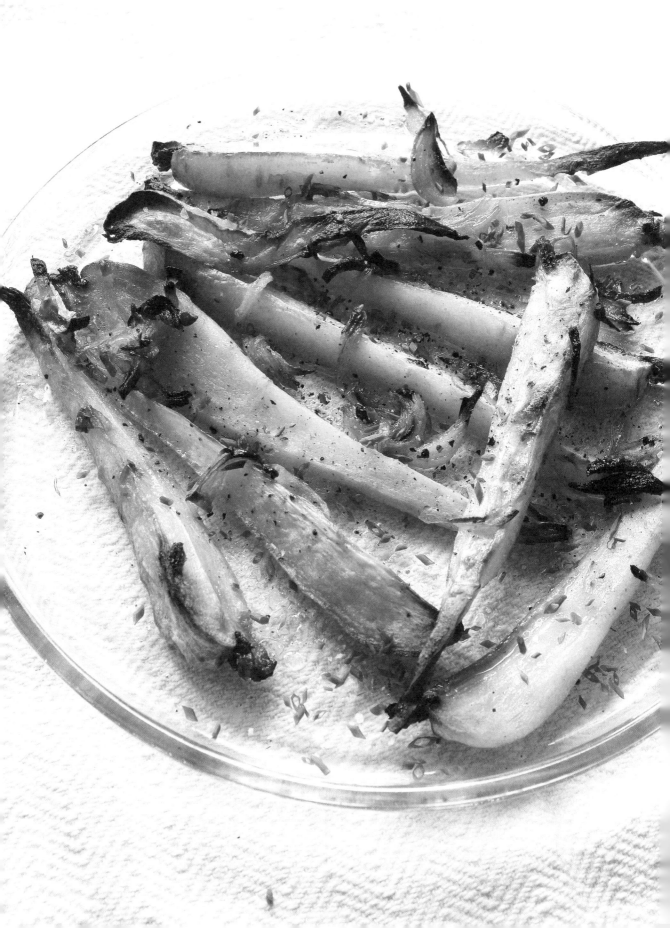

Roast parsnip chips

I think the top-heavy cone-shape of parsnips is a vital part of their charm. Roast them like this, in long, thin 'chips', and they're crisp and caramelised at the thin ends, chewy in the middle and tender and creamy at the fat ends – really, the best of all worlds. Small or medium parsnips will give you elegant, slender, slightly curved 'chips'. Sometimes I roast some shallots or onions with them, and sometimes I don't...

SERVES 4-6

750g–1kg smallish parsnips

250–500g small onions or shallots (optional)

2–3 tablespoons rapeseed or olive oil

Sea salt and freshly ground black pepper

Preheat the oven to 190°C/Gas Mark 5. Peel the parsnips, top and tail them and quarter lengthways. Any very thick pieces should be cut in half lengthways again – you want the pieces to be no more than 2–3cm wide at the thickest end. Put the parsnips into a large roasting tray, spreading them out evenly. (If using both parsnips and onions or shallots, you'll need a pretty large tray, or two smaller ones.)

Peel the onions or shallots, if using, and trim each end, but keep them together at the root end. Halve or quarter shallots lengthways; cut onions into eighths. Add them to the tray with the parsnips. It's important not to crowd the tray – they can be snug, but in a single layer, not overlapping or piled on top of each other.

Trickle over the oil and some salt and pepper and toss the lot together. Roast for 40–50 minutes, giving them all a good stir about halfway through the cooking time. The parsnips are ready when they are tender, crispy, caramelised and well browned. The onions will also be soft in the middle and nicely browned at the edges and ends.

Roast new potatoes with two mojo sauces ᵛ

A mojo is simply an intensely flavoured, aromatic sauce that hails from the Canary Islands. These lovely condiments are generally served with potatoes – often boiled in very salty water so that a fine crust of salt clings to their skins. However, I also like them with simply roasted new spuds, as here.

SERVES 4–6

1kg small new potatoes

2–3 tablespoons olive oil

Flaky sea salt and freshly ground black pepper

FOR THE MOJO PICÓN

2 mild, dried chillies, such as poblano

2 flame-grilled or roasted red peppers (from a jar if you like, or cooked as on page 336), roughly chopped

1 garlic bulb, cloves separated and peeled

¾ teaspoon ground cumin

½ teaspoon sweet smoked paprika

100ml white wine vinegar

180ml extra virgin olive oil

FOR THE MOJO CILANTRO

1 garlic bulb, cloves separated and peeled

¾ teaspoon ground cumin

100ml white wine vinegar

A big handful of coriander, finely chopped

180ml extra virgin olive oil

First make the sauces, to allow time for their flavours to develop. For the mojo picón, put the dried chillies in a bowl and cover with just-boiled water. Leave to soak for 45 minutes, then drain and chop. If you have a good, large pestle and mortar, pound the chopped chillies in it with the red peppers, garlic, cumin and paprika until smooth. Stir in the wine vinegar and then slowly mix in the extra virgin olive oil until you have a thick sauce. Alternatively, you can blitz everything together in a blender, but leave it with just a bit of texture. Season with salt and pepper to taste, adding a touch more vinegar too, if you like.

For the mojo cilantro, put the garlic cloves in a large mortar with the cumin and a good pinch of salt, then pound with a pestle until you have a smooth paste. Stir in the wine vinegar, then the chopped coriander. Finally, stir in the oil slowly until you have a smooth, herby dressing. Alternatively, you can do this in a blender. Season with salt and pepper to taste, adding a touch more vinegar too, if you like.

To roast the potatoes, preheat the oven to 200°C/Gas Mark 6. Parboil the potatoes in salted water for 5 minutes. Drain well and leave to steam in the colander for a few minutes to drive off excess moisture. Cut any larger spuds in half or into quarters, so they are roughly the same as the smaller whole ones.

Toss the potatoes with the olive oil in a roasting dish. Season well with salt and pepper and roast for 25–30 minutes until golden and crisp. Serve the potatoes hot, with the mojo sauces for dipping.

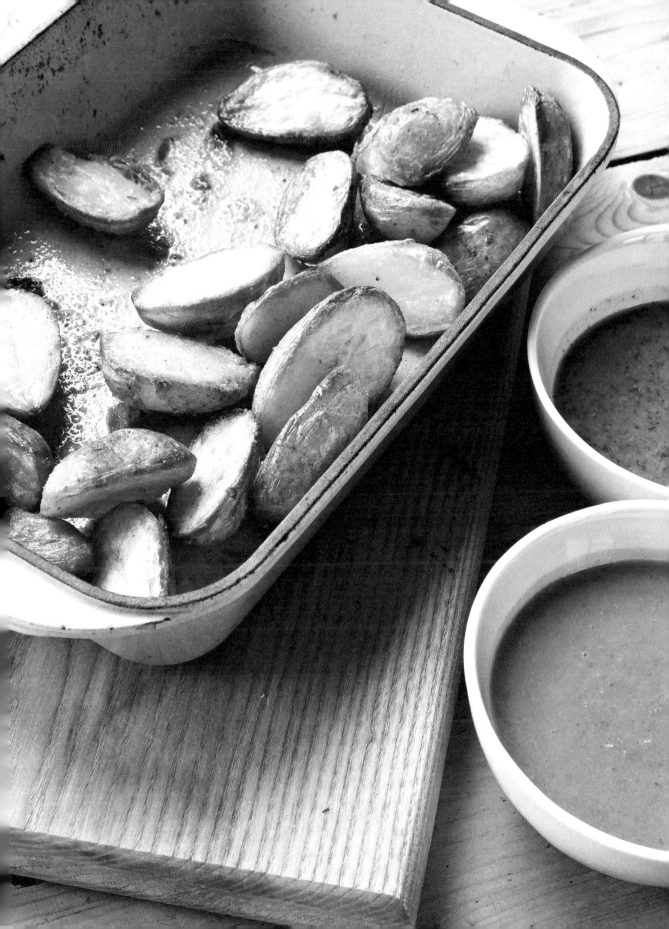

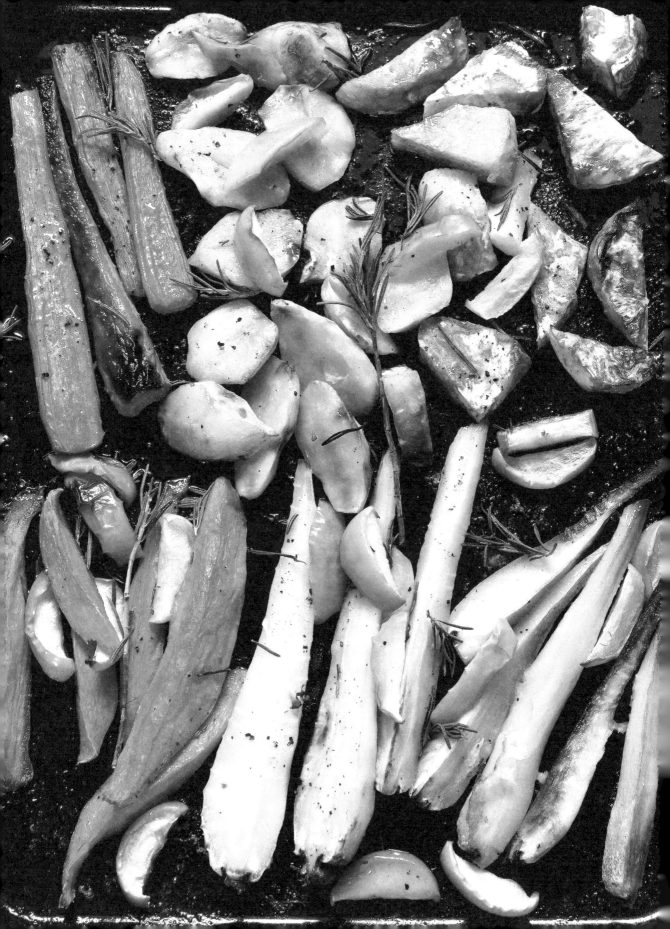

Roasted roots with apple and rosemary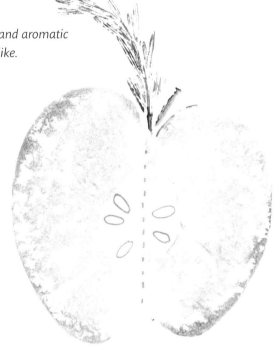

This dish produces a lovely commingling of rooty, fruity, sweet and aromatic flavours. You can include some squash or pumpkin too, if you like.

SERVES 4

1kg mixed root veg, such as parsnips, celeriac, carrots, Jerusalem artichokes and potatoes

3 tablespoons rapeseed or olive oil

3 medium or 2 large crisp, tart eating apples, cut into eighths, core removed, skin left on

A couple of sprigs of rosemary, roughly torn

Sea salt and freshly ground black pepper

Preheat the oven to 190°C/Gas Mark 5. Peel all the veg and cut into medium chunks. Put into a large roasting tin with the oil and some salt and pepper. Toss well and roast for about 35 minutes, stirring halfway through, until the veg are tender and starting to brown.

Add the apple wedges and rosemary, toss with the roots and roast for a further 15–20 minutes, until the apples are golden. Serve at once.

Oven-roasted ratatouille ♥

Roasting intensifies the flavours of the veg in this modern interpretation of the classic niçoise dish. The rich, garlicky tomato sauce that ties it all together could very deliciously be replaced by one quantity of my roasted tomato sauce (see page 366). Serve the ratatouille with bread and salad to make a main course, or as a side dish or part of a spread.

SERVES 4

2 onions

2 red, orange or yellow peppers, halved, cored and deseeded

400g courgettes

1 large aubergine (about 350g)

5 tablespoons olive oil

Sea salt and freshly ground black pepper

FOR THE TOMATO SAUCE

2 tablespoons olive oil

3 garlic cloves, slivered

2 x 400g tins plum tomatoes, chopped, any stalky ends and skin removed

1 bay leaf

A large sprig of thyme

A pinch of sugar

TO FINISH

A small handful of oregano or thyme sprigs, leaves only, chopped

Preheat the oven to 190°C/Gas Mark 5. Cut the onions into thick slices, from root to tip. Cut the peppers into 2–3cm pieces. If the courgettes are very thick, halve them lengthways before slicing them thickly. Cut the aubergine into 2–3cm cubes.

Tip the vegetables into a large roasting dish, add the olive oil and plenty of salt and pepper and toss well together. Roast for 1–1½ hours, giving it all a good stir once or twice, until the veg are tender, reduced and starting to brown in places.

Meanwhile, make the tomato sauce. Heat the olive oil in a large frying pan over a medium-low heat. Add the garlic and let it sizzle gently for a minute, without browning, then add the tomatoes with their juice, the bay leaf and thyme. Cook at a gentle simmer for about 45 minutes, stirring often and crushing the tomatoes down with a fork. When you have a thick, pulpy sauce, season with salt, pepper and the sugar.

When the veg are cooked, add the tomato sauce, mix well, then return to the oven for 10 minutes until bubbling and fragrant. While still hot, stir in the chopped oregano or thyme. Serve the ratatouille warm or cold, but not chilled.

VARIATION

Dry-roasted ratatouille ♥

This is a lovely variation, using oven-roasted cherry tomatoes instead of the tomato sauce. It's great served on bruschetta, or with couscous or rice. Arrange 500g halved cherry tomatoes snugly in a single layer in a roasting tray (slightly smaller than the one you're roasting the veg in). Trickle with a little olive oil and season with salt and pepper. Roast the tomatoes at the same time as the veg, on a lower oven shelf for at least an hour (but not as long as the veg), until reduced, wrinkled and lightly charred. Once the roasted vegetables and tomatoes have cooled a little, toss them very gently together in a bowl. Trickle with a little best olive oil and serve at room temperature.

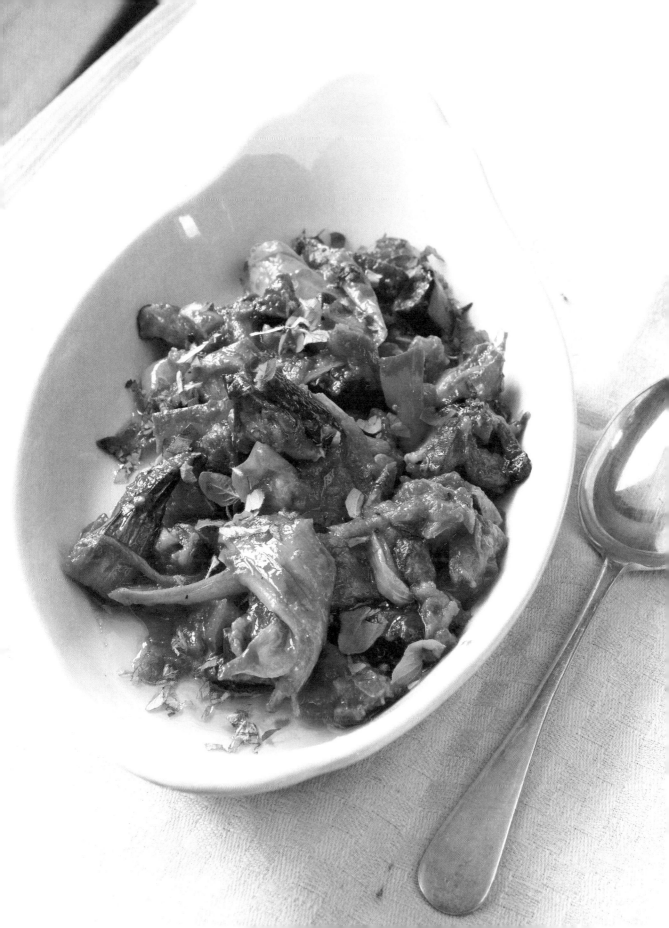

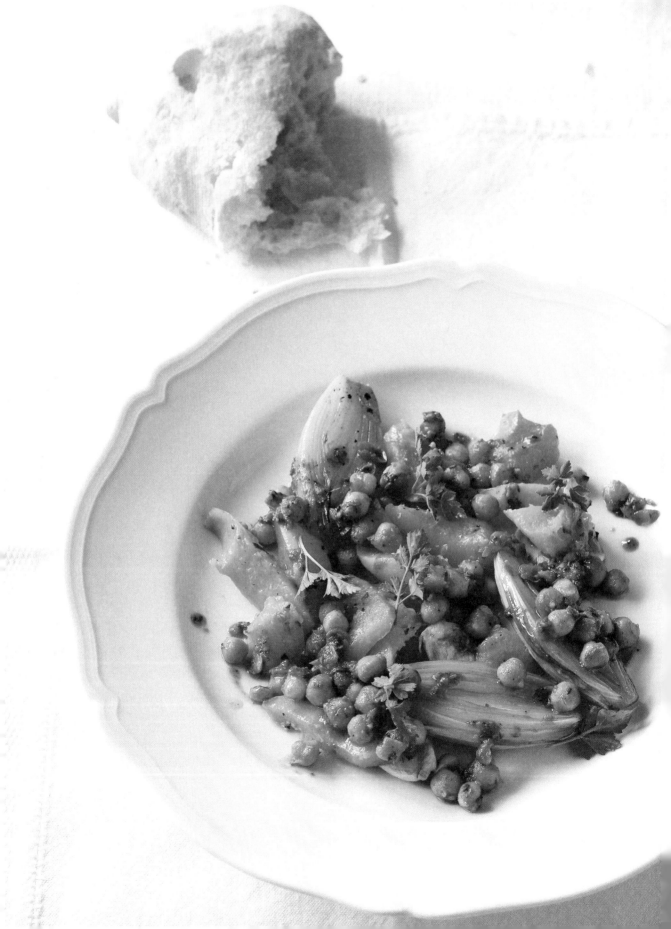

Roasted squash and shallots with merguez chickpeas ♥

I like to cook dried chickpeas from scratch for this dish. Mixed with the spicy oil while still hot, they absorb the flavours beautifully – and home-cooked chickpeas have such a lovely, nutty texture. But this is still a sterling dish if made with tinned chickpeas – use two 400g tins, drained and rinsed. Actually the merguez chickpeas are a lovely tapas dish in their own right – worth plonking on the table with any spread of veg dishes.

SERVES 4

About 1kg squash or pumpkin

About 300g shallots or small onions, peeled

4–5 garlic cloves (unpeeled), bashed

3 tablespoons olive oil

Sea salt and freshly ground black pepper

FOR THE MERGUEZ CHICKPEAS

200g dried chickpeas, soaked overnight in plenty of cold water

2 bay leaves

1 teaspoon cumin seeds

1 teaspoon fennel seeds

1 teaspoon coriander seeds

1 teaspoon caraway seeds (optional)

10–12 black peppercorns

1 garlic clove, finely chopped

1 teaspoon finely chopped rosemary

1 teaspoon sweet smoked paprika

A good pinch of cayenne pepper

¼ teaspoon fine sea salt

4 tablespoons extra virgin olive oil

TO FINISH

A handful of flat-leaf parsley

First, drain the chickpeas and put them into a large saucepan. Cover with lots of cold water, bring to the boil and boil hard for 10 minutes, then lower to a gentle simmer. Skim off any scum and add the bay leaves. Simmer for 1–1¼ hours, topping up with more boiling water if necessary, until tender and crushable.

Meanwhile, preheat the oven to 190°C/Gas Mark 5. Peel and deseed the squash or pumpkin and cut into roughly 4cm chunks. Halve or quarter the shallots or onions, depending on size. Put the squash, shallots and garlic cloves into a large roasting dish. Trickle over the olive oil and sprinkle generously with salt and pepper. Toss well and roast for about 50–60 minutes, stirring and jumbling once or twice, until soft and caramelised.

Meanwhile, for the chickpea dressing, toast all the spice seeds and the black peppercorns in a dry frying pan for a few minutes until fragrant. Crush to a coarse powder, using a pestle and mortar or spice grinder. Combine with the garlic, rosemary, paprika, cayenne, salt and extra virgin olive oil in a small saucepan. Warm gently for 1 minute (the oil should barely sizzle), then remove from the heat and set aside.

When the chickpeas are cooked, drain them well, return to their hot pan and toss while still hot with the spicy dressing. (If using tinned chickpeas, heat them through in the spicy oil, then leave to cool a bit.)

Divide the roasted squash and shallots between warmed plates. Top with the warm chickpeas, spooning over any extra oil left in the pan. Finish with a scattering of parsley leaves.

Roasted tomato sauce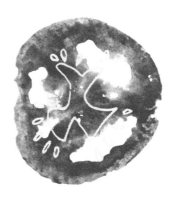

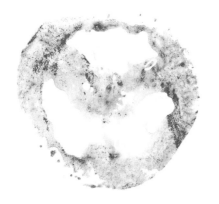

This intense tomato sauce is a River Cottage classic and an absolute mainstay of my cooking. I prepare tray after tray of it from the tomatoes I grow at home, and freeze batch after batch for use in the coming months. I make no apologies for including the recipe again here because it's such a useful and delicious thing – and elsewhere in this book you will find several new ideas for using it. The consistency of the sauce can vary quite a bit, depending on the tomatoes you use – sometimes you end up with a thick purée, and sometimes with a rich liquid. The flavour should always be good, though. Simmer the sauce to reduce and thicken it as necessary.

MAKES ABOUT 500ml

1.5–2kg ripe tomatoes, larger ones halved

3 garlic cloves, finely chopped

A few sprigs of thyme

A couple of sprigs of marjoram (optional)

2 tablespoons rapeseed or olive oil

Sea salt and freshly ground black pepper

Preheat the oven to 180°C/Gas Mark 4. Lay the tomatoes, cut side up if halved, on a baking tray. Scatter over the garlic and herbs, and trickle over the oil. Season with plenty of salt and pepper.

Put the tray in the oven for about an hour, maybe a bit longer, until the tomatoes are completely soft and pulpy, and starting to crinkle and caramelise on top.

Set the tomatoes aside to cool off for half an hour or so. Then tip them into a large sieve and rub through with a wooden spoon, or use a traditional mouli. Discard the skin and pips. Your tomato sauce is now ready to use.

RECIPES USING ROASTED TOMATO SAUCE

Aubergine and green bean curry (page 29) • Oven-roasted ratatouille (page 362) New potato gnocchi (page 284) • Tomato and mozzarella risotto (page 272) Beetroot pizza with cheddar (page 180) • Roasted tomato ketchup (page 392)

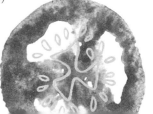

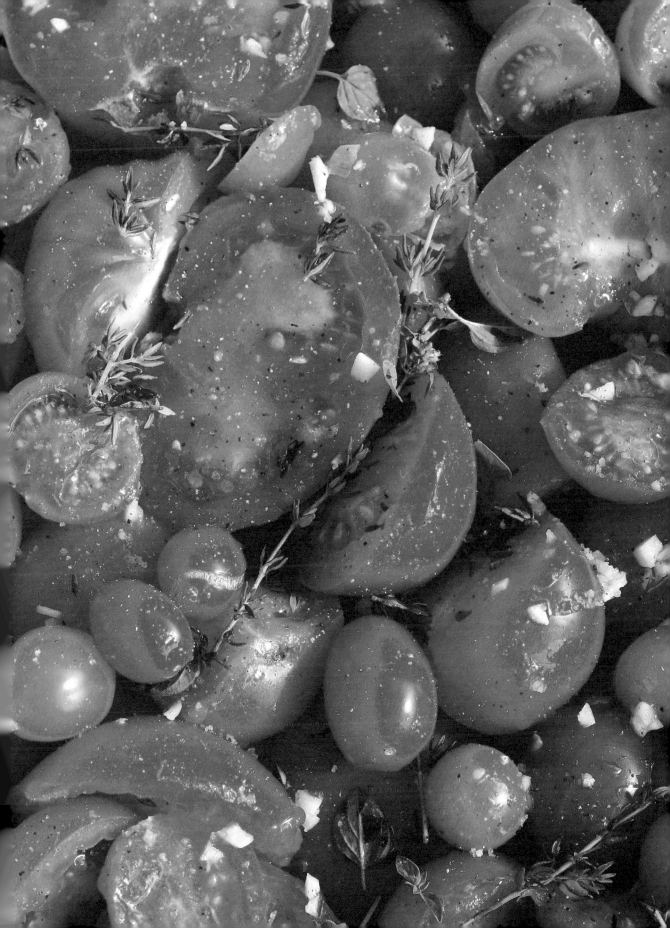

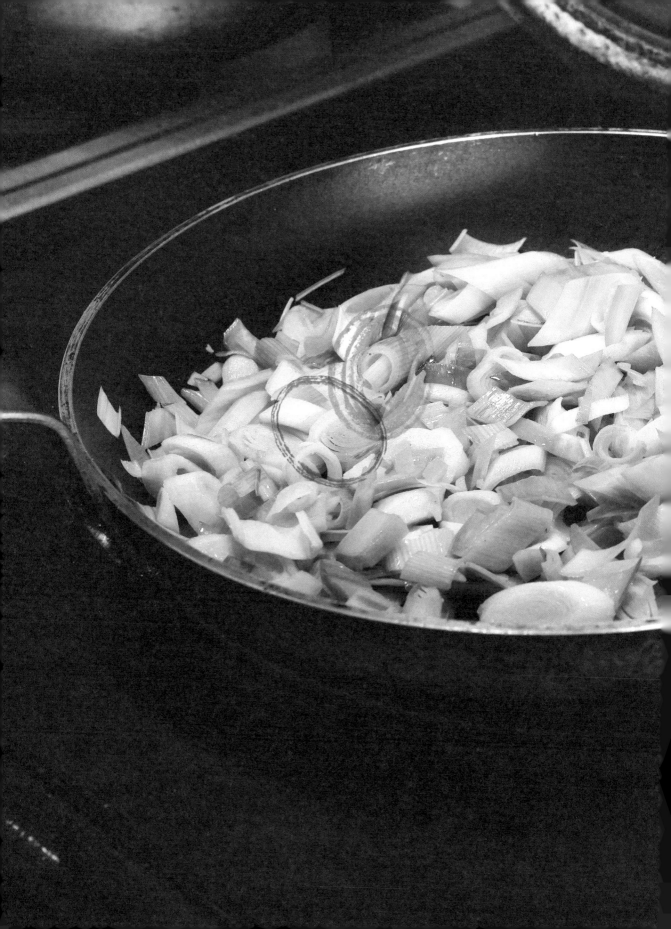

Side dishes

The recipes in this chapter are among the simplest in the book, and many are among my oldest favourites, having done years, even decades of service. Some of these ways of giving plainly cooked veg 'a bit of a lift' were devised to nudge younger members of the family towards more avid consumption of vegetables – and they worked a treat.

Indeed the enduring successes – steamed veg with a hint of garlic (see page 372) and creamy potato and celeriac mash (see page 388) – are now perceived as a treat. And some of the newer recipes – swede with onion and sage (see page 382) and leeks (and greens) with coconut milk (see page 378) – look set to achieve the same 'firm family favourites' status.

So the term 'side dishes' does not in any way diminish the recipes you will find here – it simply describes how they are usually deployed. To be honest, I often serve them beside fish or meat. And I'd be delighted to think that you'd want to do that too, from time to time. But increasingly, I dish them up alongside other more substantial veg dishes. In this context, they seem less like side dishes, more like pass-around dishes in their own right.

While few of these dishes are sustaining enough to constitute a whole meal, they have other virtues. The simple cooking allows the flavour, texture and colour of the veg to shine through; they unambiguously celebrate the principal ingredients. I like that. It's a bit of a cliché of food writing these days to note that, if you have some beautiful, plump, fresh leeks or some sweet, earthy, just-dug carrots – or even some very nice potatoes from the farm shop or supermarket – doing as little as possible to them is often the best approach. But it's a cliché for good reason – because it's absolutely true. The first few recipes here prove the point – these are just very plainly cooked veg, given the merest twist of spice, or the most basic of dressings, to enhance their flavours and to indicate that they deserve your attention.

All that's required is a little mind-shift. I realise it might seem slightly odd to put a plate of mash on the table, unaccompanied by bangers – but if it's good mash, it will go as quickly as any other dish. The same is true of stir-fried sesame cauliflower (see page 376), or a bowl of garlicky, minty mushy peas (see page 387), or golden potato rosti (see page 391). All you need is one or two complementary dishes to bring the meal together.

The recipes here are perfect foils to the more complex and often more highly seasoned ones in Mezze and tapas (pages 290–327), and many of my comments in that chapter apply here too. These are dishes that suit that generous, communal, mix-and-match way of eating that feels so wonderfully appropriate when vegetables are at the heart of your cooking. In that sense they pretty much have honorary mezze or tapas status anyway.

The reason why I've called them 'side' dishes is that they can also do sterling service as the single extra element that rounds out a 'big dish' meal. You might, for example, consider runner beans with tomatoes and garlic (see page 375) alongside a creamy potato dauphinoise (see page 60), or big baked mushrooms (see page 385) with a hearty frittata (see pages 232 and 234).

The chapter ends with a quirky flourish, which I'll happily admit is a bit of an indulgence. A handful of sweet recipes, whose primary ingredients are also vegetables feels like a fun way to finish. They are not side dishes, I'll grant you, they're definitely 'afters'. But they are not afterthoughts, nor are they mere novelties. On the contrary, they are lovely examples of the way in which vegetables can find their way into every corner of our diet.

We are all familiar with the carrot cake, and those of you who are familiar with my other work may be au fait with the chocolate and beetroot brownie, and the mashed potato lemon trickle cake. The treats with which I've chosen to round off this book fall into the same category: indulgent sweet recipes that just happen to be based on veg. And, I promise you, the duo of vegetable ice creams is an absolute revelation. Maybe even a revolution.

So, perhaps surprisingly, this is the broadest chapter in the book, ranging from the very simplest dish of garlicky, buttered green veg, through a selection of luxurious, creamy root veg purées, to a splendid dessert tart that you might choose to serve with a glass of sticky pudding wine. What it demonstrates again, I hope, is just how adaptable vegetables can be. Whether you are tired and pushed for time, or you have an entire afternoon free to spend pottering about in the kitchen, vegetables delicious, wholesome, enticing and infinitely various and versatile – are perhaps the most useful and rewarding of all ingredients.

Steamed veg with a hint of garlic

This is possibly the simplest recipe in the book, but it's one I turn to often.
It's an easy way to take any green veg up a notch. I've found it particularly
successful for encouraging younger family members to eat their greens...

SERVES 4

400–500g green veg
(peas, beans, broccoli,
cauliflower, shredded
cabbage etc)

25g butter

1 tablespoon rapeseed
or olive oil

1 fat garlic clove, crushed

Sea salt and freshly ground
black pepper

Prepare the veg: peas are fine as they are, of course. Trim beans (removing the strings from the sides of runner beans, if using, with a potato peeler), then cut into 3–4cm lengths. Cut broccoli or cauliflower into small florets. Remove tough stalks from cabbage, greens or kale and shred their leaves.

Now steam the veg over boiling water until just done – tender but with a bit of crunch left. The time taken depends on the vegetable.

While the veg is cooking, heat the butter and oil in a saucepan over a low heat. Once melted, add the garlic. Cook very gently for a couple of minutes, letting the fat just fizz slightly but taking care that the garlic doesn't colour. Remove from the heat.

Toss the hot, steamed veg in the garlicky butter, along with some salt and pepper, and it's ready to serve.

VARIATIONS
Garlic and caraway greens
Steam greens, kale, cabbage or Brussels tops as above, or wilt in a scrap of water and drain well. Add ½ teaspoon lightly bashed caraway seeds to the butter and oil at the same time as the garlic.

Garlic and cumin roots
For lightly steamed carrots, parsnips or beetroot: prepare as above, peeling and cutting the veg into slices or batons before steaming, and adding ½ teaspoon lightly toasted and ground cumin seeds to the butter and oil with the garlic. (If you haven't time to toast and grind cumin seeds just before you cook, pre-ground is still good.)

Garlic and mint peas and beans
For lightly cooked, just-picked peas or French or runner beans: prepare as above, adding 1 tablespoon finely chopped mint and 1 teaspoon balsamic vinegar, right at the end. Toss the peas/beans thoroughly with the minty, piquant butter.

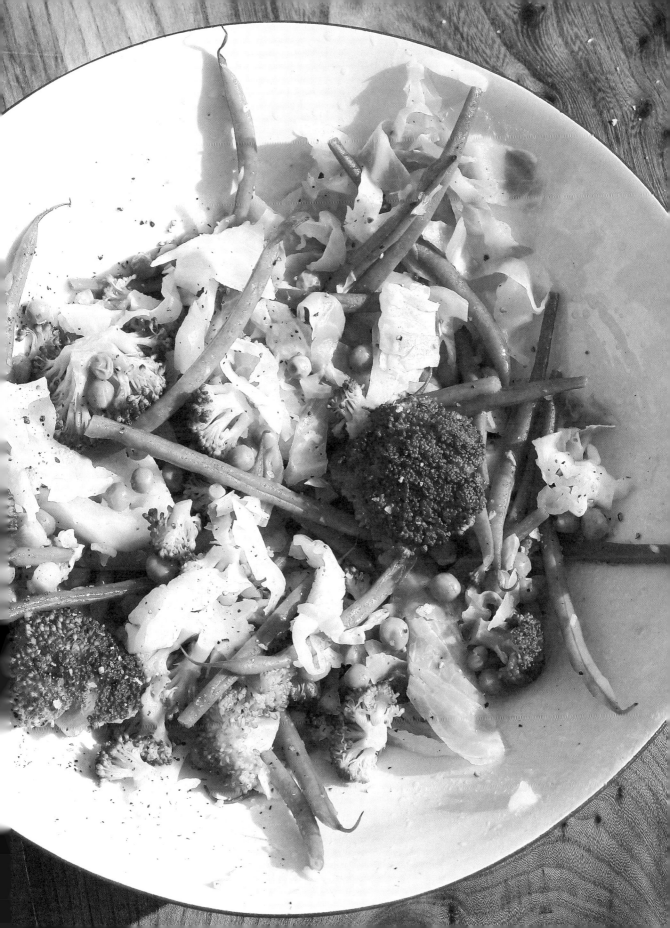

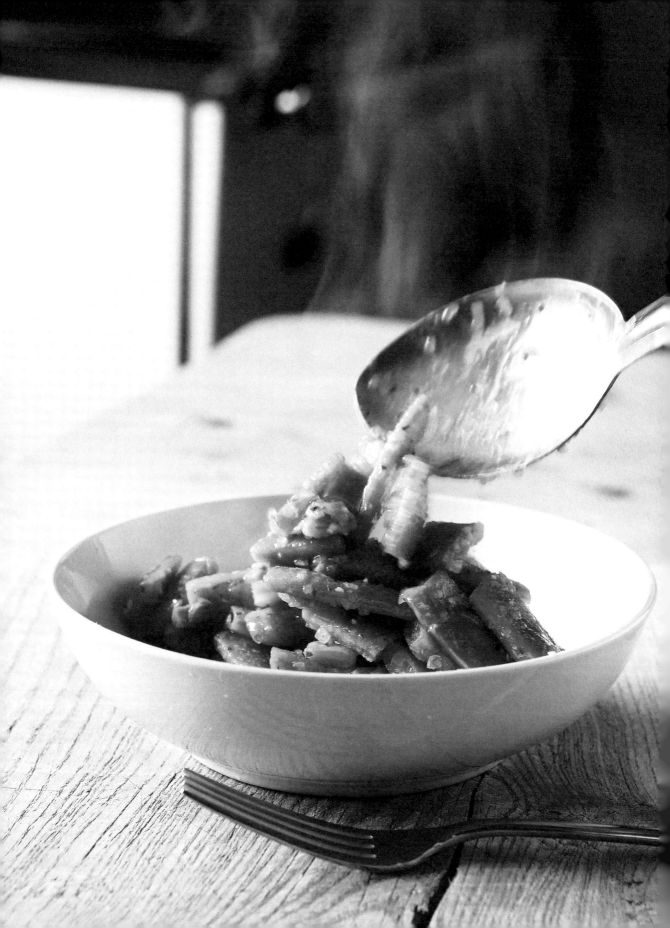

Runner beans with tarragon and lemon ♥

This is a lovely, fresh-tasting way to prepare runner beans – or French beans.

SERVES 4

500g runner beans

2 tablespoons rapeseed
or olive oil

2 shallots or 1 small onion,
finely chopped

1 small garlic clove,
finely chopped

Juice of 1 lemon

A handful of tarragon,
finely chopped

Sea salt and freshly ground
black pepper

Use a potato peeler to remove the stringy fibres from the edges of the beans, top and tail them, then cut into 2–3cm pieces.

Heat the oil in a large saucepan or casserole over a medium heat. Add the shallots or onion and sweat down for about 10 minutes, until soft.

Add the garlic and beans. Cover the pan, reduce the heat and sweat for another 10 minutes. Add about 100ml water and continue to cook, uncovered, for another 10 minutes or so, stirring from time to time. You want the beans to be just tender but still with a bit of crunch, and just a little liquid to remain at the end of cooking.

Remove from the heat and stir in the lemon juice, tarragon and some salt and pepper. Serve warm or at room temperature.

Runner beans with tomatoes and garlic ♥

Grating tomatoes is an easy way to peel them – as you rub the halved ripe tomato firmly against a box grater the skin will remain in your hand while the pulp and juices fall into the bowl. This dish works well with French beans too. Eat it hot as an accompaniment or cold as a part of a selection of mezze.

SERVES 4-6

500g runner beans

500g large, ripe tomatoes

2 tablespoons olive oil

1 onion, finely chopped

1 large garlic clove,
finely chopped

A small handful of basil
(or a mix of parsley and basil),
finely shredded

Sea salt and freshly ground
black pepper

Use a potato peeler to remove the stringy fibres from the edges of the beans, top and tail them, then cut into 6cm pieces.

Halve the tomatoes. Using the large-holed side of a box grater, grate the tomatoes into a bowl. Discard the skins.

Heat the olive oil in a large frying pan over a medium-low heat, add the onion and sauté gently, until soft, about 10 minutes. Add the garlic and sauté for a further minute.

Stir in the beans, then the tomato pulp and some salt and pepper. Bring to a simmer over a medium heat and cook for 10 minutes. Add the herbs and simmer for another 5 minutes until the sauce has thickened and the beans are tender. Check the seasoning and serve hot, warm or cold.

Stir-fried sesame cauliflower *v*

Cauliflower takes strong seasonings exceptionally well and this easy stir-fry – flavoured with chilli, garlic and ginger – is a good example. This is a great side dish, but you can also serve it with rice or noodles as a supper in itself.

SERVES 2-4

1 medium cauliflower
(about 700g), trimmed

2 tablespoons sesame seeds

2 tablespoons sunflower oil

1 onion, halved and thinly sliced

2 garlic cloves, sliced

1–2 green chillies, deseeded
and thinly sliced

2 teaspoons freshly grated
ginger

1 teaspoon toasted sesame oil

2 teaspoons soy sauce, plus
extra to serve

A small handful of coriander,
chopped, plus extra sprigs
to finish

Break the cauliflower into small, neat florets. Place in a bowl of cold water and leave to soak for 10 minutes.

In a small frying pan, dry-fry the sesame seeds for a minute or two until toasted and fragrant. Tip on to a plate and set aside.

Heat the sunflower oil in a large frying pan or wok over a medium heat and add the onion. Sauté until pale golden, then add the garlic, chilli(es) and ginger and fry, stirring, for a minute.

Drain the cauliflower. Raise the heat under the frying pan, then tip in the cauliflower and 100ml water. Cook, stirring, for 5–10 minutes until the florets are browning around the edges, adding a splash more water if they start to stick. Stir in the sesame seeds, sesame oil, soy sauce and chopped coriander.

Serve scattered with coriander sprigs, and with soy sauce to hand for people to add as they choose.

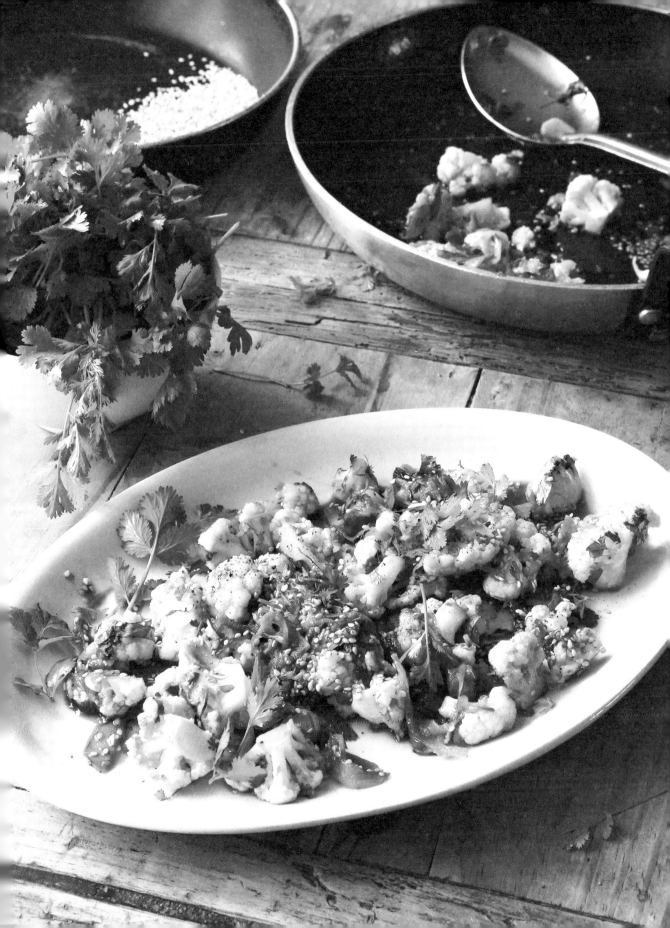

Leeks (and greens) with coconut milk ꙮ

I've been cooking this a lot recently – with or without greens. It's great with spicy roast roots or squash, rice, and maybe some dhal (see page 238) on the side. In early summer when leeks are out of season, I sometimes make it with spring onions or young green onions instead.

SERVES 4

4–5 medium leeks, trimmed of tough leafy ends, washed

About 250g spring greens, kale or cabbage (optional), tough stalks removed

2 tablespoons sunflower oil

3 garlic cloves, sliced

1 teaspoon good curry powder or curry paste

400ml coconut milk

Sea salt and freshly ground black pepper

50g roasted peanuts or cashews, roughly chopped or crushed, to finish (optional)

Cut the leeks into 1cm slices on the diagonal. If using greens, shred into 1cm ribbons and set aside.

Heat the sunflower oil in a large frying pan over a medium-low heat and sweat the garlic for a couple of minutes, being careful not to let it burn.

Add the leeks and sauté for a few minutes, then add the curry powder or paste and cook, stirring occasionally, for another couple of minutes, until the leeks are becoming tender but still have a bit of bite.

Add the greens, if using, and sweat down for 3 minutes or so until wilted but still slightly crunchy.

Pour in the coconut milk and heat through, letting it bubble for just a minute. Serve at once, sprinkled with peanuts or cashews if you like.

Cheat's cauliflower cheese

There's no need to make a béchamel for this quick and easy cauliflower gratin, yet it's still delicious and filling. A good distribution of the cheesy, crumby topping is the key to success. Serve as a side dish or alone.

SERVES 2–4

1 large cauliflower (about 1kg), trimmed

A large knob of butter

1 tablespoon cream (optional)

100g mature Cheddar or other flavoursome hard cheese, grated

40–50g breadcrumbs

Sea salt and freshly ground black pepper

Cut the cauliflower into very small florets. Put into a pan, cover with lightly salted water, bring to the boil, then simmer for about 5 minutes, or until *al dente*. Drain well and toss with the butter, the cream if you like, and plenty of salt and pepper.

Preheat the grill to medium-high. Tip the cauliflower florets into a gratin dish or shallow ovenproof dish in which they fit snugly in one layer. Combine the cheese and breadcrumbs and scatter thickly and evenly over the top. Place under the grill until golden brown and nicely toasted. Serve straight away.

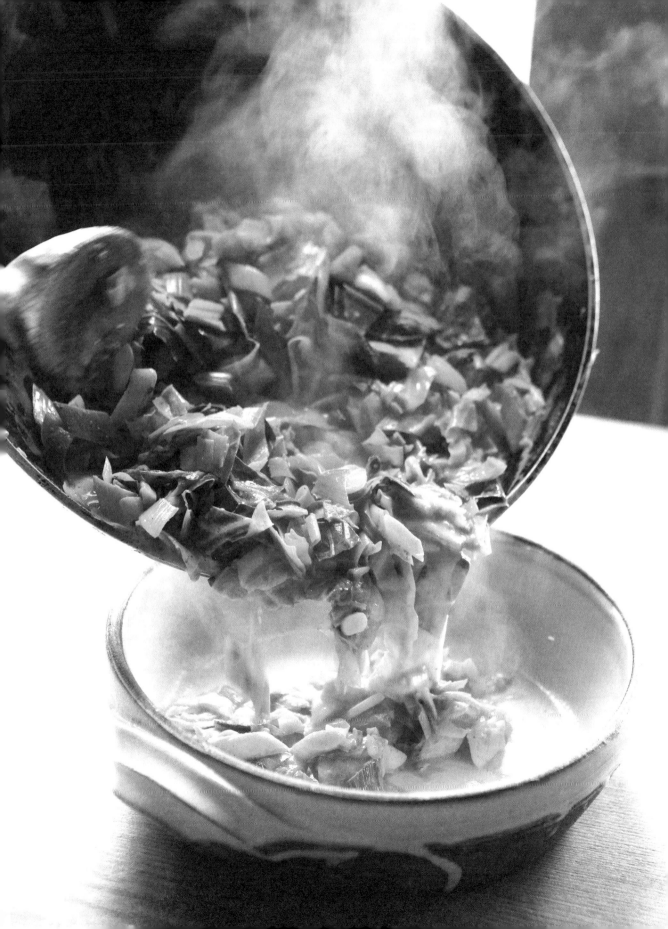

Celery gratin

It's easy to think of celery as a mere 'flavouring' vegetable, crucial to soups and stocks, but not a star in its own right. This deeply flavoured dish shows how delicious it can be when given centre stage. Try it with dressed lentils (see page 237), or even a simple frittata (see pages 232 and 234).

SERVES 4

1 head of celery

1 bay leaf

1 sprig of thyme

25g butter

About 100ml double cream

75g breadcrumbs

30g Parmesan, Gruyère, hard goat's cheese or other well-flavoured hard cheese, finely grated

Sea salt and freshly ground black pepper

Preheat the oven to 160°C/Gas Mark 3. Break the celery into stalks, and put aside the outer stalks if they look coarse, or a bit hollow – to use for stock (see page 130). Cut any leaves from the remaining stalks and save these for stock too (they would go brown in the oven). Cut all the sticks into 10cm lengths.

Put the celery into a shallow ovenproof dish and tuck the bay and thyme among the stems. Pour over 3 tablespoons water, dot over the butter and sprinkle on some salt and pepper. Cover with foil and bake for about 40 minutes or until the celery is tender. Take the dish out of the oven and turn the setting up to 200°C/Gas Mark 6.

Discard the bay and thyme and carefully pour off the liquid from the celery dish into a jug. Add enough cream to make up to 150ml and whisk together. Taste and add more salt and pepper if needed, then pour back over the celery in the dish.

Mix the breadcrumbs with the grated cheese, sprinkle over the celery and return to the oven for 15–20 minutes, until the crumb topping is golden brown and crispy. Grind over some black pepper and serve.

VARIATION

Gratin of chard stalks

If you've used chard leaves in a recipe, this is an ideal way to serve up the delicious, tender-crunchy stalks. Cut the stalks from a 1kg bunch of chard into roughly 1cm slices. Heat 1 tablespoon oil and a knob of butter in a large frying pan over a medium heat and fry the chard stalks with some chopped garlic, stirring often, for 10–15 minutes, until tender. Stir in the chopped leaves from a handful of thyme sprigs, some salt and pepper and 100ml double cream. When bubbling, transfer to a gratin dish and scatter over 25g grated Parmesan or Gruyère mixed with 25g breadcrumbs. Put under a hot grill until golden brown. Serve as a side dish, or with dressed Puy lentils (see page 237) or perhaps some new potatoes as a supper.

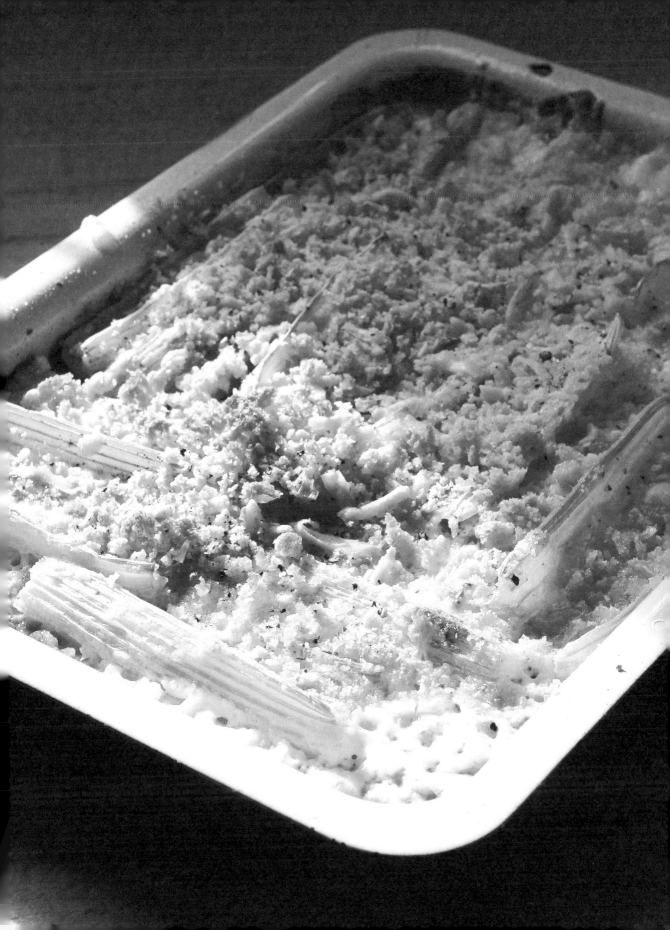

Swede with onion and sage

*This is a delicious way to serve swede: the sweetness of the onions softens
its pungency and the sage adds an extra layer of flavour.*

SERVES 4

50g butter

About 500g swede, peeled
and cut into 1cm cubes

1 large onion, chopped

About 12 sage leaves, finely
shredded

Sea salt and freshly ground
black pepper

Heat the butter in a wide pan over a medium heat. Add the swede,
onion, half the sage and some salt and pepper. Stir well. When the
vegetables are sweating nicely, cover the pan and reduce the heat
a little.

Cook, stirring from time to time, for 40–45 minutes, until the swede
is tender and the onion is sweet and caramelised.

Stir in the remaining shredded sage, taste and adjust the seasoning
if necessary, and serve.

Jerusalem artichoke frying pan gratin

*Jerusalem artichokes make an excellent gratin. For a less substantial dish,
you can just simmer them with the onions and thyme, but the addition
of crème fraîche and cheese turns this into a really luxurious treat.*

SERVES 4

25g butter

1 tablespoon rapeseed
or olive oil

1 large onion, cut into thin
wedges

500g Jerusalem artichokes,
peeled and cut into 3mm slices

A handful of thyme sprigs,
leaves only, chopped

4 tablespoons crème fraîche

About 40g mature Cheddar,
grated

Sea salt and freshly ground
black pepper

Heat the butter and oil in a large frying pan over a medium heat.
Add the onion and sweat for about 10 minutes, until soft and just
beginning to colour.

Add the sliced artichokes, thyme, some salt and lots of black pepper.
Pour in 100ml water, bring to a simmer, then cover and turn the heat
down low. Simmer, stirring from time to time, for about 20 minutes,
until the artichokes are nice and tender throughout, adding a little
more water if you need to. Remove the lid and simmer for a further
few minutes if necessary to reduce the liquid to a thick glaze.

Preheat the grill to high. Check the seasoning of the artichokes, then
dollop the crème fraîche over them evenly. Scatter over the cheese
and grill for a few minutes until bubbling. Serve straight away.

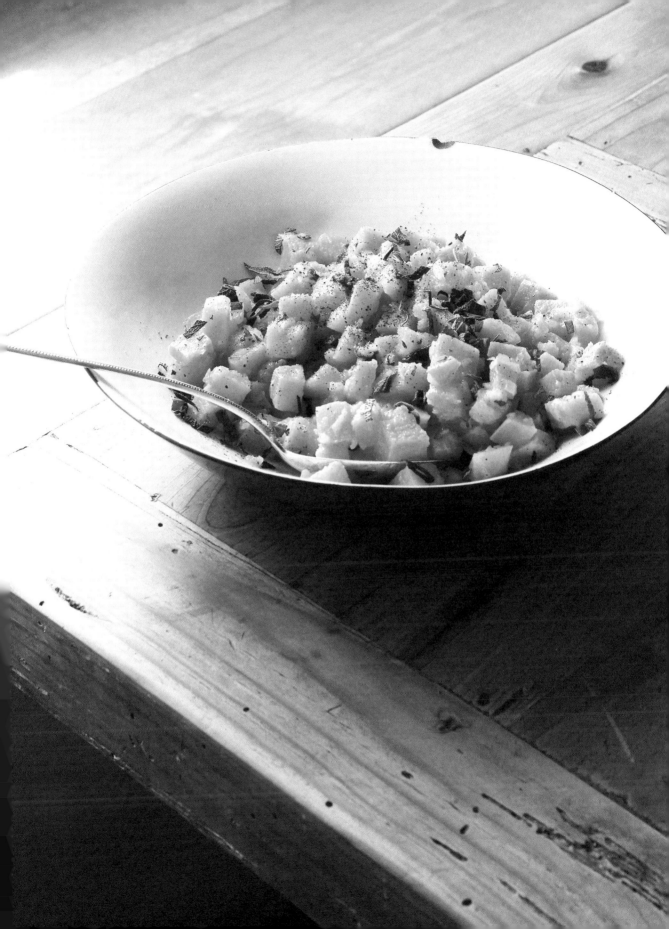

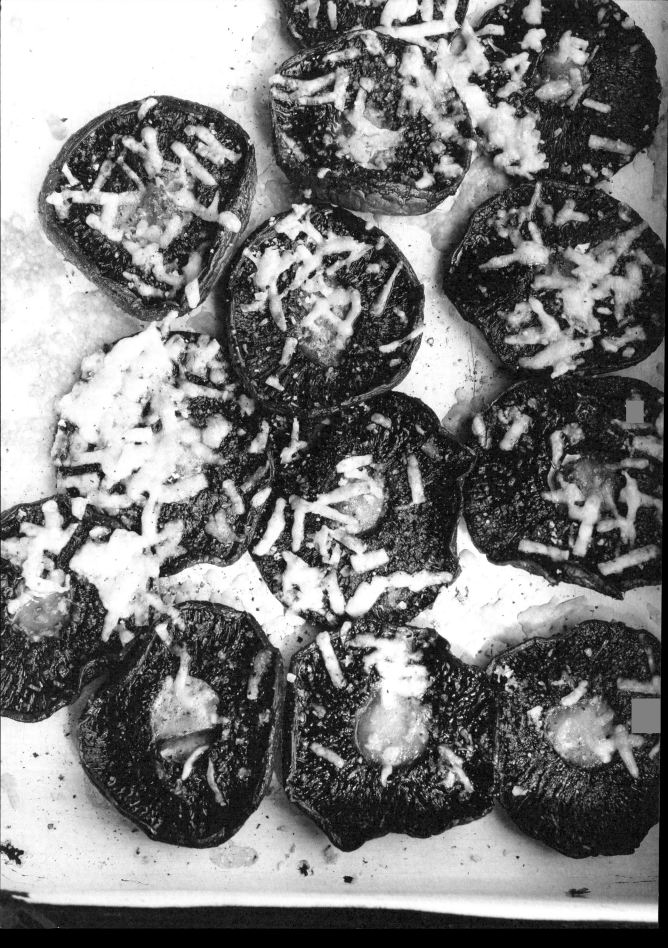

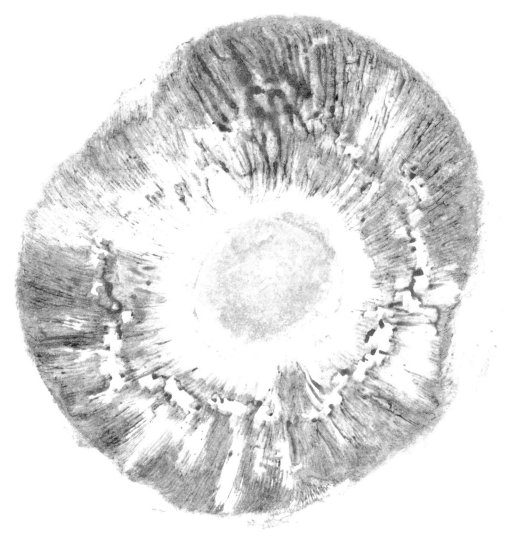

Big baked mushrooms

This is such an easy way to cook big, flat fresh mushrooms, and they make a surprisingly 'meaty' accompaniment to anything from a potato gratin to a spelt salad. You could serve them with the cheesy topping as a starter, but they are very good just as they are.

SERVES 2

4 large, flat open-capped mushrooms

A knob of butter

1 garlic clove, finely chopped

About 30g well-flavoured Cheddar or hard goat's cheese, grated (optional)

Sea salt and freshly ground black pepper

Preheat the oven to 190°C/Gas Mark 5. Put the mushrooms, open side up, into a small, lightly oiled roasting dish. Dot with the butter, scatter on the garlic, then dust with some salt and pepper. Bake for about 15 minutes, until the mushrooms are tender and juicy.

Serve the baked mushrooms as they are, or sprinkle over the grated cheese and return to the oven for another 5 minutes or so, until golden and bubbling.

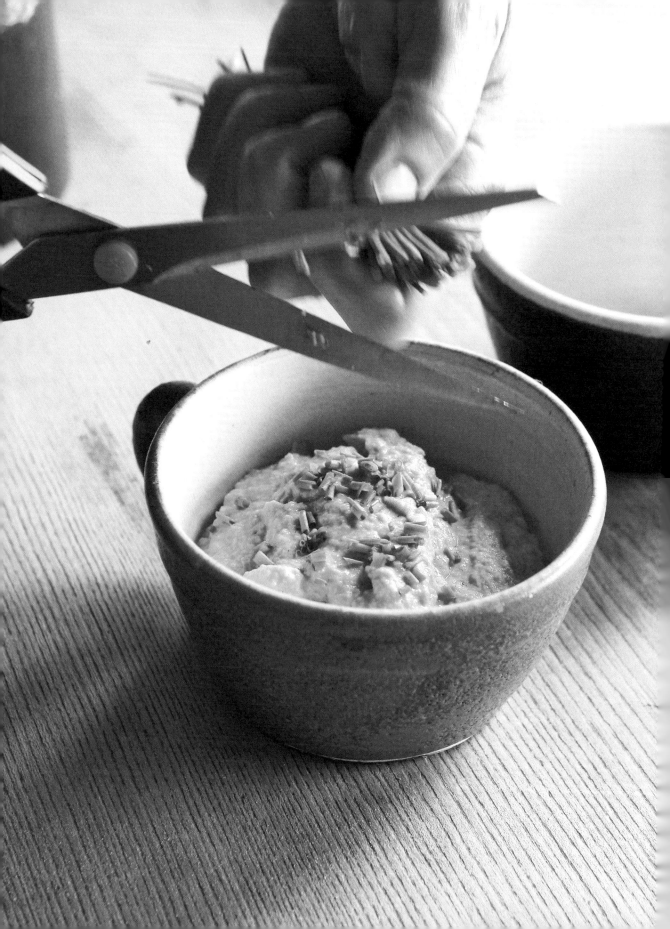

Garlicky, minty mushy peas

*This is another one of those highly seasoned, blitzed vegetable purées that I am
so fond of. They are great as a side dish, or as part of a mezze spread, or they
can be eaten as a snack or starter with some toast soldiers or flatbread wedges.*

SERVES 4

20g butter

3 shallots or 1 medium onion,
finely chopped

3–4 garlic cloves, finely chopped

A good handful of mint, finely
chopped, plus a sprig

500g fresh or frozen peas

Sea salt and freshly ground
black pepper

A handful of chives (optional)

Melt the butter in a saucepan over a low heat. Add the shallots or
onion and sauté for 15–20 minutes, until very soft. Add the garlic and
sauté for a couple more minutes, then set aside.

In a separate saucepan, cook the peas with a sprig of mint in enough
lightly salted boiling water to cover them by 2–3cm, until tender.
Drain, saving some of the cooking water.

Using a food processor, blender or a stick bender, blitz the peas with
the shallots, garlic, chopped mint and a twist of pepper, adding just
a little of the pea cooking water, to obtain a coarse purée.

Taste and adjust the seasoning. Serve warm, scattered with chopped
chives, if you like.

Salsify purée

*Salsify is a root veg with a delicate earthy flavour. It's lovely just boiled
and tossed with butter and pepper, but this turns it into something rich and
comforting. Scorzonera, which is closely related, would work well here too.
Serve as a side dish, or with flatbreads (see page 176) or toast as a starter.*

SERVES 4

About 500g salsify or
scorzonera

30g butter

3 tablespoons double cream

A handful of thyme sprigs,
leaves only, chopped (optional)

Sea salt and freshly ground
black pepper

Peel the salsify, dropping the roots directly into a pan of water (they
discolour extremely quickly on exposure to air). Chop the peeled roots
into large chunks and return to the pan. Add salt to the water – which,
for cooking, should just cover the roots by 1cm or so. Bring to the boil,
reduce the heat and simmer for 15–20 minutes, or until the salsify is
completely tender. Drain, reserving the cooking water.

Transfer the salsify to a blender and add the butter, cream, thyme
if using, and a generous few twists of black pepper. Process to a thick
purée. You can add a splash of the cooking water to loosen it if you
like, but it's best when thick enough to hold its shape. Check the
seasoning. Serve straight away, or leave to cool, then reheat gently.

Creamy potato and celeriac mash

This makes a gorgeous smooth and velvety mash – worth the little extra effort of passing the cooked potatoes through a ricer or mouli. Don't be tempted to blitz them in a processor as this makes them gluey and will spoil the texture of the mash.

SERVES 6

1kg floury potatoes, peeled and cut into even-sized chunks

700ml whole milk

400g celeriac, peeled and cut into 3cm chunks

50g unsalted butter, plus extra to taste

A few gratings of nutmeg

Sea salt and freshly ground black pepper

Add the potatoes to a large pan of salted water, bring to the boil and cook until tender, about 20 minutes. Drain well and leave to steam in a colander for a few minutes to drive off excess moisture.

While the potatoes are cooking, bring the milk to the boil in a separate pan. Add the celeriac and simmer until very soft, about 20 minutes. Drain, reserving the milk; keep it warm. Purée the celeriac in a food processor with the butter and about 150ml of the hot milk. Place the celeriac purée in a warmed large bowl.

Press the potatoes through a potato ricer or pass through a mouli legumes into the bowl with the celeriac. (If you don't have a ricer or mouli, mash them separately until they're very smooth.)

Using a wooden spoon, beat the celeriac purée with the potatoes until smooth and well combined, adding a little more of the hot milk and/or some more butter until you get the consistency you like. Season with salt, pepper and nutmeg to taste and serve immediately.

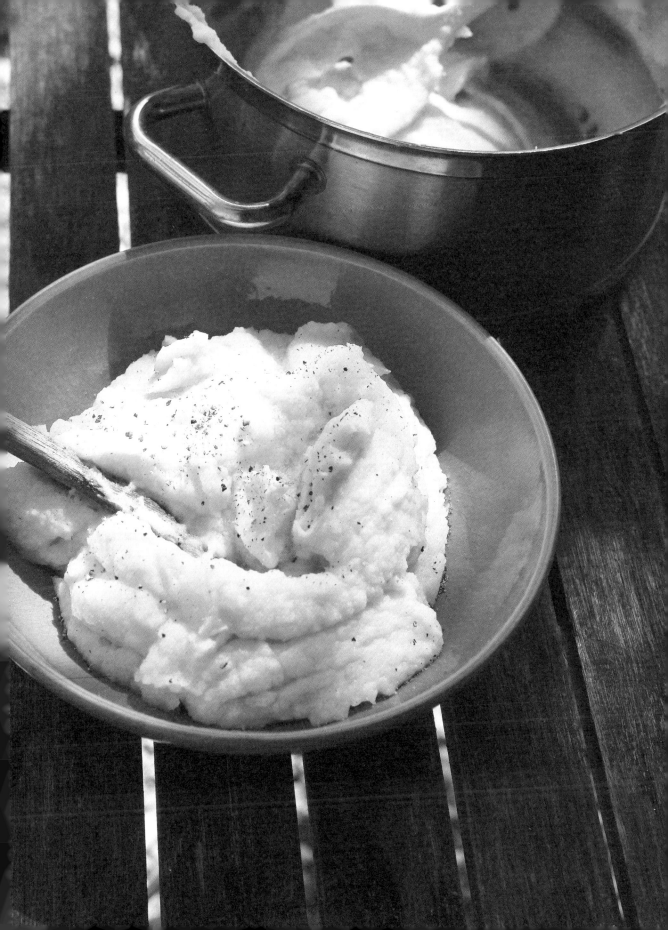

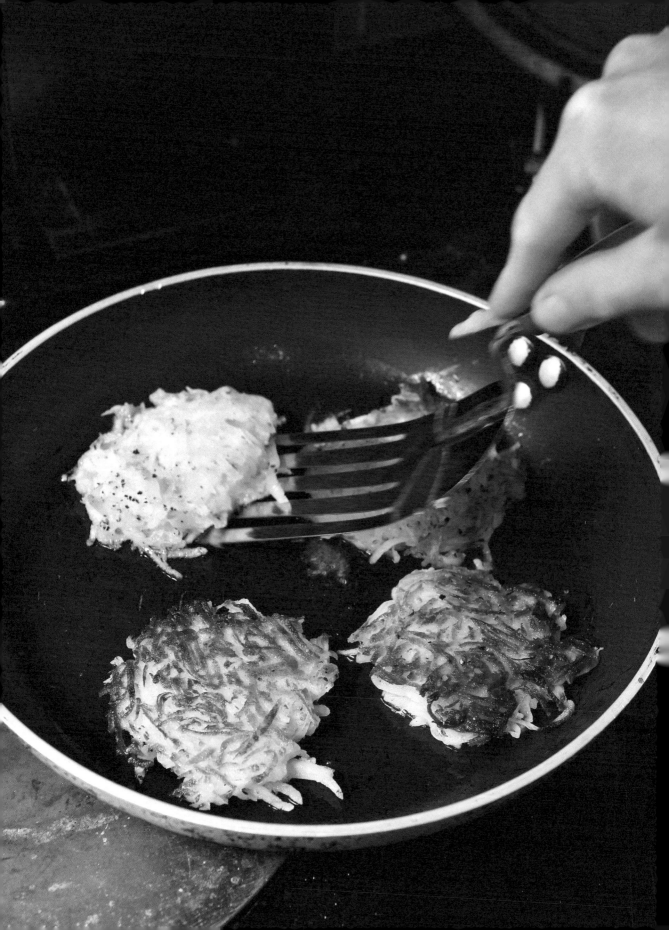

Potato rosti ♥

A simple rosti – well-seasoned grated potato, fried until golden and crunchy – is hard to beat, but do try the variations below. Sometimes, rather than making individual rosti, I put all the mixture in the pan at once to form a single giant rosti cake. Serve as a side dish, or with a poached egg (see page 210), or a pile of dressed lentils (see page 237) or beans – for lunch or supper.

MAKES 6 SMALL
OR 4 LARGE ROSTI

500g floury potatoes, such
as Maris Piper

Rapeseed oil, for frying

Flaky sea salt and freshly ground
black pepper

Peel the potatoes. Leave small ones whole, halve medium ones and quarter large ones – they should be an even, large-roast-potato size. Put into a pan, cover with water, add some salt and bring to the boil. Lower the heat and simmer for just 5 minutes – they should be just underdone. Drain and leave to cool completely (otherwise they will crumble as you grate them), then grate coarsely. Season generously with salt and pepper, tossing thoroughly to mix.

Heat enough oil in a non-stick frying pan to cover the base by about 1mm and place over a medium heat. Form handfuls of the grated potato into shallow cakes, no more than 1cm thick. Don't worry if they are prone to falling apart at this stage – the cooking will sort that out.

Add the potato cakes to the hot pan and fry without moving for about 5 minutes, so they form a golden brown crust underneath. Carefully flip them over. Continue to cook until golden brown and crisp on each side, turning once or twice more if you need to. They will take about 12 minutes in all. Remove and drain off any excess oil on kitchen paper. Sprinkle over a little salt and serve the rosti on warmed plates.

VARIATIONS
Potato and onion rosti ♥
Fry 1 finely sliced onion in 1 tablespoon rapeseed oil for 10 minutes, or until soft. Stir into the grated potato and continue as above.

Potato and seaweed rosti ♥
Simmer a good handful of fresh dulse seaweed in water for about 10 minutes until tender, drain well and chop roughly. (Or, soak about 15g dried seaweed such as dulse, wakame or arame according to the pack instructions, usually about 10 minutes, then squeeze out excess liquid and chop roughly.) Fry 1 sliced onion in 1 tablespoon rapeseed oil for about 10 minutes, until soft. Mix the seaweed and onion with the grated potato and some salt and pepper, before forming the cakes (or one big cake). These are good sprinkled with a little soy sauce before serving. For tips on gathering fresh dulse and other seaweeds, see John Wright's *River Cottage Edible Seashore Handbook*.

Roasted tomato ketchup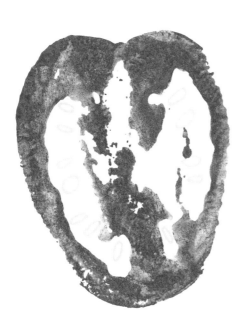

This is a lovely, loose ketchup with a deep rich flavour acquired from roasting the tomatoes. For a bit of heat and a smoky tang, include the smoked paprika. Use this sauce whenever you might think of using ketchup – it's perfect with chips.

MAKES 300–500ml

1 litre roasted tomato sauce (see page 366)

50g soft brown sugar

50ml cider vinegar

¼ teaspoon ground mace

¼ teaspoon ground mixed spice

1 teaspoon hot smoked paprika (optional)

Sea salt and freshly ground black pepper

Put the roasted tomato sauce into a fairly large, heavy-based saucepan and add all the rest of the ingredients, except salt and pepper. Bring to a merry simmer, stirring occasionally.

Cook down over a medium-low heat for 20–40 minutes, maybe longer, stirring regularly to prevent it catching on the bottom of the pan. You'll want to reduce the sauce by at least half, up to three-quarters, depending partly on how loose the sauce was to start with, and partly on how thick and intense you want your ketchup to be. So when you think you're pretty much there, take a teaspoon and blob some on to a cold plate, leave it to cool and then taste it. Add salt and pepper to taste.

The finished ketchup will keep in a sealed jar in the fridge for a couple of weeks. Alternatively, if you want a long-keeping, store-cupboard version, you can pot it while still piping hot into warm, sterilised jars or ketchup bottles. Fill them right to the brim and seal immediately with metal, vinegar-proof caps.

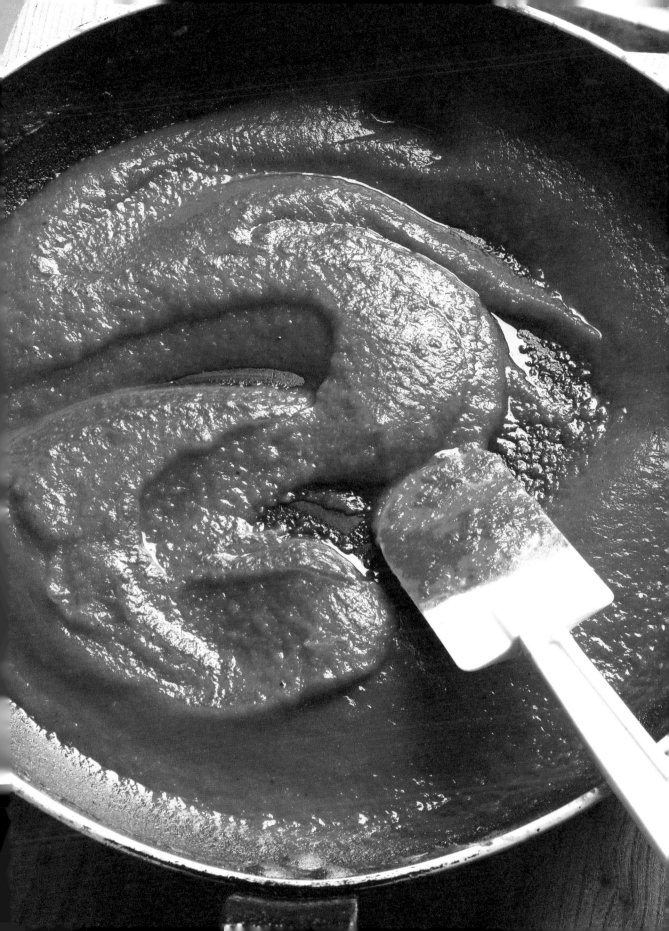

Pumpkin and raisin tea loaf

This delicious tea loaf is rich and sweet, but also quite light because it doesn't contain any butter or oil.

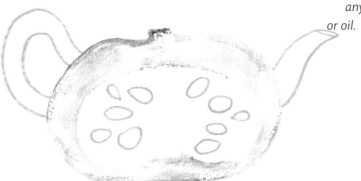

MAKES 12 GENEROUS SLICES

A little butter or sunflower oil, for greasing

200g light muscovado sugar

4 large eggs, separated

200g finely grated raw pumpkin or squash flesh

Finely grated zest and juice of 1 lemon

100g raisins

100g ground almonds

200g self-raising flour

A pinch of fine sea salt

1 teaspoon ground cinnamon

A generous grating of nutmeg

Preheat the oven to 170°C/Gas Mark 3. Lightly grease a loaf tin, about 20 x 10cm, and line with baking parchment.

Using an electric whisk, beat the sugar and egg yolks together for 2–3 minutes until pale and creamy. Lightly stir in the grated pumpkin or squash, lemon zest and juice, raisins and ground almonds. Sift the flour, salt and spices together over the mixture and then fold them in, using a large metal spoon.

In a large, clean bowl, beat the egg whites until they hold soft peaks. Stir a heaped tablespoonful of the egg white into the cake mixture to loosen it a little, then fold in the rest as lightly as you can.

Tip the mixture into the prepared loaf tin and gently level the surface. Bake for about 1 hour, or until a skewer inserted into the centre comes out clean.

Leave to cool in the tin for 10 minutes, then transfer to a wire rack to cool completely before slicing.

VARIATIONS

Courgette, carrot or beetroot tea loaf
Replace the pumpkin with 200g finely grated raw courgette, carrot or even beetroot (which produces a striking purple-marbled effect).

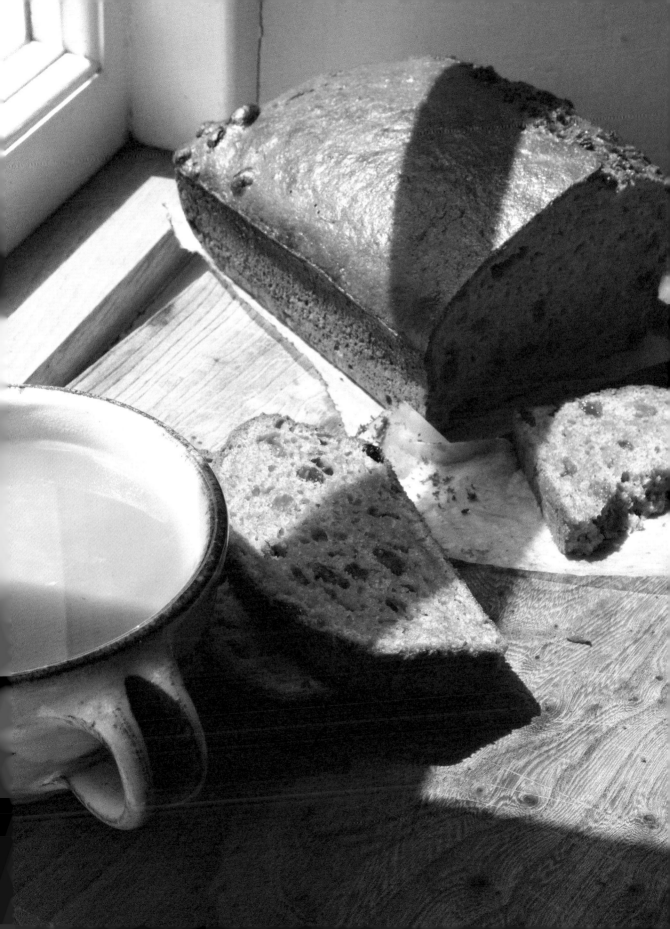

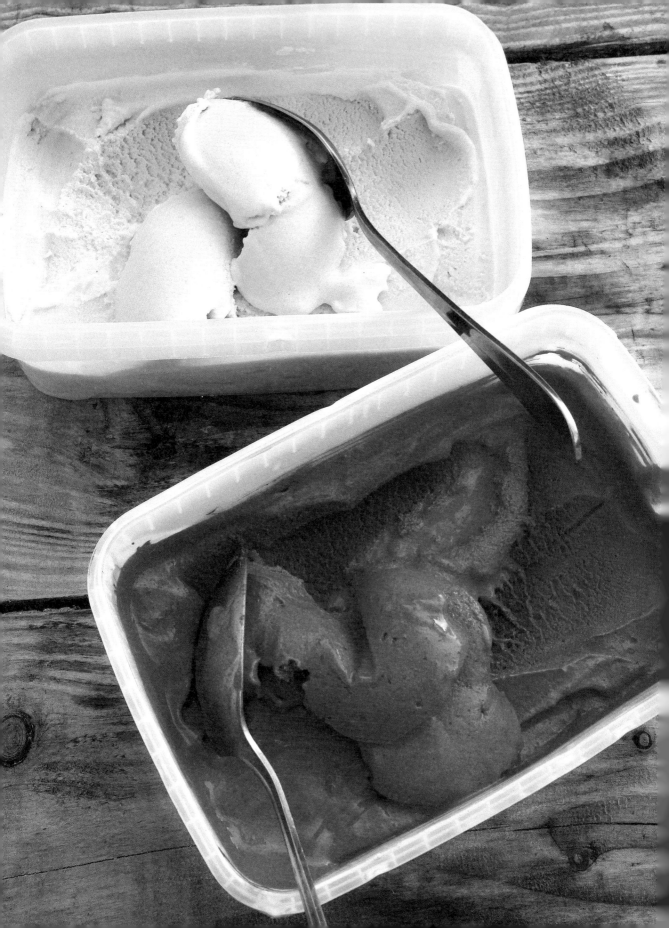

Chocolate and beetroot ice cream

This pairing works brilliantly in an ice cream – the velvety beetroot purée contributing a subtle, earthy-sweet flavour and excellent smooth texture. Go on, give it a go... And once you're in the swing of vegetable ice creams, try the variation. It's a stunner – cool, minty and gorgeous.

MAKES ABOUT 800ml

300g beetroot

300ml whole milk

200ml double cream

4 large egg yolks

100g caster sugar

100g dark chocolate, broken into small pieces

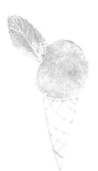

Preheat the oven to 200°C/Gas Mark 6. Put the beetroot into an ovenproof dish, add a 1cm depth of water, cover with foil and roast until tender: at least 1 hour, possibly longer. Leave to cool completely. Peel the beetroot, chop it roughly and purée in a blender with 100ml of the milk. Measure the purée. You should have about 300ml; it does not matter if there's a little less, but you don't want more. Set aside.

To make the custard, heat the remaining milk and cream in a pan to just below boiling. Cool a little. Whisk the egg yolks and sugar together in a bowl, then pour on the hot milk and cream, whisking till smooth. Return to a clean pan. Cook gently, stirring all the time, until the custard thickens. Don't let it boil or it will 'split'. Remove from the heat and leave to cool until tepid, stirring often to stop a skin forming.

Meanwhile, melt the chocolate in a heatproof bowl placed in a larger bowl filled with just-boiled water, stirring from time to time. Stir the melted chocolate into the custard (don't worry if it looks a bit grainy at this point). Stir in the beetroot purée. Pass the mixture through a fine sieve into a jug, leave to cool, then chill.

Once cold, churn the mixture in an ice-cream maker until soft-set, then transfer to a suitable container and freeze until solid. (If you don't have an ice-cream maker, freeze in a shallow container, mashing with a fork three times at hourly intervals before the mixture is solid.) Transfer to the fridge 20–30 minutes before serving, to soften a little.

VARIATION

Pea and mint ice cream

Make the custard as above, but use all 300ml milk with the cream. Strain the cooked custard into a bowl, cover with cling film and cool, then chill. Make a minty pea purée: simmer 350g peas with 2 mint sprigs until just tender. Drain, rinse under cold water and discard the mint. Blitz the peas in a blender with 4 tablespoons finely shredded mint and 2 tablespoons crème fraîche until smooth, adding a dash of milk if necessary. Stir the chilled custard and pea purée together. Taste and add a little icing sugar if necessary – the ice cream will seem less sweet once frozen. Chill, then churn or freeze as above.

Tourte de blettes

Based on a traditional niçoise recipe, this sweet pie makes a lovely dessert, and it's a great way to use Swiss chard. You only need the leaves; use the stems for another dish, such as a gratin of chard stalks (see page 380).

SERVES 8

FOR THE SWEET PASTRY

300g plain flour

50g icing sugar

A pinch of fine sea salt

175g chilled unsalted butter, cut into cubes

1 large egg yolk

About 75ml cold milk (or water)

A little milk or beaten egg, for brushing

FOR THE FILLING

50g raisins

3 tablespoons cider brandy

Leaves from 1kg Swiss chard

2 large eggs, lightly beaten

50g pine nuts, lightly toasted

Finely grated zest of 1 lemon

35g caster sugar

2 dessert apples (about 250g)

Icing sugar, to dust

For the filling, combine the raisins and brandy in a small bowl and leave to soak for a few hours.

For the pastry, put the flour, icing sugar and salt in a food processor and blitz briefly to combine (or sift into a bowl). Add the butter and blitz (or rub in with your fingertips) until the mixture resembles breadcrumbs. Add the egg yolk, and enough milk or water to bring the dough together in large clumps. Tip out on to a lightly floured surface and knead lightly into a ball. Wrap and chill for 30 minutes.

Preheat the oven to 200°C/Gas Mark 6. Put the chard leaves into a saucepan with just the water that clings to them from washing. Cover the pan and cook over a medium-low heat until the leaves have wilted in their own steam – about 5 minutes. Tip into a colander and leave to drain. When cool enough to handle, squeeze out all the liquid from the leaves, then chop them.

Combine the chopped chard with the beaten eggs, pine nuts, lemon zest, sugar and raisins, plus their soaking liquid. Grate the apples, avoiding the core, squeeze out as much liquid as you can from them with your hands, then stir these into the mixture too.

On a floured surface, roll out two-thirds of the pastry fairly thinly and use to line a loose-bottomed 24cm flan tin. Trim the excess pastry away from the edge. Spread the chard mixture in the pastry case. Brush a little milk or beaten egg around the rim of the pastry. Roll out the remaining pastry to form the lid, place over the tart and press the edge down lightly to seal. Trim off the excess pastry.

Make a couple of slits in the pastry lid for steam to escape. Bake for 30 minutes, or until golden brown on top. Leave to cool for a few minutes in the tin, then lift out the tart, keeping it on the tin base, and slide on to a wire rack. Dust the surface generously with icing sugar. Serve warm.

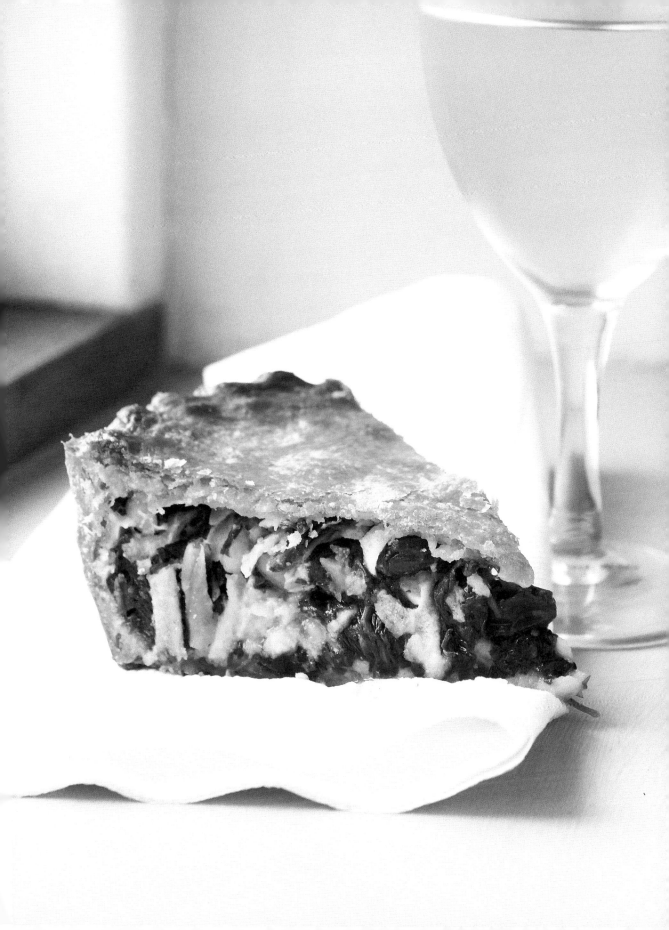

Store cupboard

Many of these ingredients are hugely useful for on-the-hoof veg-based cooking, and you'll find all of them referred to several times, at least, throughout this book. Some, I think, are pretty essential if you're looking to go meat-free at least some of the time. Others are perhaps not quite so crucial, but extremely useful.

Oils for cooking For frying, I like sunflower (*not* cold-pressed) and rapeseed oil; both can be heated to a high temperature. I sometimes also use an inexpensive (generally refined) olive oil, but it's not suitable for very high temperature frying. For salads, extra virgin rapeseed oil and a good, peppery, extra virgin olive oil are my usual choices, although intense, grassy hempseed oil makes a welcome change.

Vinegars Organic cider vinegar is my default option here, while apple balsamic is my favourite when a slightly sweet, rich vinegar is called for. I use red and white wine vinegars too, and brown rice vinegar for oriental salad dressings and marinades.

Mustards Occasionally, I dabble in fancy, seedy mustards but I always have a good, strong English mustard to hand.

Nuts I like to have at least one or two of the following standing by: walnuts, pine nuts, almonds, pistachios, cashews and peanuts.

Seeds I'm never without pumpkin, sesame and sunflower seeds at the very least.

Flour Between them, organic white bread flour, plain white flour and wholemeal cake flour cover most of my needs, though I do like to try out different flours when bread-making, including spelt and rye flours.

Yeast These days, I mostly use instant or 'easy-blend' dried yeast – the kind that goes straight in with the flour – as I find it gives very good results. However, I do sometimes pick up fresh yeast when I'm visiting the local health food shop.

Tinned pulses Chickpeas, some kind of white bean such as cannellini, and tinned brown lentils (which can be used to make a very quick dhal) are store-cupboard essentials for me.

Dry lentils I keep Puy lentils, mostly for using 'whole' in salads and soups, and red (actually orange) lentils for cooking to a purée, or dhal.

Tinned tomatoes I never have fewer than four tins in the cupboard. I prefer whole plum tomatoes, rather than chopped, because I think you get more tomato for your money and a better, richer flavour.

Spices It's lovely to have a whole range of spices in your cupboard, but inevitably a lot of them stand idle for months on end. In my kitchen, the ones that get used pretty much every week are cumin seeds, coriander seeds, cayenne pepper, smoked paprika (sweet and hot), caraway seeds, black peppercorns, dried chilli flakes and/or dried chillies, and a good blended curry powder (I keep a mild blend handy and spike it up with extra chilli if I want more heat).

Salt A good, fine-grained, free-flowing sea salt for salting cooking water and for instantly seasoning dishes is a must. For finishing dishes and to have on the table, I favour a good, flaky British sea salt, such as Cornish, Maldon or Halen Môn.

Vegetable stock cubes I favour the organic, yeast-free ones produced by Kallo, which are not overly salty. Marigold bouillon granules are also worthwhile.

Lemons and bay leaves Although not exactly store-cupboard items, I'd say never be without either of these, if you can help it.

Excellent extras

You might not have all of these items in your larder (or freezer) all of the time but I like to have most of them, most of the time. They all place you that much nearer to a truly satisfying, relatively fuss-free veg-based meal.

- Couscous
- Pasta
- Noodles
- Basmati rice
- Risotto rice
- Pearled spelt and/or pearl barley
- Quick-cook polenta
- Quinoa
- Coconut milk
- Oil-preserved artichoke hearts
- Tomato purée
- Capers
- Olives
- Frozen puff pastry
- Tahini
- Peanut butter

Veg on the go

Meat-free midday sustenance doesn't have to mean endless cheese sandwiches. Think outside the (lunch)box when it comes to packing up a portable meal and you'll find workday lunches can be just as exciting as your evening repast. All of these recipes will serve well…

Dips, spreads and sandwich or wrap fillings These are so versatile – in a straight-up sandwich or wrap, maybe with a few crunchy salad leaves, or in a sealed jar or box as a portable dip for crudités, tortilla chips or even a bag of crisps. If you're making flatbreads for wraps (using the recipe on page 176), remember to wrap them immediately after cooking in a clean tea towel and they will stay soft as they cool. Try the following tasty fillers:

- Garlicky broad bean purée, ricotta and mint (page 196)
- Cannellini bean hummus ♥ (page 300)
- Oven-roasted ratatouille ♥ (page 362)
- Caponata ♥ (page 307)
- Broad beans with herbed goat's cheese (page 316)
- Baba ganoush ♥ (page 303)
- Artichoke and white bean dip (page 303)
- Carrot hummus (page 296)
- Beetroot and walnut hummus ♥ (page 300)

Big salads Most of the recipes in Hearty salads (pages 66–95) will be delicious eaten cold from a tub, but my lunchbox favourites are:

- Herby, peanutty noodly salad ♥ (page 71)
- Spelt salad with squash and fennel (page 72)
- Summer spelt salad ♥ (page 72)
- Tahini-dressed courgette and green bean salad ♥ (page 74)
- New potato, tomato and boiled egg salad (page 76)
- New potato salad 'tartare' (page 79)
- Rocket, fennel and puy lentil salad ♥ (page 82)
- Fish-free salad niçoise (page 85)
- Couscous salad with herbs and walnuts ♥ (page 89)
- Summer couscous salad ♥ (page 89)
- Roasted baby beetroot with walnuts and yoghurt dressing (page 92)
- Green beans, new potatoes and olives ♥ (page 222)
- Quick couscous salad with peppers and feta (page 231)
- Tomato and olive couscous ♥ (page 231)
- Moroccan spiced couscous ♥ (page 231)
- White bean salad with tomatoes and red onion ♥ (page 240)
- Broccoli salad with asian-style dressing ♥ (page 316)

Raw salads and coleslaws When you take a leafy salad in a lunchbox, you'll want to take the dressing separately and dress it just before you eat, as dressed leaves are inclined to wilt as your lunchbox sits around. As the following are not leafy, they can be taken pre-dressed. You may lose a little crunch in some cases, but the dressing has a marinating effect on the ingredients, which is rather nice. Try these tasty options:

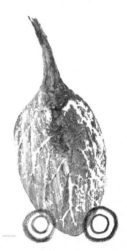

- Fennel and goat's cheese (page 102)
- Carrot, orange and cashews ♥ (page 107)
- Celeriac with apple, raisins and parsley ♥ (page 107)
- Cauliflower with toasted seeds ♥ (page 108)
- Red cabbage, parsnip, orange and dates ♥ (page 110)
- Beetroot with walnuts and cumin ♥ (page 113)
- Asian-inspired coleslaw (page 115)
- Marinated cucumber with mint ♥ (page 122)

Tarts, pasties, pies and frittatas
All of these sustaining choices are highly portable when cold:
- Lettuce, spring onion and cheese tart (page 44)
- Beet top (or chard) and ricotta tart (page 47)
- Swede and potato pasties (page 52)
- Spinach and thyme pasties (page 326)
- Frittata with summer veg and goat's cheese (page 232)
- Oven-roasted root frittata (page 234)

Cold, cooked veg These are a really satisfying addition to a lunchbox, along with a lubricating dip or hummus, or something a little 'saucy' such as a coleslaw. Try a sprinkle of seeds or dukka as well...
- Dressed puy lentils ♥ (page 237)
- Honey roasted cherry tomatoes (page 343)
- Roasted cauliflower with lemon and paprika ♥ (page 352)
- Roasted potatoes and aubergines ♥ (page 351)
- Roasted roots with apple and rosemary ♥ (page 361)
- Roast parsnip chips ♥ (page 357)
- Spiced spinach and potatoes ♥ (page 321)
- Grilled aubergines with chilli and honey (page 340)
- Roast squash wedges ♥ (page 346)
- Roast baby potatoes with two mojo sauces ♥ (page 358)
- Roasted squash and shallots with merguez chickpeas ♥ (page 365)

And, of course...
- DIY 'pot' noodles (page 248)

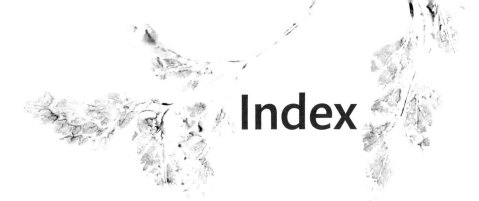

Index

Acknowledgements

A huge amount of work has gone into *River Cottage Veg Every Day!* and I am indebted to the many dedicated and talented people who've made it happen.

Among the skilled cooks who contributed to this book was Philippa Corbin – 'Pip' to all of us – a highly valued member of the River Cottage team and a dedicated advocate of local, seasonal food. She tragically died before it was completed. She is greatly missed by us all.

I want to thank Gill Meller, who has led the River Cottage kitchen from the start and from the front, and has always been a great pleasure to work alongside. I'm grateful not just for his delectable recipe ideas, but also for the immense work he has put into preparing the dishes for photography. He has been ably supported by the whole River Cottage kitchen team and I'd especially like to thank Neil Matthews, Oliver Gladwin and Bryan Johnson. Thanks also to Tim Maddams, James Whetlor and their kitchen team, for upping the veg ante at the River Cottage Canteen.

And of course it's the images generated by the extremely talented Simon Wheeler that bring all these dishes to life on the page. Simon and I have now celebrated our tenth anniversary, and our seventh book together. I say 'celebrated', I guess I mean that metaphorically, but it's high time we did it literally. Thank you so much, Simon.

I would not have been able to pull all these dishes together without the hard work and inspiration of two dedicated and knowledgeable writers, Debora Robertson and Nikki Duffy. Their work in brainstorming, developing, testing and editing recipes has been invaluable. Nikki's thoroughness and enthusiasm in 'bringing this book home' has been unrelenting and highly professional.

Away from the kitchen, there are many people who've put in a huge amount of effort to bring this book to fruition. To my truly wonderful PA, Jess Upton, a thousand thanks for working her cool, calm, level-headed organisational magic on everything from photo shoots to the sourcing of ingredients, to the seventh circle of hell that is my schedule. And a big thanks to all the other members of the team at Park Farm (and beyond) who have worked with and supported me during the making of this book, including Lucy Brazier, Cat Bugler, Sally Gale, Liz Murray, Steve Lamb, Mark Diacono, Victoria Moorey, Ali Thomson, Kate Colwell, Pam Corbin, John Wright, Murry Toms and Simon Dodd. Particular thanks to Rob Love, for his continuing partnership, support and encouragement in all things River Cottage.

For providing some lovely extra veg for the photo-shoots, thanks to all at Trill Farm, Fivepenny Farm, Washingpool Farm and Millers Farm Shop. And a special thanks to Mary Hugill for helping us to nurture all the wonderful vegetables here at home.

At Bloomsbury, my heartfelt thanks go to my editor Richard Atkinson for his continuing commitment to all my book projects, and superb editing and guidance from start to finish. Huge thanks to Natalie Hunt and Janet Illsley who have put so much careful thought – and so many hours – into honing the text from raw to nicely done. Lawrence Morton's clever design work and Mariko Jesse's beautiful illustrations make an elegant and witty marriage, which has truly done the recipes and text proud – it's been great fun working with you both. I'm grateful also to Penny Edwards who has guided the book so efficiently through the production stages.

To the team at Keo Films, especially Claire Lewis, Callum Webster, Kim Lomax, Aidan Woodward, Sancha Starkey, Jade Miller Robinson, Mark Davenport, Maria Norman, Tom Zynovieff and, of course, my Keo partners Andrew Palmer and Zam Baring, a big thank you for 'RC Veg Every Day TV'.

To Antony Topping, my agent, and the third member of the 'ten years and counting' club, a million thanks for your amazing work behind the scenes, on this and every other project I'm involved in.

Last, and the opposite of least, thank you to the people who continue to inspire, nourish and support me (and share wonderful food with me, mainly vegetables) every single day: my wife Marie and our fantastic children Chloe, Oscar, Freddie and Louisa.

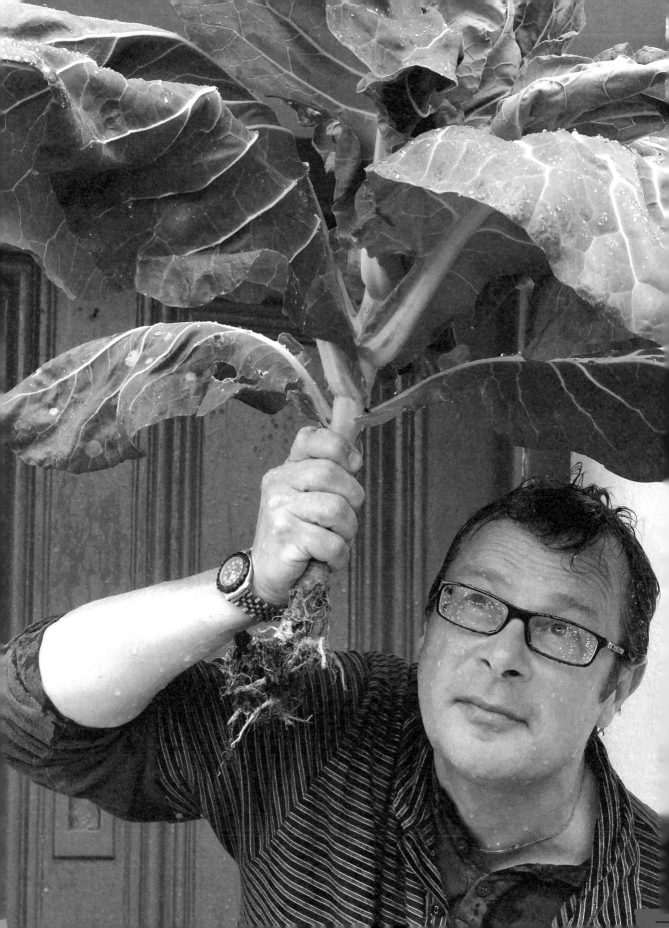